Please remember that this is a library book,
and that it belongs only temporarily to each
person who uses it. Be considerate. Do
not write in this, or any, library book.

Power and the Profession of Obstetrics

Karen,

I was very glad to have Doug and you serve as midwives to this project. May you have many successful deliveries.

Bill Amey

William Ray Arney

Power and the Profession of Obstetrics

The University of Chicago Press
Chicago and London

William Ray Arney is a Member of the Faculty (Sociology) at The Evergreen State College.

The University of Chicago Press, Chicago 60637
The University of Chicago Press, Ltd., London

© 1982 by The University of Chicago
All rights reserved. Published 1982
Printed in the United States of America
88 87 86 85 84 83 82   1 2 3 4 5

Library of Congress Cataloging in Publication Data

Arney, William Ray.
    Power and the profession of obstetrics.

    Includes bibliographical references and index.
    1. Obstetrics—Social aspects.   2. Obstetrics—
Practice.   3. Midwives.   4. Physician and patient.
5. Power (Social sciences).   I. Title.
RG526.A76   1982   362.1'982   82-8410
ISBN 0-226-02728-7   AACR2

To **Debbie** with love

Contents

Preface   ix

1 Introduction   1

Part One   Forming the Profession   19

2 Midwifery vs. Obstetrics
  Themes in the Development of a Profession   20
3 Residual Normalcy and Pathological Potential   51

Part Two   Re-forming the Profession   87

4 Monitoring and Surveillance
  A New Order of Obstetrical Control   99
5 Maternal-Infant Bonding
  Monitoring and the Problem of
  Falling in Love with Your Child   155
6 Medicine, Ethics, and the Reformulation
  of the Doctor-Patient Relationship   175
7 Modern Women and Modern Obstetricians
  The Development of a Univocal Discourse   208

Notes   243
Index   281

vii

Preface

It is a fair question, one that I consider seriously no matter how many times it has been asked before: "How did *you* get interested in *this?*" I am not sure that I can provide a satisfactory answer even now, but it is worth a try. Over the past four years I have followed a number of lines of work. I have always had an interest in methodology. Perhaps that should be Methodology, with a capital "M," since I mean that I have always had an interest in the relationships among the rules for producing knowledge, knowledge, and the uses of knowledge. I gained some experiences operating in the interstices of these three aspects of methodology as the director of evaluation for the Vermont/New Hampshire Regional Perinatal Program. During my three-year tenure with the program, an old interest in medicine was reawakened and I learned a great deal about obstetrics and perinatology under the patient tutelage of George A. Little, Director of the Program in New Hampshire, and G. Millard Simmons, a practicing high-risk obstetrician and teacher *extraordinaire*. Also, during my time with the program some excellent histories of medicine and critical analyses of other social institutions began to appear. I was fortunate enough to be able to use some of that material in teaching a number of different courses and to have students who, for the most part, were willing to let me struggle with the material at the same time they were. They did not demand that I necessarily *teach them* something, and so I had time to learn with them.

ix

During a sabbatical leave in England and Scotland I tried to bring together all these disparate threads—an interest in methodology, experience in a medical setting, a new knowledge of obstetrics and perinatology, and my understanding of new directions in sociology—and this book is the result.

This book is primarily about the profession of obstetrics, but it is about more than just that. It is an exploration of the deployment and transformation of power. In part, it is a study of the way conflict—in this case, between women and obstetricians—can transform itself into a conjunction of interests and still be cloaked in a language of conflict. It is a study of knowledge and practice, their creation, their use, and the changes they sometimes undergo.

Any book benefits from the advice and support of many other people, and this one is no different. I have already mentioned Drs. Little and Simmons.

Several students wrote especially provocative papers in my courses on health care and, to one degree or another, influenced my thinking. I would like to mention, in particular, Deborah Nissley, Sue Kahil, Jane Neill, and Ross Jaffee. Robert Charles did some excellent background research for Chapter 6.

My work was facilitated by a fellowship from the Marion and Jasper Whiting Foundation. Their support allowed me to travel to Great Britain on two occasions. In Britain the following libraries provided valuable assistance: the library of the Royal College of Obstetricians and Gynecologists, the library of the Wellcome Institute for the History of Medicine, the Wills Library of Guy's Hospital Medical School, the British Library, Senate House Library of the University of London, and the libraries of the University of Edinburgh. Closer to home, the Dana Biomedical Library of Dartmouth Medical School provided considerable assistance. Diane Kaufman and the Dartmouth Time Sharing System helped prepare the manuscript.

Colleagues and friends are important critics and sources of support. Una Maclean and Professor Sir John Brotherston made my stay in Edinburgh most pleasant. David Armstrong provided an intellectually challenging three months in London and read drafts of several chapters. Others who read the manuscript and provided useful comments include Elise Boulding, Diana Scully, William Young, Barbara Ehrenreich, Peter Conrad, and Charles Bosk.

As will become obvious, the work of Michel Foucault served as a point of departure for much of my work. Thanks go to him for providing such a stimulating and provocative oeuvre—even though he would be the first to wish that such a term be depersonalized—and for reading the manuscript prior to publication.

Professor Bernard Bergen deserves special mention. He has been a friend, a kind critic, and a supportive colleague since we started teaching together two years ago. I could not begin to list all the ways he influenced this project. He knows how much he contributed, and that will have to suffice.

Finally, my wife Deborah Henderson Arney has been with me throughout my work over the last nine years. She has tolerated much and given more than I ever expected. Thanks, champ.

During the delay between completion of the manuscript and publication of the book a new edition of *Williams Obstetrics* appeared. After reading it I concluded that the revisions in this central text did not call for revisions in my manuscript. Those who follow my argument will appreciate the totalizing character of these paragraphs from the introductory chapter of the sixteenth edition of *Williams Obstetrics* which I offer without comment:

> Obstetrics is related also to certain fields that are not strictly medical. Since nutritional requirements are altered by pregnancy, obstetrics requires knowledge of the science of nutrition. In studies of fetal malformations, genetics is obviously of prime importance. Since the mother-child relationship is the basis of the family unit, the obstetrician is continually dealing with psychologic and sociologic problems. Economics plays a prominent role in obstetrics since health care may be quite expensive, and especially so when those who provide it have little concern for costs. In addition, obstetrics has important legal aspects, especially in regard to the increasing number of malpractice suits. . . .
>
> The concept of the right of every child to be physically, mentally, emotionally ''well-born'' is fundamental to human dignity. If obstetrics is to play a role in its realization, the specialty must maintain and even extend its role in the control of population. . . . This concept of obstetrics as a social as well as a biologic science impels us to accept a responsibility unprecedented in American medicine (Jack A. Pritchard and Paul C. MacDonald, *Williams Obstetrics,* 16th ed., [New York: Appleton-Century-Crofts, 1980], pp. 8, 9).

1 Introduction

There are two histories of the profession of obstetrics. The profession has one interpretation of its past; critics of the profession have a different one. The two histories share certain ideas, such as the notion that the recent period of obstetrical history was characterized by exponential advances in technology; but they differ on other points, such as their explanations of the disappearance of the female midwife early in this century. Besides ideas, the two histories share a characteristic of all theory and all history in that their substance is conditioned by the social interests of the theoretician or the historian. People write history to shape the present or fashion the future, and to one degree or another the social location of the historian—his or her social interests—causes the historian to choose selectively those parts of the past on which his or her interpretation will be based.

Power and the Profession of Obstetrics is a third kind of history of the profession. It is neither pro-obstetrics nor anti-obstetrics. It offers no beautiful or apocalyptic vision of the future nor does it offer a political program for the reform of obstetrics. It uses the historical archive of the profession to examine the problems of, first, how the profession seized childbirth and staked it out as the exclusive domain of a new profession; and, second, how obstetrics protected childbirth, the basis of the obstetrical project, in the face of internal and external challenges to the profession's autonomy and privilege to practice as it wished. This social history seeks to lay bare the nature of professional power, how it was acquired by obstetrics, and how it was retained through its reformulation.

This history differs from the two extant histories in that it shows the profession of obstetrics suffered a significant discontinuity in its social development during the post–World War II period, a time which the other histories have characterized as simply an era of accelerated, but continuous, technical development. The discontinuity is obvious in the obstetrical literature, but the other histories have overlooked it either because they have not payed sufficiently close attention to the archive, or because the historians' visions of the present or dreams for the future were heavily dependent on having the history of obstetrics accumulate continuously and relentlessly, driving obstetricians and women along more or less unwittingly, to an either exceptionally good or exceptionally bad (depending on the history) present. This book differs from previous histories in that it has no investment in making a history continuous when the record shows it was not.

This history is like the others, though, in that it was written by a person with his own understanding of the present who wishes to reshape others' understanding of the present by elaborating the contemporary character of professional power as expressed in the practice of obstetrics. Though I intend to reveal the misunderstandings of professional power in both pro- and anti-obstetrics histories I refuse the temptation to offer a vision for the future. Speaking for others is not the job of a social analyst, and to offer one's own vision of the future is to do precisely that, albeit in a seemingly benign and academically acceptable way. In what follows I will try to make my interests and intentions clear, but I realize that, just as I have interpreted others' accounts of the past with an eye to revealing their interests and intentions, my "true" interests will be revealed only in the interpretations of future historians of histories.[1]

Three Histories of Obstetrics

The profession's understanding of its past focuses on the scientific, cumulative nature of knowledge and emphasizes the notion that there is a direct link between knowledge and practice. Theodore Cianfrani, in his book *A Short History of Obstetrics and Gynecology*,[2] represented the history of the profession with the graph shown in figure 1.1. He did not supply a vertical axis, but his title for the figure makes it clear that the exponential rise occurs on a dimension of "progress" or "achievement." There are lulls in the development of the profession during certain periods (at points h and r, during the 1830s and the 1920s) and periods of rapid advance (around points f, i, o, and s, during the early nineteenth century, following the discovery of anesthesia in mid-century, during the first decade of this century as the profession was securing its license and mandate, and following the discovery of antibiotics and the expansion of endocrinology around 1929), but the general impression conveyed is that of a profession driven along on a tide of technological progress, rising to higher and higher crests of professional achievement, all to the benefit of patients. Cianfrani alludes to the disappearance of the midwife, but he was more concerned with the question of how men could possibly have contributed so much to obstetrics and gynecology in the face of the embarrassment and ridicule heaped upon them by their colleagues and the public for their participation in these fields than he was about the meaning of the male takeover of the profession.[3]

The loose amalgam of theoretical perspectives known collectively as feminist scholarship rewrote the history of obstetrics paying close attention to the fate of the female midwife. Authors like Barbara Ehrenreich and Deirdre English[4] and other scholars before them read the obstetrical archive closely enough to see what, in fact, is self evident: the profession, in its early days, saw the midwife as a problem, a social, political, and economic impediment to the development of obstetrics along the lines members of the profession wished to pursue, and the profession implemented a political program to solve the "midwife problem," as the profession knew it. Feminist scholarship did not reject the profession's model of its own development, but it examined closely the effects, the human meaning, of that development. Feminist scholarship discovered that there was someone, the female midwife, who helped to launch the profession on its climb, and it sought to revive memories of her. It did history the favor of putting people—women and men—back in where the profession's history had sought to exclude them, and it recited a litany of the human uses and abuses of the knowledge and practices which even today remain prominent in the profession's histories. Feminist scholarship, along with other critical sociology of the last decade, transformed science from the driving force behind the

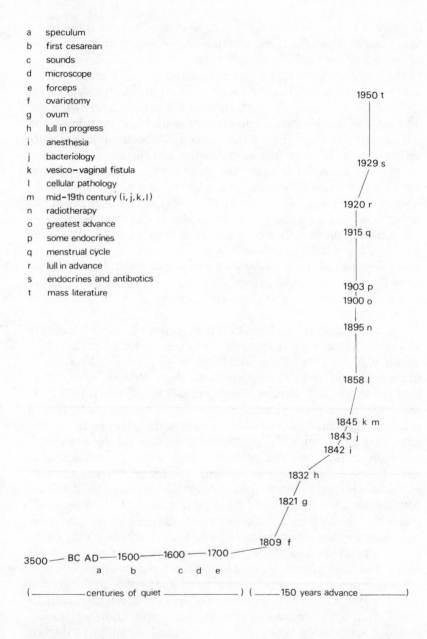

a   speculum
b   first cesarean
c   sounds
d   microscope
e   forceps
f   ovariotomy
g   ovum
h   lull in progress
i   anesthesia
j   bacteriology
k   vesico–vaginal fistula
l   cellular pathology
m   mid–19th century (i, j, k, l)
n   radiotherapy
o   greatest advance
p   some endocrines
q   menstrual cycle
r   lull in advance
s   endocrines and antibiotics
t   mass literature

1950 t

1929 s

1920 r

1915 q

1903 p
1900 o

1895 n

1858 l

1845 k m
1843 j
1842 i

1832 h

1821 g

1809 f

3500 — BC AD —1500——1600 —1700
          a   b   c   d   e

(——————centuries of quiet ——————) (——150 years advance ——)

Figure 1.1. The profession's history of itself. From Theodore Cianfrani, *A Short History of Obstetrics and Gynecology* (1960). Courtesy of Charles C. Thomas, Publisher, Springfield, Ill.

beneficial expansion of the profession into a "force to which doctors looked to lift medicine out of the mire of commercialism" into which it descended during the nineteenth century, a resource to be used by "any group which hoped to establish itself as the 'experts' in a certain area,"[5] a social utility which worked to the disadvantage of some and the advantage of others.

Even though revisionist histories of obstetrics have directed attention toward the human effects of the development of the profession and have insisted that the people affected by history be considered in the writing of it, revisionists still rely on the profession to provide the outline of the general course of its development. The second history of obstetrics, written primarily by critics of the profession, accepts and focuses on the view that knowledge and the technology it spawns increase at an ever more rapid rate. It differs from the profession's history, though, in the meaning it attaches to that development. The profession argues that knowledge and technology benefit women, babies, and society generally; critics argue that increased technology and an expanded knowledge base *medicalize* pregnancy and birth to the detriment of women's experiences and families' freedoms during a period of life that need not be treated as a medical problem. Ann Oakley, for example, adopts this view in her book *Women Confined,* where she says, "The process of medicalization has accelerated particularly in the last ten years, as pharmacological and technical innovation has been introduced to obstetric work on the untested assumption that more means better."[6] Oakley is especially critical of the thoughtless application of new technology which, she says, is a characteristic of the profession. Mary Daly, likewise, sees the history of obstetrics as one long, episode of increasing brutality in male-dominated world history. She says of obstetrics and gynecology, "the doctored diseases have spread. . . . the mutilations and mutations masterminded by the modern man-midwives represent an advanced stage in the patriarchal program of gynocide."[7] Daly says the advanced and improved violence of modern medicine is a directly repressive response to the rise of modern radical feminism,[8] but the underlying image she offers is that of a profession whose knowledge and practice have expanded systematically and relentlessly to the decided disadvantage of women.

There is no doubt that technological advance has accelerated recently, but to link the development of the profession to the expansion

Table 1.1 Characteristics of Obstetrical Care in Three
           Historical Periods

	Preprofessional—to End of Nineteenth Century	Professional Period, 1890–1945	Monitoring Period, Post–World War II
Metaphor and Logic	Birth as mystery Aristotelian order	Body as machine Scientific rationality	Body as open system of communication Ecological order/ systems theory
Conceptualization of Pregnancy	Normal/abnormal	Potentially pathological Dichotomous categories still applicable but boundaries blurred	Pregnancy as process Two-dimensional childbirth: psychological and physiological
Division of Labor	Symbiotic relationship of midwife and obstetrical attendant Midwife attends normal births Barber-surgeons and obstetricians attend abnormal births Terms controlled by midwife	Terms controlled by obstetrical specialist Midwives attend normal birth in Britain Debates over proper division of labor in America	Well-integrated, continuously hierarchical, ubiquitously present obstetrical teams Parents are team members

of technology and knowledge, regardless of whether one thinks progress is good or bad, is a mistake. Close reading of the obstetrical literature reveals that the social development of the profession underwent a severe and probably irreversible disruption near the end of the Second World War. The discontinuity in development was more than a change in the rate of technological advance. Instead, the profession experienced (and was partly responsible for bringing about) a qualitative transformation in its mode of social control over women, pregnancy, and childbirth generally. The second transformation of obstetrics was just as profound and perhaps ultimately more significant than the first, which occurred as men seized control of birth a century ago.

	Preprofessional—to End of Nineteenth Century	Professional Period, 1890–1945	Monitoring Period, Post–World War II
Attendant/Patient Relationship	Midwife "attends" birth Midwife calls for obstetrical intervention in difficult cases	Obstetrical specialist dominant Specialist presides over birth Patient is vehicle of obstetrical material	Collegial Patient responsible for psychological aspects of birth Obstetrical attendant responsible for physiological aspects of birth
Professional Organization	Localized	Centralized production of knowledge Localized care	Widely dispersed, geographically penetrating, regionalized care centered on medical centers Flexible system of obstetrical alternatives
Who controls birth?	No one Birth is attended and is "uncontrolled"	Obstetricians	The structure of monitoring No agent in control
Technology	Mild relief for normal deliveries Destructive intervention in abnormal deliveries	Technology of domineering control (e.g., forceps, anesthesia, operative intervention)	Technology of monitoring and surveillance

Table 1.1 outlines the dimensions of the two changes obstetrics has undergone in this century.[9] The first change, the roots of which can be traced back to at least the seventeenth century, culminated in the success of modern obstetrics' program to eliminate the traditional midwife. This is the transformation of the profession on which feminist scholarship has concentrated. Birth had been part of the general moral order, something that was "attended" exclusively by women. It followed a rule of dichotomies: birth was normal or abnormal; female midwives attended normal births and called male midwives in abnormal ones; female midwives' technology was rudimentary and oriented toward easing birth, male midwives' tech-

nology was destructive and oriented toward the fast termination of birth, and usually of life. As men succeeded in eliminating their female competition, their approach to birth spread throughout the profession and society at large. The "body as machine" metaphor, which originated with the rise of rationalism, came to inform all of medicine, and the logic of medical inquiry changed.[10] All births, like all machines, carried in them the potential for pathology, the potential for breaking down. Technology that controlled and dominated the forces of birth, just as one dominated and controlled the forces of a machine, replaced midwives' attendance of birth. The boundary between normal and abnormal births became fuzzy, as did the division of labor organized around old dichotomies. In America, "normal" births disappeared along with the female midwife, and all births became potentially pathological. In Britain, men assumed control of the right to designate births normal and abnormal and rose to dominate the social organization around childbirth.

Near the end of World War II another transformation of the profession occurred. A new logic and a new metaphor changed the conceptual basis of medicine. The body was no longer looked upon as a machine which was made of up of other machines; instead, it became a system composed of systems articulated at many points and levels. Furthermore, the body existed as a single component in other, higher-level, systems. An ecological metaphor replaced the mechanical one. Obstetrics reconceptualized pregnancy as a process which had a trajectory, the "normal" course of which was known to obstetrics but which was influenced by the many systems with which the body articulated and communicated—the neurohormonal system, the social system, the economic system, and so on. Birth became less circumscribed anatomically, temporally, and geographically. All the events in a woman's life up to the point of birth became important obstetrical data; all the events after birth became potential obstetrical material worthy of study and incorporation into the obstetrical project; the whole community, extending over large geographical spaces replaced the hospital as the field of obstetrical operation. Technology changed from a technology of domineering control to a technology of monitoring, surveillance, and normalization. The social organization around birth, including the nature of the doctor-patient relationship, changed. Obstetrics organized itself as a continuously hierarchical, ubiquitously present team which included patients as team members and on which doctors were not necessarily team leaders, but just team members. Each team member had his or her responsibilities with respect to some aspect of birth and was accountable to the team for the proper performance of his or her duties. Birth became something to be *managed* in order to optimize the experience rather than something to be attended or dominated. The social organization of obstetrics extended outwards from the hospital over large areas, putting in place a flexible system of obstetrical alternatives as it went. Even so, every aspect of birth became more carefully controlled, as a structure of control I call "monitoring" was deployed across a greatly expanded obstetrical space. Everyone—women, husbands or significant others, and obstetricians—got caught up in monitoring's webs of power and so became more and more alienated from the event and experiences of childbirth.

The two transformations of the profession follow a dialectical track as illustrated in figure 1.2. Birth in the preprofessional period was dichotomized at the symbolic and material levels. Female midwives and male midwives practiced symbiotically to care for normal

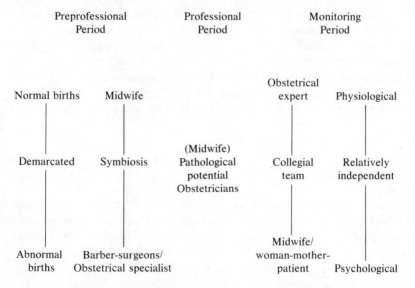

Figure 1.2. The dialectic of childbirth and obstetrical care. The "normal" pole of childbirth was dissolved and submerged in the professional period. The pole reemerged as the "psychological" side of childbirth in the postprofessional period under monitoring.

and abnormal births respectively. The professional period of obstetrics was characterized by the submersion of one pole, the normal pole, of the prevailing characterization of birth. Birth became "potentially pathological," and the professions in Britain and America differed in the way they deployed themselves around this new conceptualization. In the monitoring period the submerged pole reemerged. Birth did not become normal or abnormal again, but birth did acquire a second, nonphysiological, dimension. It was reconceptualized as a process having physiological and psychological components which were related to one another in complex ways even though they were relatively independent, relatively distant, components of birth. The social organization around birth changed to follow and mirror its new conceptual base, and the nature of obstetrical power changed dramatically.

In this brief explanation of the transformations of childbirth and of obstetrics few people appear. It sounds as if birth followed, more or less unwittingly, some grand theoretical plan. It did not. To this point I have merely outlined the results of a long history of human struggles—political battles big and small in which scheming and shrewd maneuvering combined with serendipity to create winners and losers and some who occasionally had to settle for a draw. There is no logic inherent in birth or in the deployment of power which forced obstetrics along the path it took. The history described here was created by people who were engaged in social activity. The body of this book is about people and the way they created, challenged, and defended a profession. First, though, I must say something more about theory and history.

The Place of Theory and the Task of History

Theory, and knowledge generally, are often thought to exist in an ideational realm, different from and usually hovering above the material realm, the level of social action. The sociology of knowledge is a branch of the parent discipline that treats knowledge as a social entity, a creation of and in culture, "something which is actively developed and modified in response to practical contingencies."[11] Recently, even scientific knowledge has lost its privileged character at the hands of sociologists of knowledge. All knowledge, including scientific knowledge, "has the character of a *resource, communally* exploited in the achievement of whatever interests actors decide. And precisely because of this, knowledge is always linked, in its generation and initial evaluation, to an interest in prediction and control." In addition, knowledge develops in response to "a covert interest in rationalization and persuasion," according to Barry Barnes.[12] Linking the production of knowledge to social interests— particularly to externally oriented interests of control and prediction and to internally oriented interests of rationalization and persuasion—is the major contribution of the sociology of knowledge. According to this approach all knowledge must be treated "symmetrically." That is, the sociologist is obligated to treat knowledge derived according to the rules of science in precisely the same analytical way as he treats knowledge derived through divination or mystical revelation or knowledge received from authority. The theories of the scientist that explain why the universe is held together are equivalent in the eyes of the social analyst to the explanations of the same phenomenon given by the Balinese priest.

That we must treat all knowledge and all theories identically, because all knowledge is a social product and a social resource, and that we must not accord certain knowledge and certain theories a privileged place are both methodological rules. Neither tells us what knowledge and theory are. Some claim that knowledge and theory are socially conditioned representations that are generally understandable in terms of the objectives of some social group. This is certainly Barnes' view.[13] This materialist view posits the group with its history, interests, and current situation as somehow prior to and initiative of knowledge. The material world is separable from and causally prior to the ideational world of knowledge and theory. Others claim the opposite: that the ideational world precedes and conditions (or determines) the social world.

The work of Michel Foucault, the French historian of ideas, provides an escape from the materialism/idealism debate. Foucault agrees that "knowledge is an 'invention' behind which lies something completely different from itself: the play of instincts, impulses, desires, fear, and the will to appropriate." But knowledge cannot be distinguished from a situation that conditions its production. "Knowledge is produced on the stage where these [other] elements struggle against one another." Not only are all forms of knowledge symmetrical, but, according to Foucault, knowledge itself is symmetrical with everything in the material world; it is produced *on the same stage* where the struggles of materiality occur. "It is not a permanent faculty, but an event, or at the very least, a series of events."[14] According to this view, practice is not the application of theory and theory the abstraction and representation of practice. Instead, "representation no longer exists; there's only action—theoretical action and practical action which serve as relays and form networks."[15] "In this sense theory does not express, translate, or serve to apply practice: it is practice."[16] Theory is not the benign, humoral substance that accumulates in libraries. "A theory is exactly like a box of tools. It has nothing to do with the signifier. It must be useful. It must function."[17] Theory is produced by a signifier, a theoretician, but it is instantly separated from him. It exists fleetingly as practice, equivalent to all other forms of practice.

According to this view, theories and knowledge take on a brutality that most theoreticians, especially social scientists, are reluctant to admit they have. The idea is not absolutely new, though. During the 1960s Thomas Cottle of Harvard had members of various ethnic groups read academic essays about their own groups. An editor of an anthology in which Cottle's report of his research appeared called the reactions of Cottle's informant-friends "estranged." I would call them enraged. Cottle described one woman as "steaming mad, . . . a time of uncontrolled anger had overtaken her." Why? She had read what academicians had said of her and the people who lived around her. She called it a "pack of lies" with "not a morsel of truth" in it. The only reason her anger was somewhat mollified was that Harvard students renting her upstairs apartment had told her that they had read something academic which said just the opposite about her and her kind. Her anger was transformed into the humor of bewilderment as she said, "Either these are real facts or they're make-believe, and scientists don't make things up, at least the ones on TV I see don't make things up." Cottle described the reactions of his informants this was:

> To read the essays, documented as they were with figures of
> certainty and authenticity, was to be invaded, molested, as it
> were, swallowed up by the rough-grained pictures of
> professionals who, in a funny way, had no business being there
> at all. It was not the explicit political position of these articles

that hurt as much as the sense that sacred properties had been ignored.[18]

Invaded. Swallowed up. Molested. This is a language of violence. And it is a language of violence that must be used to describe what theory does. Gilles Deleuze, speaking to Foucault, said,

> In my opinion, you were the first . . . to teach us something absolutely fundamental: the indignity of speaking for others. We ridiculed representation and said it was finished, but we failed to draw the consequences of this "theoretical" conversion—to appreciate the theoretical fact that only those directly concerned can speak in a practical way on their own behalf.[19]

Theory silences those who are able to speak for themselves and on their own behalf. That is why, in this book, I try to avoid speaking either for obstetrics or for women as I outline my understanding of the history of obstetrics. Obstetrics has spoken for itself for more than a century and women have recently regained the voice that the profession silenced for so long. To avoid speaking for others is also why I refuse to present a vision of the future. To presume to speak on behalf of women or on behalf of us all by putting forward a particular political program would be to engage in just that kind of behavior—the creation of new knowledge and new theories because of an interest in prediction, control, rationalization, or persuasion—which is found in the darkest recesses of the history of obstetrics, which informs so many of the obstetrical reform movements of the day, and against which the criticism of this work is directed.

We must not become paralyzed by the proscription against taking sides, though, for there is an alternative. The alternative is to assume the role of social analyst, of the intellectual. What is that role in the modern age? Again, Foucault is helpful. He described the de facto position of the intellectual, the position of which he and I are critical, and the alternative in this way:

> In the most recent upheaval [the events of May, 1968, in France], the intellectual discovered that the masses no longer need him to gain knowledge: they *know* perfectly well, without illusion; they know far better than he and they are certainly capable of expressing themselves. But there exists a system of power which blocks, prohibits, and invalidates this discourse and this knowledge, a power not only found in the manifest authority of censorship, but one that profoundly and subtly

penetrates an entire social network. Intellectuals are themselves agents of this system of power—the idea of their responsibility for "consciousness" and discourse forms part of the system. The intellectual's role is no longer to place himself "somewhat ahead and to the side" in order to express the stifled truth of the collectivity; rather it is to struggle against the forms of power that transform him into its object and instrument in the sphere of "knowledge," "truth," "consciousness," and "discourse."[20]

Foucault has put forward as a "hypothesis" the notion that

> The essential political problem for the intellectual is not to criticize the ideological contents supposedly linked to science, or to ensure that his own scientific practice is accompanied by a correct ideology, but that of ascertaining a new politics of truth. . . .
> It is not a matter of emancipating truth from every system of power (which would be a chimera, for truth is already power) but of detaching the power of truth from the forms of hegemony, social, economic, and cultural, within which it operates at the present time.[21]

The proper role of the intellectual is to use whatever tools are at hand to expose and elaborate those systems of power and control that would make him their agent. The goal is *not* to rage against those systems on behalf of those who are subject to them but to lay them bare so that the nature and effectiveness of their silencing mechanisms are revealed, made visible, and thereby attenuated.

We must be clear on one point. The alternative intellectual described by Foucault does not adopt a "value-free" or even "neutral" position. In fact, he or she does just the opposite. In this work I presume to speak only for myself; this book is my own interpretation of history conditioned by my own life and interests. My intention is to describe, not explain, mechanisms of power. My description, though, is offered as a resource, like all other knowledge, to be used by others as they see fit.

How does one begin to elaborate structures of power? Are there methodological rules, besides the rudimentary ones of the sociology of knowledge, to be followed in this endeavor? Unfortunately, the answer is "not very many." Recently Arthur L. Stinchcombe has taken American sociology to task for its rush to be theoretical without being attentive to the details of history. He is very direct in his criticism:

> Social theory without attention to details is wind, the classes it invents are vacuous, and nothing interesting follows from the fact that *A* and *B* belong to the same class; "theoretical" research appears as a species of wordy scholasticism, arranging conceptual angels in sixteenfold ranks on the head of a purely conceptual pin.[22]

Stinchcombe insists that sociology must return to the Weberian tradition of scrupulously examining the details of the historical record and deliberately withholding the urge to impose on history a theoretical scheme. He says, "people do much better theory when interpreting the historical sequence than they do when they set out to do 'theory.' "[23] He urges sociology to develop theory only by construction of "deep analogies" between historical sequences. Fruitful, useful, theoretical concepts are derived only by the "piecemeal deepening of analogies."[24] Stinchcombe might not agree, but according to this perspective constructing theory seems to become the task of developing metaphors. Barry Barnes, speaking of scientific reasoning, says that science uses "characteristic procedures and techniques to further the metaphorical redescription of an area of experience in terms of a characteristic, accepted set of cultural resources."[25] This understanding of theory contains no clear rules for research except perhaps these dicta: study closely, reason carefully, stay close to the data, and recognize the constraints your culture and language place on your capacity to reason.

Particularly when we wish to study the development of a profession, its transformation, and changes in the deployment of professional power, we are at a loss for rules of inquiry. The historical record indicates that all aspects of obstetrics—its mode of inquiry, its field of interest, its underlying metaphor, its social organization, its technology—changed around World War II. Foucault would say that the "discursive practices" of the profession changed. Discursive practices are the manifestations of the social choices made by actors and groups in the production of knowledge. They designate certain parts of the world as objects of knowledge and inquiry and exclude others from view. They, together with practices and institutions in which they are embedded, constitute a field of power, and fields of power can transform themselves. Transformations of fields of power occur autonomously and are not necessarily linkable to any specific agent of change. How to study such transformations is especially problematic since "the tools that permit the analysis of the will to knowledge [formulated by discursive practices embedded in social institutions] must be constructed and defined as we proceed, according to the needs and possibilities that arise from a series of concrete studies."[26] To write about discontinuities of a profession like obstetrics is not a theoretically conditioned choice. One must not approach history with a model built on the idea of discontinuity; rather discontinuity "is something that one cannot deny once one has looked at the text with sufficient attention."[27] The message is unambiguous, if somewhat troubling to those interested in developing general social theory: study a *specific* field and try to let the archive speak. Do not silence the texts with theory.

This book is in the tradition of Foucault's "histories that are not history."[28] It is a study of the profession of obstetrics. In the same way that Ann Oakley[29] listened closely to women who were going to have babies, in order to pave a path toward a sociology of childbirth, and Charles Bosk[30] listened closely to his surgeon-informants in a major medical center, in order to understand how one branch of medicine manages medical mistakes, this study listens closely to the obstetrical archive to hear what it has to say about the development of a profession.

I want to make clear that this is not a book about the practices of all obstetricians, nor is it about women's experiences at the hands of obstetricians. Diana Scully wrote a fine book about obstetrical practices and obstetrical training, and others have written equally fine books about women's experiences.[31] I have tried to expose the development of the profession as a whole as it is reflected in the profession's literature. Debates in the literature may or may not indicate that a diversity of practices exists in hospitals and clinics. Likewise, consensus in the literature does not necessarily mean that all obstetricians practice as the journal editors, published authors, and other opinion leaders of the profession would have them practice. For every statement in this book that could possibly be interpreted as pro-obstetrics I have heard a dozen or more horror stories that show "obstetrics is just not like that." I have had to respond, "Obstetrics *is* like that; some obstetricians are not." Similarly, for every statement which could possibly be interpreted as anti-obstetrics I have had pointed out to me two or three obstetricians who are "just the opposite." I have had to respond to this criticism in the same way as I responded to the other criticism. To repeat, my task is to uncover the nature of obstetrical power, how it was acquired and how it changed; I am not choosing sides in the current debate so much as I am offering my own, admittedly personal view of the debate.

Part One

Forming the Profession

> I believe that it is not to the great model of signs
> and language that reference should be made, but
> to war and battle. The history which bears and
> determines us is war-like, not language-like.
> Relations of power not relations of sense. History
> has "no sense," which is not to say that it is
> absurd or incoherent. On the contrary, it is
> intelligible and should be able to be analyzed to
> the slightest detail: but according to the
> intelligibility of struggles, of strategies, and tactics.[1]

The profession of obstetrics did not result from technological imperatives or the accumulation of scientific advances. It was a strategic success. The first chapter of this
section outlines developments in the struggle between female midwives and male midwives, later to be called obstetricians. The formation of the profession gave obstetrics a
degree of autonomy and privilege that would be useful in
struggles against future critics. Also it left the profession a
repertoire of socially successful strategies that would be
deployed again and again throughout the profession's history. Thus, I have subtitled the chapter "Themes in the
Development of a Profession."

Once formed, the profession turned inward to problems
of organization and practice. What the profession would
look like was a matter to be fought out on a field conditioned
by history and surrounded by potential challenges to the
profession's social position. The internal struggles of obstetrics were the second phase in the formation of the profession and the topic of the second chapter of this section.

2 Midwifery vs. Obstetrics
Themes in the Development of a Profession

The midwife, traditional attendant of all births, became an anomaly in America in this century. Now the terms on which childbirth is conducted are under the control of men. How this situation came about is a question to which there is no simple answer. The decline of the female midwife was not just the result of "market forces" (increased demand for better care from a better-educated public). Nor was the elimination of the midwife a case of technical superiority of men over women. In no sense was the disappearance of the midwife inevitable, since in Britain, which experienced parallel though somewhat different developments in medicine, medical men were unsuccessful in their attempts to eliminate completely the female midwife. Midwives in Britain secured legal sanction for their profession under the Midwives' Act of 1902, were established as a Royal College in 1941, and play a role, albeit a significantly diminished one, in the delivery of obstetrical services today. The different paths which men practitioners followed in gaining control of childbirth on the two sides of the Atlantic suggests that the ascendancy of men must in each case be understood as a complex interplay of social forces and events. This chapter shows how serendipity, political maneuvering, shifting alliances, and keen rhetoric all contributed to the early professional development of obstetrics.

It is not my intention to write a history of midwifery in this short chapter. That history is much too rich, too convoluted, too "textured"—to use the historian's word—for such an attempt. Instead, I wish to use the histories[1] which are available for my own sociological ends. In the history of midwifery we may see the precursors to and analogues of the more recent professional developments, and the primary purpose of this chapter is to point out these themes, which will be repeated later. For example, the decline of midwifery resulted in part from the creation of a boundary, a social boundary, around a new "profession" of obstetrics. The later history of the profession can be understood as the defense, the patching, the manipulation of that boundary in order to protect the interests that it encircled. Many strategies of contemporary "boundary work" have their counterparts in the early development of the profession.

In bold strokes, the argument of this chapter is this. Throughout most of history women having babies were attended by women. The "midwife," meaning "with-woman," was ensconced in the rituals of virtually every culture. For many and varied reasons male midwives, later to be called "obstetricians," from the Latin *obstare* meaning "to stand before," tried to replace women as birth attendants. Changing such a significant part of culture is never an easy task nor does it proceed simply. In general, though, changes on at least two levels are required. One must effect change in the *symbolic order* and in the *material aspects* of society, the level of meaning and the level of social practices. Changes in the symbolic, conceptual aspects of culture are used to bring about change at the material level, and vice versa. One does not necessarily precede the other. Inevitably, it seems, there are false starts, missed opportunities, scuttled attempts, and unexpected occurrences at both levels and in the strategic interplay between them. In the case of birth, men had to reconceptualize the phenomenon of birth and bring to it a meaning different from the one it had in the hands of midwives. Then they had to be able to act on that new meaning. Action required organization, social support in various forms, and the acquisition of a capacity to fend off or ignore critics, all in ways that were culturally acceptable. Action influences meaning, changes in meaning influence or require changes in action, and cultural change proceeds in complex and usually gradual ways. Essentially, the battle for birth was a battle over livelihood, but not livelihood in the restricted economic sense of that term. It was a struggle at many levels: a struggle over the control of birth attendance with its economic implications, over the terms and conditions of birth, over the meaning of birth, and over the very experience of women delivering babies. It was a struggle over life as it is organized around the singular event of childbirth.

Midwifery in Britain

Birth, it seems, is always construed as a mysterious event loaded with spiritual and religious significance. It is not surprising, then, that early birth attendants should come under the purview of the church and that there should be a generalized concern for morality surrounding childbirth. The church in England and elsewhere exercised authority over midwives and imposed certain requirements on them. The midwife was to be of good character and of good religious standing. She could be prosecuted for practicing abortion, concealing births, switching children, and she could be barred from practice for failing to baptize properly a child who could not be baptized by a priest before it died. Attending childbirth gave one access to the material used by witches, so there was an association between midwives and witches that was of concern to the Church.[2]

In 1511 Parliament placed licensure of physicians under the direct control of the church[3] and thereby demonstrated its interest in centralization of control over medicine. Midwives came under legal purview of the church one year later. The act that granted licensing authority simply formalized arrangements already in effect in many parishes throughout England, although the act did remove authority from the local level and place it higher—at the level of the bishop—in the bureaucracy of the church. As before, concern was directed more at the moral standing of midwives than at their competence, although they did have to produce clients who could testify to their skill before they could be licensed.[4]

Experience was the teacher of most midwives. Graduates of Oxford and Cambridge, institutions that admitted only men, automatically had license to practice "physick," but it is unlikely that any men entered midwifery, itself, through this route. Women gained knowledge of labor and delivery by participating in the social events carried on around birth. Typically, several women would be in attendance at a birth even though there might be only one midwife. Women who had had children themselves or who had attended several births might begin their practice as a result of being called by women in labor and might gain their reputations thereby, or they might enter practice through hope of supporting themselves financially. Those who entered the profession for economic reasons often engaged in informal apprenticeship with an established midwife. Midwifery was a ubiquitous institution with its practitioners being drawn from all but the uppermost classes and with midwives attending births of women in all social strata.

The institution of midwifery was based on a conception of birth as a natural and normal process. Birth was simply part of the moral order of the universe. Midwives were "to be with" a laboring woman. They might administer some simple folk medicines—herbal teas, cordials, or the like—or, with highly skilled midwives, they might attempt rudimentary interventions including versions—turning of a fetus in utero. In general, though, birth was thought to be normal and was to be "attended," not hurried along or interfered with.

The concept of "crisis" was attached to birth but in a very different way than is used today. Birth was a moral crisis through which women had to pass. That is to say, the delivering woman's behavior in birth was thought to reveal her moral character. There was no proper, consensually endorsed way to deliver a child. A woman's behavior was to be observed for what it revealed of her character; behavior was not prescribed and proscribed for the benefit of her attendants. If the child had not been fathered by a woman's husband, it was thought that during her labor pains or during expulsion she might shout out the name of the real father. A child born dead or deformed might be taken as a reflection of the mother's and perhaps even the father's low moral standing or diminished stature in the sight of God. But even the moral crisis of childbirth was "natural." It was simply one manifestation of humankind's standing in relationship to God and of woman's inferior standing in society. It was, in other words, one aspect of the natural order and one aspect of the nature of woman.

Occasionally, something would go awry in the birth process. Cases of cephalo-pelvic disproportion, malpresentation, some intrapartum deaths, and extremely prolonged labors were considered "abnormal" cases which the midwife was bound not to treat. By her oath and common practice, the midwife was forced to call a surgeon to extract a child that was not expelled normally within a reasonable amount of time. The barber-surgeons, members of a guild formed in the thirteenth century, were men who owned instruments. They used their hooks, knives, levers, saws, and other tools to pull a fetus from the womb either whole or in parts. Their techniques were usually fatal for the fetus and often for the mother as well.[5]

Midwives and barber-surgeons practiced symbiotically in Britain against a backdrop of Continental obstetrics. In France, public hospitals chartered in the sixteenth century,[6] the Hotel-Dieu being the most notable, provided instruction for midwives and, perhaps more important, provided an opportunity for midwives and doctors to observe many births. (Britain did not open lying-in wards in public hospitals until late in the seventeenth century.) The systematic observation of birth that the hospital allowed proceeded apace and culminated in the pelvimetry—instrumental measurement of the female pelvis—of Levret in the mid-eighteenth century.[7] With their instruments of description rather than intervention the French set the stage for a "rational" or "scientific"[8] approach to childbirth. As the Wertzes indicate in their history of childbirth, birth was considered a "normal" process by the French, just as it was in England, but physiological processes, including birth, were more carefully conceptualized through use of the metaphor of the body as machine. Each part of the body was a machine unto itself and a component of a larger machine. The task of the physician was to keep the machine running and to make it work more efficiently. This new conception of birth stripped away much of the magical and emotional baggage attached to childbirth in Britain and elsewhere. It permitted intervention in the birth process, but it disallowed intervention of the utterly destructive sort practiced by the barber-surgeons. One might try to enlarge the vaginal opening a bit to ease the passage of the baby or try to change an abnormal presentation so that the baby followed the "proper," scientifically known angle through the birth canal. But the machine metaphor restricted intervention of the sort most commonly available to practitioners of the day since the metaphor required medical practitioners to concentrate on the outcomes of their efforts. Clearly, one would not want to stop a machine's functioning completely, as intervention in birth often did. So, somewhat ironically, the theoretical[9] basis of most modern obstetrical practice served as a constraint on practice, i.e., on active intervention, for the French who originally developed the theory.[10]

In the seventeenth century, the French influence made its way to Britain where invasive treatments were already accepted. The

French approach to birth came in books. Even though the texts were written for female midwives and physicians in France, their audience in England was almost completely male. Hugh Chamberlen, two generations removed from Peter Chamberlen the Elder, who invented the obstetrical forceps, said that he translated a midwifery text by Mariceau, the famous French obstetrician who practiced at the Hotel Dieu, "for the benefit of our midwives." This and a few other books were available, but it is unlikely that any were widely read by their intended audience, the female midwives. Many midwives could not get an education, and as Jane Donegan observes, prudery and modesty may have kept literate female midwives from reading such texts anyway.[11] For those who did read the texts, there were significant omissions—plates or descriptions of female anatomy, for example—that reduced their value. The authors invoked their own modesty and decorum to justify such omissions.[12]

The "rational" approach to childbirth which crossed the Channel into Britain undermined the symbolic basis of the traditional midwives' practice by blurring the demarcation between "normal" and "abnormal" births. This was crucial, and many histories of obstetrics have overlooked its importance by concentrating on technological developments of the period, particularly the invention of the obstetrical forceps. This reformulation of the ideological basis of midwifery was essential to the ultimate success of male midwives in their struggle against women practitioners.

Normal births had been the province of the female midwife, but in an odd way abnormal births had been, too. The midwife had control, ecclesiastically sanctioned control, over the distinction between normal and abnormal, and it was on the control of this distinction that her power rested. Birth was not well understood by anyone, so no one had any basis for infringing on the privilege of the "mysterious office" of midwife to decide when a birth had crossed the line from "normal" to "abnormal." Of course, a midwife could be prosecuted if she failed to call a surgeon at all or if she delayed in seeking the assistance of a man and something drastic happened. But prosecution was a *post facto* procedure. Until the scientific approach to birth appeared in England, no one besides the midwife had a theory, an a priori basis, by which to judge the normality or abnormality of a given birth. The French "science" of midwifery provided the conceptual basis for the development of such a theory. It is not important that it did not provide a specific theory. What is important is that the concepts of "normal" and "abnormal" took on a new relationship to one another. No longer was there a clear demarcation between the two; a gray area had been created that was capable of taking on added dimensionality. A machine is not "normal" or "abnormal"; it is either "effective" or "ineffective." Almost all uteri are "effective" eventually, but this issue was displaced by the mechanical metaphor. A machine can work well, or work poorly, or not at all. With a new metaphor informing childbirth, one could "do well" or "do poorly." Rationalism freed birth from the constraints of nature and opened it to improvement, and the boundary between normal and abnormal births became a matter for dispute and contention.

This ideological change had important social structural implications. The boundary between "normal" and "abnormal" had been reflected in the institutional arrangements of the time. Midwives cared for normal births and called barber-surgeons to assist in abnormal ones. With the conceptual basis of midwifery changed, the stage was set for a change in the institutional configuration as well.

It is in this context that the "secret instrument," the obstetrical forceps, of the Chamberlen family became important. The story has been told many times and need not be recounted in detail.[13] Briefly, two sons of William Chamberlen, both named Peter, were members of the Barber Surgeons' Company and both practiced midwifery. They were an obstreperous pair fined or cited often by the Barber Surgeons' Company and cited on several occasions by the Royal College of Physicians for illegally practicing medicine. Peter the Elder was once sent to prison by the Royal College but was able to secure his release by appealing to well-placed friends. It was this same Peter who invented the forceps, an instrument passed down as a proprietary family secret for more than a hundred years. The Chamberlens sold their secret to a Dutch practitioner early in the eighteenth century, but when it came time to turn over the instrument they delivered only half the forceps, which in this form amounted essentially to a lever that had been used for years by many barber-surgeons. Jean Palfyn, a Belgian, created forceps that may have been inspired by the Chamberlen forceps, and displayed them for the Academie Royale de Sciences in 1720. After that, the forceps went through many revisions, but the instrument must have gained wide acceptance quickly, since as early as 1733 Edmund Chapman described the forceps as "now well known to all the principal men of the profession, both of the town and country."[14]

It is true that "It was the surgeons' possession of the forceps that enabled them to challenge directly the women midwives' traditional role as the attendants at all normal cases."[15] However, no technology carries the force to change institutional arrangements automatically. Nor does a "scientific advance," by itself, effect change. No technology will gain widespread acceptance and be the basis for reform of culture unless it is introduced into an ideologically fertile social field or unless such a field can be cultivated around it. The forceps was used initially as simply another instrument in the barber-surgeons' armamentarium. It was less destructive than other instruments, but this alone would not permit penetration of the institutionalized province of the midwife by men. Even had the forceps been a matter of public knowledge, its use would have been constrained by the social relationships between the two major kinds of birth attendants. Forceps bearers could encroach on normal births and effect a major social reorganization of midwifery only because of the conceptual reorganization of the field which had occurred earlier. So it may have been the case that the obstetrical forceps accelerated the decline of the midwife, but this decline was facilitated by the conceptually unsettling influence of "scientific midwifery" imported earlier from France.

The revised view of birth which might permit the use of the forceps in deliveries that midwives would otherwise consider normal only created the potential for the ascent of the male midwife over the female. How this potential was realized and why it was realized in different forms in America and Britain require an analysis of the organizational developments in and around the profession which occurred from the late seventeenth century onward.

Men had made some early attempts to invade the province of the midwife. In the first edition of his obstetrics text, Edmund Chapman urged women not to attempt versions and claimed that successful maneuvers by women were only a matter of luck. If Culpepper's *Directory* is any indication, however, some women had been doing versions for a very long time. Chapman and others were trying to expand the practice of men to the detriment of women, but their success was probably limited.

William Smellie was the person who, in the eighteenth century, led the vanguard of male practitioners to attendance at normal births.

Smellie trained as a surgeon in Scotland and used all the instruments of that trade. He learned of the forceps from a 1735 essay by Alexander Butter and began using the instrument immediately if somewhat cautiously. He traveled to London and Paris to become the student of the male masters of midwifery. Then, in 1740, when he took his first student into his house, Smellie became an instructor. Over the next few years Smellie gave organized courses on midwifery to both men and women and became, probably, the most successful of the several lecturers on the subject in London. He claimed to have taught more than nine hundred men, but he did not record the number of women in his classes. The courses were notable because students were allowed to observe deliveries of women (Smellie paid the women for the privilege of observing them). It is significant, also, that he segregated his courses by sex, thereby contributing to rather than ameliorating the division and antagonism between the two classes of birth attendants. He taught men and women at different times of the day and gave them different courses of instruction, as did other teachers of midwifery of his day.

An equally important contribution of Smellie's was his continuation of work in the "scientific" vein. He was the opposite number in Britain of Levret, Baudelocque, and others in France, for he, too, measured normal pelvises and fetal heads, and noted deformities that could impede the "correct delivery" of women. Others like William Hunter, the author of *Anatomy of the Gravid Uterus,* carried on this tradition later in the century and firmly established midwifery as a "scientific" discipline in Britain.

Both the increased number of male practitioners with experience in midwifery and their continued development of the scientific approach to birth augmented the potential for men to take over normal deliveries, but men faced a major impediment to wholesale takeover of the field. They did not have access to the "material," the laboring women, they needed to ply their trade. Men had a strategic social resource in this regard, though, in that hospitals and lying-in charities were their domain. Most public hospitals in Britain were philanthropic ventures established to provide a modicum of medical care for the poor. Those who had founded them thought it their humanitarian duty to do so, but the hospitals in no small way responded to the interests and needs of a growing, affluent middle class as well as to the needs and interests of scientific medicine. The early hospitals provided services primarily for the indigent, but some married women of means did deliver there. Middlesex Hospital, for example, reserved some of its beds for the "better sort" of women. Only men attended upper-class women in hospitals and no teaching was done using these women as models. Men who attended women of the upper classes in public hospitals, William Hunter among them, gained notable reputations thereby and attracted other upper-class women to their private practices as well. In this way, the hospital proved to be a strategic organizational resource for the emergent male practitioner.

The hospital was the scene of a significant social alliance as well. Men taught female midwives in hospitals but they aligned themselves with the "monthly nurses," women who stayed with postpartum women and their babies but who played no part in delivery. This cooperation was significant because, as Philip Thickness wrote in a caustic review, *Man-Midwifery Analysed,* "[the monthly nurse] sounds the Doctor's trumpet far and near; and all her kind mistresses, and indulgent masters are sure to have the warmest recommendation of Dr. Blowbladder's art of touching."[16] Enlisting on the side of men women who posed no threat to obstetricians must have had tremendous symbolic value.

In a short time medical men were able to make significant inroads on the practice of midwifery. A new technology facilitated by a new science of birth, together with the capability of expanding the new male role through education and the control of key resources and foci of organization, put men in the ascendance.

What of the midwives? Why were they unable to resist? The midwives were not well-organized nor did they have an institutionally recognized body of knowledge for which they could claim a privilege and which they could use to argue against the approach offered by men. Midwives, by and large, were local practitioners who had little reason to communicate with each other. Practical knowledge was passed on locally, and until the seventeenth and early eighteenth centuries the midwife's role was unquestioned. Yet the only sense in which her knowledge was institutionally recognized worked to her detriment. She had no franchise on her practice, no prescribed and sanctioned duties. Instead she had proscriptions imposed upon her by ecclesiastical authority. Midwives as a group had no body of prescriptive knowledge with which they could mount a rebuff to the ideological and practical advances of men armed with their new science.

There were early attempts to organize midwives, but they came from men and were designed in the interests of men. In 1616, both Peter Chamberlens, the Elder and the Younger, petitioned Sir Francis Bacon, a member of the Privy Council, and the king for the incorporation of a Society of Midwives. The petition was referred to the Royal College of Physicians, which suggested that the petition be denied, not a surprising result given the Chamberlens' relationships with the College. Later, another Peter Chamberlen, son of Peter the Younger, and first in the line to take the title "Doctor," also tried to establish an organization of midwives. His interests were clear: he wanted to establish a corporation with himself as governor. Midwives resisted this overture, claiming that Chamberlen wanted to gain the sole right to instruct and license midwives. To drive home their point midwives told the College that Dr. Chamberlen had claimed to have greater knowledge of midwifery than "all the grave and learned Physicians in the Kingdom." Even though Dr. Chamberlen was a member of the Royal College of Physicians, his impudence and audacity must have been too much for his colleagues, for the College recommended the petition be denied; thus the midwives were successful in their resistance to his efforts. The bishops who finally heard the midwives' petition added insult to injury when they ordered Dr. Chamberlen to apply for a license in midwifery himself.[17]

The main form of resistance to the encroachment of men was pamphleteering directed mainly against the use of forceps. An especially strong advocate of female midwifery was Elizabeth Nihell, author of a *Treatise on the Art of Midwifery*. Her five-hundred-page book was a vehement attack on male midwifery in general and on William Smellie in particular. She protested the unequal pay for male and female midwives. She claimed that men used their forceps and other instruments unnecessarily and on occasion used them just to impress the patient or her husband with their "superior" skill. She recognized that men had successfully revised the conceptual and the instrumental aspects of birth. Nihell appealed to the "naturalness" of women occupying the office of midwife,[18] but the power of this argument had been attenuated since men had managed to change the terms of the debate. No longer was "nature" an effective argument since birth was no longer a "natural" matter to be overseen by its "natural" attendants. Birth was now a subject of science and was within the purview of scientists. Nihell understood this. In fact, she perhaps more than anyone else at that time clearly recognized the ideological character of this new "science." She saw that "science" was for the most part a political device being used by men in a struggle against women:

> May the women then, for their own sakes, for the sake of their children, cease to be dupes, sure as they are to be in some measure the victims of that scientific jargon, employed to throw its learned dust in their eyes, and to blind them to their danger or perdition! May they, in short, see through that cloud of hard words used by pedants, whose interest it is to impose themselves upon them: a cloud, which is oftener the cover-shame of ignorance, than the vehicle of true knowledge, and perhaps oftener yet the mask of mercenary quackery, than a proof of medical ability.[19]

But this was a period of enlightenment, and science held sway over keen sociological rhetoric of this sort. Nihell dropped into obscurity and the writings of her male competitors flooded the market.

The midwives' position was a difficult one. Their traditional position was being challenged in terms quite foreign to their practice—the terms of the scientist. The solutions available to women practitioners were few and the problem was profound: "the women would need to find new definitions for themselves and their art if they hoped to continue in their mysterious office."[20] In the culture of the time, rhetoric, polemics, and astute political commentary like that of Nihell would take them only so far. They either would have to assert their absolute social and conceptual independence from male practitioners, refuse the gauntlet, and let the market decide, or they would have to engage in the conflict on the scientists' terms. There was a historical precedent for the first course in the midwives' dispute with the Chamberlens. It also had a contemporary basis in the assertion of some midwives that they needed no sophisticated knowledge of anatomy to deliver women safely. But after the middle of the eighteenth century, to attempt such a course would have been disastrous. Well-respected midwives, including Elizabeth Nihell, had acknowledged the need for anatomical knowledge and had started to make claims concerning the efficacy, actually the inefficacy, of using instruments in childbirth. They argued that the instruments had deleterious effects on the "machine" it was designed to assist. It could be argued that simply by beginning to argue in this way—in the terms of the scientists—they had lost the battle before it had started. Such a hasty and automatic conclusion would be unwarranted in this instance, though, because, while some people were busy with rhetoric, others were examining claims and counterclaims empirically. They collected data that to the embarrassment of men practitioners and often to the embarrassment of the researchers themselves showed midwives were "better" birth attendants than men. They were not "better" because they were more "natural"; they were "better" in the framework of the rationalistic, scientistic view of birth proffered by men.

Dr. Charles White, for example, states his intentions and orientation in the preface to a book devoted to reducing maternal deaths from childbirth:

> We are too apt to neglect what is simple and evident, for the sake of those creations of the mind which may be produced at pleasure; but a single argument drawn from a certain fact, is a surer ground to rest upon than an entire system of speculative invention. . . .
>
> At a time when reasoning from real facts and accurate observation has taken the place of idle theory in almost every other science, and has with particular advantage been applied to many branches of medicine, no apology is necessary for trying the same method of reasoning, on this important subject, which has hitherto been too much governed by arbitrary custom, and ignorant prejudice.

After this solemn invocation of the scientific muse, White compared maternal mortality rates in London, Manchester, and Northhampton, with those in lying-in hospitals. He found that death rates for the cities were lower than those for the hospitals. He notes that those delivering in cities are mostly poor, many are attended by "very ignorant" midwives and are "destitute of proper assistance, and of even the necessities of life"; yet they have lower maternal mortality rates than those "where all proper assistance is supposed to be at hand." Such findings seem to support the claims of Nihell and the female midwife advocates, but, understandably, White did not see it that way. Instead, he presented his embarrassing data in an apologetic way and said that he expected the "mismanagement" that must be occurring in hospitals would be remedied.[21] Even if the midwives' detractors would not see the importance of their own data, midwives and their advocates were able to use these figures and others to their benefit, and such arguments would continue well into the nineteenth century. But if the data had any effect at all, it was only to postpone the demise of the female midwife; for other, more powerful forces were at work.

Midwifery was a lucrative practice for men. They could charge higher fees than women even though they spent less time at their tasks than their female counterparts. Also, midwifery gave men an important entrée to general practice. As men learned to use their instruments and not damage women or babies, they probably became more acceptable as birth attendants and as healers generally. Most authors have also attributed the late nineteenth-century rise of men in this profession to increasing affluence—more people could afford male accoucheurs—and to fashion—the upper classes started using male attendants and other people imitated them. I suspect these factors played a role in the increased use of men, but I also suspect a more subtle, and ultimately more important, process was at work as well. Birth practices of earlier times created an atmosphere of fear and dread at the periphery of the mysterious phenomenon of childbirth. These two aspects—the mysterious and the fearsome— had separate reflections in institutional forms. Midwives filled the mysterious office, while men with their instruments were the bearers of the terrifying in birth. The use of hooks and craniotomy to extract fetuses drew these comments from notable male practitioners: Hugh Chamberlen—"where a *Man comes one or both [the mother or the child] must necessarily die.*"[22] William Smellie (who recommended that instruments for craniotomies be concealed from patients)—"this expedient [craniotomy] produced a general clamour among women, who observed that when recourse was had to the assistance of a man-midwife, either the mother or the child, or both were lost."[23]

With educational programs like Smellie's urging men to be more conservative in their practice and with men attending more normal births and the births of more publicly "visible" upper-class women, the idea of death was, no doubt, partially dissociated from men. However, the veil of fear surrounding pregnancy and birth remained, judging from the religious recommendations that women contemplate pain and death as their confinement approached. This residual fear facilitated the development of the idea that all pregnancies were pathological, a concept which would be used by men in their struggle to gain control of normal births in the following centuries. Public acceptance of men which proceeded swiftly at the end of the eighteenth century was due, then, to a constellation of factors. Fashion and affluence played their part, but during this period the embryonic notion of pregnancy as pathological arose out of vestigial institutional forms and practices.

Early attempts to organize men to take over birth were supplemented by the development of ethical arguments concerning obstetrical practice. Ethics is sometimes considered to be a set of "eminently reasonable" statements or principles that are designed to guide action and that tend to develop in those circumstances where difficult decisions are required. A difficult decision is simply a decision for which no widely accepted, culturally prescribed resolution has been found. Therefore, groups involved in such decisions often develop codes of ethics in order to legitimate the practices of their group and to keep outsiders from scrutinizing those practices too closely. If one can successfully declare one's actions "ethical" and make them seem "reasonable," then there is no problem in proceeding along one's chosen course of action. Ethics viewed in this way becomes a rhetorical device designed to unify a social group.[24] Smellie, Chapman, and Benjamin Pugh were among those prescribing dress and demeanor and suggesting answers to the question of whether or not to accept hopeless cases as parts of informal ethical codes. They were concerned about the reputation of male midwives and the acceptability of procedures associated with them, and they saw appealing to ethics as a way to obtain social privilege.[25] Ethics was used as a means to secure political advantage in the early days of the profession just as it would be used later.

Organizationally, male and female midwifery followed rather serpentine paths which intersected in important ways. In the first half of the nineteenth century many groups wanted to gain the right to license midwives. Several petitions to the Royal Colleges were unsuccessful. An attempt by the Apothecaries to gain the right to penalize unqualified midwives also failed. Beginning around 1826, the Obstetrical Society, an organization of male practitioners, began to make its case for the regulation of unqualified midwives and had some small success. But all of these efforts occurred in an atmosphere which stressed free trade and derided anything resembling a monopoly or government intervention. This atmosphere, together with a fair degree of provincialism, made the Royal Colleges cautious when they considered anything that might appear to enlarge their franchises over the practice of medicine. In this context, however, men scored an indirect coup near mid-century when the Colleges established examinations for men in midwifery and other aspects of medicine and began the *Medical Register.* Unqualified practitioners were not regulated out of business by the General Council for Medical Education and the *Medical Register,* both set up in 1858, but they could not appear on the *Register.* Thus, unqualified practitioners did not have the legitimacy accorded those practicing with a diploma or by examination. As Jean Donnison notes, "because the Universities and corporations admitted only men to their examination, the [registration] Act appeared to put the final seal on the exclusion of women from the profession."[26]

In the last half of the nineteenth century, several things happened that sent female midwifery on a completely new tack. A new definition for midwives would be found in this period, and the occupation would emerge at the end of the century in a form that embodied interests different from those of traditional midwives. The profession would be on the verge of acceptability, but the terms for "acceptability" would have changed, and so, therefore, would the office.

It seems that the key to survival of midwifery as a separate occupation for women in England was the interest expressed in it by women of higher social standing than the typical rural midwife. Florence Nightingale envisioned the training of "Physician-Accoucheuses" and to that end she founded a school to turn out highly trained midwives. Her efforts were thwarted by outbreaks of puerperal fever in her wards and thereafter she abandoned her organizational efforts in midwifery. This did not stop other upper-class women from moving on midwifery, though. Another training institution, the Ladies' Medical College, was established by the newly formed Female Medical Society. The society professed an interest in getting women into medicine on a fully qualified basis, but their first efforts were directed toward the provision of high-quality training in midwifery. A group closely aligned with the Society, the Obstetrical Association of Midwives, proposed legislation that would admit women to the *Medical Register* as Midwives. Such an achievement would have been significant since being on the *Register* in this manner would have given at least one group of midwives, the well-educated ones, a relatively independent status. Their hopes went unrealized. Even Florence Nightingale did not support their efforts because she believed female midwives needed even better training than women were receiving in the Society's college.

The Obstetrical Society, which had scored moderate successes in its campaign for the registration of male midwives earlier, reentered the scene with its scheme for the registration of females and again scored a qualified victory. The Society set up its own examination board for midwives, male and female this time, and then proceeded to seek legitimacy for it. James Hobson Aveling took the Society's case to the General Medical Council with his book *English Midwives: Their History and Prospects*.[27] The Council ultimately decided that it had no power over the licensure of midwives, a move which left the Female Medical Society and the Obstetrical Association of Midwives without a base for their claims to license women and which left the Obstetrical Society's examining board in a position of preeminence on the licensing scene. The scheme of the Obstetrical Society to bring midwives under the control of male medical practitioners through the Society's examination remained in place almost by default as everyone's attention turned, near the end of the century, to the emergence of the female *doctor* and away from the less threatening female midwife. The Obstetrical Society revised its scheme in order to make it more acceptable to the existing medical powers, but it never gained the official recognition it needed. Ultimately, the power the Society wielded through its examination was lowered by the lack of enforcement powers and by the small number of people who voluntarily came forth for training and examination by the Society.

Then, just as the Obstetrical Society was fading into the background, a new organization of, and purportedly for, midwives was formed. This was the Matrons' Aid or Trained Midwives' Registration Society, later to be called simply the Midwives' Institute. This organization was formed by upper-class women, some of whom had taken the examination of the Obstetrical Society. They moved quickly to seek the support of the Obstetrical Society and thereby seemingly sealed the fate of midwifery as a practice subordinate to the "higher calling" of medicine. The women's Society immediately accepted the rhetoric of critics of female midwifery concerning the inferior service received at the hands of female midwives. They made the improvement of practice one of their primary goals and gave force to this intention by requiring a certificate from the Obstetrical Society for admission to their own Society. The Midwives' Institute retained a degree of independence, though. They saw fit to offer some resistance to registration bills developed jointly by the Obstetrical Society and the British Medical Association, and they resisted the overtures of the British Nurses' Association, which suggested joint registration of nurses and midwives. (The nurses later turned on the midwives, attacking their cause and urging that the nurse-midwife licensed by the BNA be recognized as the only appropriate childbirth attendant.)

There were two other players in the development of midwife legislation: the rural general practitioner and the government. The midwife threatened the practice of the general practitioner much more severely than she threatened the practice of his urban counterpart. Therefore, there was a considerable animosity between midwives and GPs that would become an important factor in the midwives' struggle for recognition after the enfranchisement of the GP into the regulatory scheme of English medicine under the General Medical Council's reorganization in 1858. Under the reorganization the GPs had a say in registration matters and could oppose the recognition of midwives with their votes as well as with their rhetoric. The conflict was not resolved finally until the GP was assured a set income from the National Health Insurance scheme two decades into the next century.

The government became involved in the registration dispute in the 1890s. In 1893, a select committee of Parliament suggested midwife registration and a two-tiered system of childbirth attendants with the recognized, well-educated practitioners being administered by government agencies. Because of the complicated organization of interests which surrounded this issue, no bill could receive broad support and, in fact, none passed until 1902.

The medical profession used the period of shifting alliances prior to the passage of midwifery legislation to solidify its "scientific" ideological framework for childbirth. Robert Barnes described pregnancy as a "natural experiment" which, when "induced" on a healthy woman, provided an opportunity "to observe and to record the effects of this change on the economy." Of pregnancy he said, "the transition from physiology to pathology, and back again, is wonderfully rapid; . . . often the boundary can hardly be defined."[28] In hearings before the select committee of Parliament, doctors anchored pregnancy within the realm of the pathological by arguing that "childbirth could no longer be regarded as a natural process, nor could 'natural' labor be accurately defined. Every birth should therefore be attended by a medical practitioner, who . . . should 'guide' and 'control' it."[29] Such rhetoric was, perhaps, even more important than the political developments that culminated in the Midwives' Act. It created a climate in which there was no chance to return to a prior time when midwives practiced in their own way, independent of doctors, the dominant figures on the medical scene at the end of the nineteenth century.

The Midwives' Act of 1902 is regarded by many as the climax of a successful struggle for the preservation of midwifery in Britain. I see it as a somewhat anticlimactic, reasonably predictable outcome of the organizational permutations of the preceding thirty years, in particular the alignment of well-educated practitioners of female midwifery with the portion of the medical profession that had struggled for midwife registration for seventy-five years. The final bill to pass Parliament was a slap in the face of the British Medical Association and the General Medical Council. The legislatively mandated overseeing body for midwives, the Central Midwives' Board, was to report to the Privy Council, an arm of the government, and was not to be under the direct control of medicine. Similarly, a rule requiring that midwives register every year with local medical authorities was dropped from the legislation. But in its original form the bill required that the Midwives' Board have its majority composed of medical men. (In the final version, a member of a nursing association—significantly, not the British Nurses' Association—was added, giving the midwives a chance to secure a majority of the Board depending on the proclivities of the nurses' representative.) Unqualified midwives were given a grace period of eight years before they had to register to practice, but midwives registered under the Act could still be dropped from the rolls of the *Medical Register* for "unprofessional" and undefined "improper" conduct. So the Act that gave midwives a professional status not enjoyed by women previously also put them in a position not suffered by any profession dominated by men. The profession could not be self-regulating, as most professions were, since it would be under the constant scrutiny of members of other, rival professions. Women were able to continue to attend births, but on very different terms from those in the past. Midwifery had become a profession for the benefit of an upper-class segment of practitioners who had aligned themselves with medicine, a development that was to the detriment of the independent practitioner on whom the responsibility of childbirth attendance had rested for centuries.

Midwifery in America

Developments in American midwifery paralleled those in Britain. This is not surprising, given that colonial culture borrowed freely from Britain. But the colonists had set out to establish a new state, a new commonwealth, and with considerable struggle had done so. Thus, it would seem reasonable that the crucial differences in the social and political development of obstetrics depended largely on the different role the state played in the two countries.

Until the time of the American Revolution, American practitioners of medicine were technically under the jurisdiction of the medical governing bodies in Britain, but there were some early shows of independence from that control.[30] All areas of life, including, or perhaps one should say especially, the practice of professions, were of concern to local authorities in the colonies, and the patriarchs saw fit therefore to regulate the practice of midwifery. In the northern colonies leaders saw their authority as derivative of their "calling." Striving for something different from a democracy, they set out to establish a theocracy. Accordingly, early licensing of midwives followed English ecclesiastical licensing to a large degree, but responsibility for administration devolved onto what we would term civil authority.[31]

The practice of medicine was not well organized. Civil authorities did nothing to encourage organization since they had a clear interest in avoiding a grant of monopoly to any particular group of practitioners. The colonists self-consciously avoided the model of the Royal Colleges. Medicine was practiced by anyone who showed a talent for it or who had acquired a modicum of training. In the middle of the eighteenth century colonists began returning in large numbers from the great medical schools of England, Scotland, and, to a lesser degree, of Europe, bringing with them the new scientific medicine, such as it was. Those who could afford foreign study became the shining stars in the newly developing, yet rather chaotic, medical profession, eclipsing all who had studied as apprentices or who had entered practice because it was a lucrative line of work.

William Smellie's counterpart in America was William Shippen, one of the several hundred practitioners able to study abroad. Like Smellie, Shippen gave courses in medicine and midwifery; also like Smellie, he allowed his students to attend indigent women who were giving birth. Shippen, too, taught women, but perhaps due to expense, perhaps due to notions of propriety, it appears that few women chose to attend his lectures.[32]

From the record it seems that increased acceptance of men practitioners of midwifery proceeded much more quickly and much more simply in America than it did in Britain. This impression may be an artifact due to the lack of organization of both medical men and midwives. Organizations are more likely than individuals to leave records that are accessible to historians and that paint a picture of large-scale social change. The small local struggles which occurred over the practice of midwifery may have been every bit as brutal and complex as those which occurred on the larger social scene in Britain. Yet the image that emerges from extant records in America is simple: male midwifery increased and female midwifery declined without all of the twists and turns experienced in Britain. Though this may be an artifact of the record, differences between Britain and America suggest that it is an apt description of just what occurred.

Medical men in America did not have an exclusive franchise over their work as their counterparts in Britain did. Therefore, they were all threatened by the existence of the midwife. All of them were in a position comparable to that of the general practitioner in England. No one enjoyed the autonomy and protection of a Royal College. Midwifery was an important entrée to family practice and it was extremely lucrative compared to other aspects of medical practice.[33] Medicine did not have an elite group of practitioners whose interests in midwifery differed from those of the rank-and-file physician. Midwifery was economically important to all physicians and became an object of their desire.

Midwifery was strategically important as well. In theory midwives could have organized to protect their interests and would have presented a major alternative to traditional medical care, but they did not do so. Practicing midwives were probably more oriented toward their practice and their patients than toward a body of knowledge or toward the organization of a profession. The decentralized nature of government, the high degree of official concern over personal deportment, and the large body of theories that objectified the inferiority of women[34] all conspired to keep "ladies" out of midwifery. So American midwives lacked the organizational basis and upper-class patronage which British midwifery had. The state played an indirect role in their lack of organization as well. Access to medical education was an entirely private venture. Going abroad was enormously expensive and apprenticing oneself locally also presented economic and, for women, social impediments. Civil authorities did nothing to reduce these barriers in the prerevolutionary period, and after the Revolution the federal government refused to make funds available to sponsor a school of midwifery.[35] Federal interest in training midwives and in the health of the populace generally was a major difference between British and American developments in this field.

There were schools of medicine for women in the nineteenth century just as there were schools for many other kinds of practitioners. Most of the schools were proprietary, money-making ventures. Women who could afford an education could attend the New England Female Medical College or the Medical College for Women in New York or a school of hydropathy or one of a number of other institutions, but graduating from a school simply allowed a woman to ply her skills in a very crowded marketplace. Certification carried little prestige unless it was conferred by one of the European medical schools or by one of the "regular," orthodox schools in the States modeled after the European ones.

To a greater degree than in Britain, women of means concentrated their efforts on gaining admission to the "regular" schools. Some succeeded. Those who did generally specialized in the diseases of women and children and tried to wage the battle for equality of admission to university training for women. Women were not admitted to any major medical school on a regular basis, though, until the 1890s. Johns Hopkins, which would become the model for American medical schools after the Flexner Report of 1910,[36] admitted women in 1893, but it opened its doors only in response to the requirements of a bequest from a woman.

For a woman to enter and graduate from medical school was difficult, but for her to effect a change in medical practice was virtually impossible. In order to get through medical school a woman had to become steeped in the language and procedures of science. Science was much more important to the social organization of medicine in America than in Britain. It was used to create privilege where none existed. It was the cornerstone of the great medical schools, and women had to accept that or not apply. Harriot Hunt, for example, had to subordinate explicitly considerations of her sex to science in a letter appealing the denial of her first application to Harvard Medical School.[37]

Science, though, was more than something that divided the sexes. It was used by male practitioners to overcome the impediments imposed by considerations of modesty and decorum, the major barriers to male attendance at birth. Science was also used to entrench pregnancy firmly in the pathological realm and ultimately to win the market by mounting arguments which stressed the safety of delivery by men instead of women.

Jane Donegan says that medical men "faced a . . . formidable obstacle to continued dominance in obstetrics in the form of the cultural mores of the period. . . . A society that grew increasingly prudish . . . could not be expected to look with equanimity upon the presence of accoucheurs in the lying-in chamber"[38] The ideal woman of the nineteenth century was sensitive, fragile, submissive, rather sickly, and above all modest. Medicine helped create this image,[39] and then had to overcome it in order to practice its art. Discussion of the place of delicacy reached a climax when Dr. James P. White, professor of obstetrics at the University of Buffalo, permitted his students to observe a delivery. He had the support of the faculty and his dean and later received an appreciative resolution from the graduating class concerning his willingness to provide "demonstrative midwifery" as part of the course in medicine. Dr. White sued one Dr. Horatio Loomis for libel, though, when the latter published a letter condemning such practices in the *Buffalo Courier*. During the trial the rhetoric necessary to overcome the modesty and delicacy of women abounded. For example, Dr. Charles B. Coventry, professor of obstetrics at Geneva College in New York, is reported to have said that he "conceives no purpose, that has for its object the saving of human life, can be either indecorous or immoral." Dr. Chandler Gilman of the College of Physicians and Surgeons in New York believed that delivering a woman while she was exposed to a class of students "should not [be considered] indelicate; when a medical man is called upon to save the lives of individuals, his position ought to raise him above such feelings of false delicacy." As Dr. John Haksteen pointed out at the trial, "The practice is what the theory teaches."[40] In order to teach in this manner and build up an ideology concerning the relative importance of safety over the constraints of modesty, medicine had to have a theory of childbirth that declared it unsafe, contrary to the general view of birth held by midwives.

Creating a theory of the pathology of pregnancy and fortifying that concept were the Americans' strong suits as indeed they had to be if Americans were to establish political dominance over female midwifery. The profession recognized that this was a political task, not a scientific one. Dr. Hugh Hodge said, "If females *can be induced to believe* that their sufferings will be diminished, or shortened, and their lives and those of their offspring, be safer in the hands of the profession; there will be no difficulty in establishing the universal practice of obstetrics."[41] Benjamin Rush termed pregnancy a "disease" and treated it as other diseases were treated, with "heroic" measures such as bloodletting and the application of leeches. Ironically, Rush had also observed that for North American Indians "nature is their only midwife." But no matter, civilization had progressed and nature had regressed, or so at least went the evolutionary arguments borrowed from England.

William Potts Dewees "systematized" existing scientific knowledge on obstetrics in his book *A Compendious System of Midwifery* that became the standard text for decades to come. Particularly because Dewees advocated conservative practice, the opening remarks of his text are worth quoting at length. They follow a familiar pattern of asserting the importance of applying "art" at the limits of "nature," the disputed boundary that had been crucial to the midwife and to the profession since the sixteenth and seventeenth centuries:

> It has often been declared, that labour, being a natural act, does not require the interference of art for either its promotion or its accomplishment. . . . This view of the subject has many followers, and has, from its influence, retarded, more perhaps than any other circumstance, the progress of improvement in the most important branch of medical science. It is so entirely comported with the theories of the fastidious admirers of nature; . . . so effectually apologized for ignorance; and so plausibly extenuated the evils arising from neglect, or the want of the proper and judicious application of skill, as to secure in its favour by far the greater proportion of the practitioners of Midwifery.

> [If labor always proceeded in an uncomplicated manner] the opinions of those who contend for the supremacy of unassisted nature, would deserve much, and perhaps exclusive attention. But, as it is but too well known, that this never has nor even can be the case, we must insist, that the powers of nature have

their limits, and that the interference of art becomes absolute necessity.[42]

Dewees acknowledges his debt to Baudelocque and other French founding fathers and then sets forth for more than six hundred pages the accumulated knowledge of the science of midwifery and catalogs the interferences available to the profession.

The middle years of the nineteenth century saw the solidification of the scientific basis of midwifery in America. Forceps had been used for a long time, not without critics, to be sure, for Americans knew of the debates in Britain and waged some of their own. The major contribution of American obstetrics was in another vein, however. Americans seemed to adopt new technical innovations quickly. These innovations depended on the idea of pregnancy being a disease and then reinforced that idea by making it clearer that the safety of delivery was dependent on attendance by doctors. In this manner medicine was able to use and at the same time fortify a conceptual cornerstone of its practice even though medicine was under attack in other quarters. For example, the use of ether, introduced in 1842, eliminated the "unbearable pains" of childbirth. It also eliminated the mother from effective participation in delivery and made necessary attendance by a person skilled in the use of instruments. Deliveries that were "abnormally long," the demarcation of which now rested with the male midwife, could be hastened by the use of ergot or, later, pituitary extract. Ergot, in turn, reinforced the need for male attendants because of the possibility of tetanic contractions and ruptured uteri, "abnormalities" for which there was no therapy but which only men could attend. Perhaps the greatest coup of scientific medicine in the eighteenth century was its finding a solution to a problem it had created: the epidemics of puerperal fever. Childbed fever was the scourge of parturient women and had a much higher incidence in hospitals than in home deliveries. On the eastern side of the Atlantic, Professor Alexander Gordon and Ignaz P. Semmelweis wrote on the contagiousness of the disease some seventy years apart. In America Oliver Wendell Holmes[43] authored the paper which caused, first, cries of outrage and indignation, and, then, rethinking of the problem of puerperal fever and its virtual elimination. The puerperal fever episode together with other "advances" of the time must have reinforced in the mind of the public the inextricably intertwined perceptions of "pregnancy as dangerous" and of the "medical man as the only practitioner knowledgeable enough to effect a safe delivery." Judy Barrett Litoff outlines other developments in American obstetrics and gynecology which similarly bolstered the position of the "scientific" practitioner. These included the ovariotomy operation and the repair of vesico-vaginal fistulas—tears between the vagina and bladder—the latter pioneered by J. Marion Sims in his experimental work on slave women.[44] The "advances" of the period made pregnancy into the pathological problem it had to be in order for it to be attended by men. Pregnancy became, literally and ideologically, more pathological.

In the last half of the nineteenth century, "regular" medicine also moved to strengthen its organizational base. During the Jacksonian era American medicine was thwarted in its attempts to secure licensing privileges. For lack of official sanction and under considerable competition from other kinds of practitioners, regular practitioners lost prestige in the public eye. At midcentury the regulars engaged in what seems now to have been a "last gasp" political and public relations campaign. Medical societies made membership entirely voluntary, a rather curious move for an institution whose membership was declining rapidly and showed no signs of improving. (The medical societies did not, however, go so far as to admit women at this time.) Publicly, medicine touted its "professionalism" and displayed the new ethical code of Worthington Hooker, who stressed the need to elevate oneself and one's profession above irregular competitors. Not so publicly, medical societies in all states placed themselves in the position of gatekeeper between medical school graduation and medical practice. By stressing the benefit to the public and denying that benefit would accrue to medical practitioners—a stance that was required given the strong antitrust sentiment of the time—regular medicine persuaded state legislatures to establish licensing boards in all states by 1898. With some variation among the states, medical societies put themselves in influential positions with regard to these boards and thereby created the potential—to be fully realized within two decades—for the regulars to become the dominant force in American medicine.[45]

Organizational developments in gynecology and obstetrics paralleled those in the profession generally. The American Medical Association was founded in 1847 but did not rise to national prominence until licensing laws were in effect in all states fifty years later. Significantly, though, the AMA structured itself so that midwifery, now routinely called "obstetrics," was part of one of its scientific divisions. Societies for medical specialties proliferated, as well, in the last half of the nineteenth century. They were competitors of the AMA and therefore a threat to general medicine, but they were a force to be reckoned with since their members occupied chairs in major medical schools and contributed significantly to the development of the profession. In 1869 the AMA gave its blessing to specialties, including the American Gynecological Society, but forbade them from advertising and bound them to the AMA's Code of Ethics.[46] Also significant during this period was the publication of the *American Journal of Obstetrics and the Diseases of Women and Children,* which started in 1868 as the first specialty publication in America. By the end of the nineteenth century, then, it appeared that midwifery was doomed by the increased security that medicine in general and obstetrics in particular had been able to achieve.

Midwives still practiced in fairly large numbers and they were especially important to people of lower classes. As late as 1910, midwives delivered more than 50 percent of all babies, more among rural residents and disenfranchised blacks and immigrants.[47] There were some notable schools for midwives, but organized medicine recognized none of them and only a few commanded the respect necessary to make their diplomas valuable.

Largely in response to public alarm over recognition of high maternal mortality rates, some states passed legislation requiring registration of midwives. New York followed its legislation by establishing a school for midwives at Bellevue Hospital. After the school had been in existence for four years, state registration requirements were revised to favor graduates of this nationally known program. With the assistance of the federal government, all states but Massachusetts made some provision for improving the lot of midwives. (Massachusetts made them illegal and at the same time required them to report any births they attended.) Public health officials advocated licensing of midwives and used cross-national comparisons of maternal mortality by prevalence of female midwifery—comparisons between states, and inter-county variations within one state—to show that trained midwives seemed to be better birth attendants than men.

Organized medicine had been too successful during the previous century, though. As soon as regular practitioners had gained the franchise, in part by promising that medicine would not try to achieve a national monopoly, they set about the task of achieving just such a monopoly. The role of the Flexner Report in this regard is well known.[48] The Carnegie Foundation financed a report by Abraham Flexner on the status of American medical education. Flexner based himself at Johns Hopkins and traveled to virtually all of the medical schools in the country in order to rate each one's quality. In judgments that paralleled the ratings of the AMA's own Committee on Medical Education, he recommended that the number of medical schools be cut by 80 percent. American medicine was too crowded, Flexner argued. Competition came not only from the "quacks" but from regular medicine itself. Using the Flexner Report as their justification, private philanthropies—most notably the Carnegie and Rockefeller Foundations—set out to eliminate competitors of "regular" practitioners.

Among the targets of the supporters of reorganization was the midwife. Exactly the same kinds of arguments that had been used for more than two hundred years were used again in this campaign. J. Whitridge Williams[49] surveyed the professors of obstetrics in all medical schools, and from surprisingly candid replies an impression of a profession in a horrible state emerged. Chairs in obstetrics were occupied by men who had relatively little experience, and students could graduate from medical school without attending a delivery. Rather than suggest the profession turn to a ready alternative, the midwife, Williams urged that the profession foster an image of obstetrics as a complicated specialty. This was precisely the path followed by Dr. Charles White in 1773 after he analyzed maternal mortality in England and apologetically expected that care in hospitals would improve. Joseph DeLee, a famous American obstetrician, followed a well-worn rhetorical path by arguing that "parturition, viewed with modern eyes, is no longer a normal function, but . . . it has imposing pathological dignity." This was the view that would be trumpeted throughout the midwife debates of 1910–30. DeLee also introduced the concept of the "prophylactic forceps operation," a move that obliterated the boundary between normal and abnormal and allowed male midwives to take over, conceptually and instrumentally, the domain of the midwife.[50]

Litoff gives an excellent summary of the attempts that were made at the federal and state levels to resuscitate midwifery or at least to preserve it as a "necessary evil" until a sufficient number of doctors could be created to attend all births. But, she concludes,

Public health advocates were unsuccessful in their attempts to convince the medical profession and lay people that the utilization of properly trained and regulated midwives would help reduce the maternal and infant mortality rates in the United States. . . . The failure of the proponents was partially attributable to the fact that their opponents were better organized and more articulate. However, social and cultural changes, only peripherally related to the early twentieth century midwife debate, also helped to bring about the midwife's downfall.[51]

Among the changes sealing the fate of the midwife were restricted immigration that lowered the demand for subculturally acceptable female birth-attendants, a lower birthrate overall, a perception of birth as a "special" event, and improved transportation which made hospital deliveries more feasible.[52]

After 1930 only midwives from recognized schools were allowed to practice. The traditional midwife was replaced by the obstetrically educated and obstetrically overseen midwife.[53] Medicine controlled her numbers and her education, and the midwife would not become a factor in American childbirth again until the 1970s.

Themes in the Development of a Profession

In the historical development of the profession of obstetrics and the concomitant demise of the midwife in America and the reformation of the terms of her practice in Britain, we can see many of the themes which will recur in future developments in the profession. The rhetorical and practical strategies used in the first 350 years of obstetrics became a resource for the professions's descendants in the twentieth century, and they merit review here.

The transformation of midwifery began innocuously enough. Two groups of people attended births, but female midwives had essential control over the conduct of the event. Critical to the midwife's existence was her control of the boundary between normal births and abnormal ones. A reasonably creative person modified the approach to birth of the other group of attendants, the barber-surgeons, not then considered serious competitors of midwives, by changing some of the tools used to deliver women having difficult labor. Barbs and hooks were removed from the ends of their instruments and two "levers" were put together to make forceps. However, with the social relationship between the groups of birth attendants and its closely associated ideology, the forceps could not play an important role in the improvement of the status of male midwives. A new conceptualization of the phenomenon of birth was needed in order to take normal births from the hands of midwives. Such a conceptual scheme had been imported to England earlier in the form of French rationalism. The scientific view of the body provided the metaphor, the theory, on the basis of which the midwives' definition of "normal" could be challenged and from which a "correct" practice of birth attendance could be devised. The assault on birth attendance began with the concatenation of the instrumentalism of England and the rationalism of France.

A successful search for an appropriate theory is important in the manipulation of professional boundaries, but once a theory is found a group must be able to organize itself around its conceptual and material bases of practice. Typically, this requires some form of patronage. In England the new practitioners of obstetrics appealed to organized medicine, which had had a legal monopoly on practice for more than three hundred years. Interestingly, the monopoly enjoyed by their colleagues worked against the interests of obstetricians. In-fighting, chauvinism, and haughty disinterest led to a failure to create a united backing for male midwifery and the placement of birth within the classical medical domain. At about the same time, female midwifery gained its own form of patronage when upper-class women who were willing to be co-opted by a concerned portion of the medical profession took an interest in midwife regulation. This coalition of forces was attractive to the government while the posturings and inaction of organized medicine were not. Thus, in 1902, the government sanctioned the efforts of the Midwives' Institute with the Midwives' Act. In America midwifery was much more crucial to the interests of the medical profession as a whole. Midwifery was one of medicine's targets in its moves to achieve social privilege and professional dominance. By shrewd politicking and the use of private and public patronage, medicine achieved its goals. It used strategies that we will see in future developments: appeals to ethics and other aspects of "professionalism," manipulation of the public's view of birth by exploitation of metaphors developed earlier, the touting of "advances" which would have been impossible but for the ideological changes and fragile structural reforms effected earlier, and the ability to rebuff or ignore critics of their practices. Medicine was abetted in all of this by developments that were seemingly unrelated to its professional interests.

Regular medicine and obstetrics entered the first part of the twentieth century with a firm hold on birth. A secure professional boundary existed around the profession in Britain and America. But owing to the different historical paths leading to the establishment of those boundaries, the professions differed. British obstetrics was still much more secure than its American counterpart. Consequently, the activities of the early years of the two professions differed significantly.

3 Residual Normalcy and Pathological Potential

Medical practice is tending ideally toward
prophylaxis. We strive to foresee and prevent
pathology rather than await its onset.
Charles B. Reed, 1920

Obstetricians used their ability to treat childbirth as pathological to create their profession, but not all births were pathological nor could they be made to seem so. The new professions in Britain and America faced a problem: What to do with the "residual normalcy" of childbirth? The problem was only partly ideological. The project of obstetrics as obstetricians originally defined it was the pathology of childbirth, but the continued existence of obstetricians depended on their ability to capture childbirth, all of it, treat it, and hold it firmly as part of their project. Until they could accomplish that, they would live with the threat, which had recent historical precedent in the midwife, that someone would offer women an alternative approach to birth, treat childbirth differently, and encroach on the obstetricians' newly secured domain of practice. The problem for the profession was to extend its influence and solidify the mandate it had written for itself. Obstetricians had to develop ways to "foresee" pathology and act prophylactically because they could not always depend on pathology being obviously present.

The professions in America and Britain were deployed in two different ways to handle the problem of residual normalcy. British obstetrics was a strongly demarcated profession; it had a clear and strong boundary around it. American obstetrics was weakly demarcated and without a strong professional boundary. Women in America were delivered by general practitioners and obstetrical specialists, but members of both groups were doctors, equals among equals. Such was the rhetoric of the profession and such was the medical profession's practice following on the American Medical Association's tactful but successful replacement of the separatist-minded specialists within the medical fold late in the nineteenth century. As a result, at the beginning of the twentieth century there was no clear demarcation between the obstetrical specialist and the rank-and-file physician who delivered babies as part of his wider practice. In contrast, British midwives still practiced, albeit under the supervision and control of doctors, and were still responsible for "normal" deliveries, although they were no longer responsible for making that determination. Midwives practiced on one side of a clear professional boundary while obstetricians were responsible for "abnormal" deliveries and remained on the other side of their professional boundary.

This difference in boundary strengths influenced the early practices of obstetrics, practices through which obstetrics extended its reach to include births which were only *potentially* pathological in addition to those that were clearly pathological. In America practices that developed in the specialty quickly diffused throughout the profession and became routine in the management of childbirth. In Britain practices developed by obstetrical specialists were differentiated from those used in "normal" deliveries and tended to remain on the specialist's side of the professional boundary. A strong boundary tends to contain practices; a weak one lets them diffuse into general practice more quickly.

The difference in boundaries had other consequences as well. Weak boundaries require more vigorous defense than stronger ones. When procedures diffused throughout American obstetrics, they tended to attract a large degree of critical attention. In response, the profession had to develop many kinds of defensive strategies to protect the procedures and, thereby, the profession itself. Criticism was ignored when possible, discounted on occasion, and parts of the profession rhetorically separated themselves from the "average man," the nonspecialist, in order to blame problems with its practices on the skills of practitioners rather than on the practices themselves. In Britain the same procedures were protected from such critical scrutiny by a strong professional boundary. Consequently the British did not have to defend their work to the degree the

Americans did. A strong boundary such as existed in Britain can cause problems, though. As the study of the history of the induction of labor in this chapter shows, once criticism of a professionally protected practice does arise, a strong boundary reduces the options open to a profession. Rigid characterizations of practices make rhetorical reconceptualization and slight amendment of the practices, in the interest of preserving a procedure, more difficult and criticism, once established, more effective. In this chapter all of these rather general propositions are illustrated through detailed studies of several practices which had their roots in the early days of obstetrics. Before examining practices, though, I will look at the profession's work on its conceptual base.

In what follows two kinds of contrasts are discussed. First, there was a difference between British and American obstetrics based on their different boundary strengths. Second, differences in rhetoric and practice appeared *within* American obstetrics in the formative years of the profession. With a weak boundary, it was almost inevitable that debates about the ultimate form of the profession should occur. One group in American obstetrics, led by Joseph B. DeLee, wanted obstetrics to be a super-profession, and all of this group's rhetoric and recommendations for practice followed from this position. Others, led by J. Whitridge Williams, wanted a more egalitarian profession which would be responsive to the needs of the average physician.

Although both sides suffered the ambivalence and uncertainty that come from having to advance a particular program in a professional milieu in which respect for fellow professionals had to be the paramount consideration, the debate within the American profession tells us just as much about the early days of obstetrics as do the differences between the British and American professions.

Ideology

Obstetricians had to confront the fact that not all births were pathological. They had ethnographies of so-called primitive peoples who delivered unassisted or with only minimal assistance. In their own midst they had the "lower sorts" still attended primarily by midwives, and these births, available data showed, were safer than those of people who could afford the obstetricians' more invasive practices. Even among the upper classes (those whose natural ability to suffer childbirth supposedly had been eroded by the advance of civilization), obstetricians found some women who could deliver without the sophistications of obstetrical art. In order to accommodate this "residual normalcy" of childbirth, obstetrics tried to cast birth in terms of *pathological potential*. Birth was an essentially normal and natural phenomenon, the profession argued, but it was overlaid with "pathological dignity," the ever-present chance that something might go wrong.

This was a new development on the blurred boundary between normal and abnormal deliveries. Birth was no longer simply "normal" or "abnormal" nor was the birth process "efficient" or "inefficient" and subject to improvement through the intervention of a skilled practitioner. Now birth was something to be watched, not through the eyes of a person like a midwife whose job it was to attend birth, read its revelatory messages, and call for help when something went wrong, but through eyes trained to be sensitive to the signs of impending pathology.

The writings of Joseph B. DeLee, a Chicago obstetrician who wore his specialist's mantle with a fierce, isolationist's pride,[1] reflect the rhetoric of the dominant school of American obstetricians and merit close examination. He is quite properly cited as the principal protagonist of the "birth as pathology" school, yet not even he claimed that all births should be treated as abnormal. He was more concerned with the possibility that any given birth might become abnormal and he tried to organize obstetrical work to respond to the often unmanifest threat of pathology. Even his polemic favoring prophylactic forceps-operations, which appeared in the first number of the *American Journal of Obstetrics and Gynecology* in 1920, makes it clear that he felt birth was only potentially pathological. In the following passage DeLee makes a bold declaration on the pathology of pregnancy, but then comments provocatively on the relativity of the normal/abnormal boundary:

> Labor has been called, and still is believed by many to be, a normal function. It always strikes physicians as well as laymen as bizarre, to call labor an abnormal function, a disease, and yet it is a decidedly pathological process. Everything, of course, depends on what we define as normal. If a woman falls on a pitchfork, and drives the handle through her perineum, we call that pathologic—abnormal, but if a large baby is driven through the pelvic floor, we say that is natural, and therefore

normal. If a baby were to have its head caught in a door very
lightly, but enough to cause cerebral hemorrhage, we would say
it is decidedly pathologic, but when a baby's head is crushed
against a tight pelvic floor, and a hemorrhage in the brain kills
it, we call this normal, at least we say that the function is
natural, not pathologic.[2]

This passage is always read as a call to arms and as the linchpin of
DeLee's views. It is always paraded about by critics who wish to
expose how obstetricians' blind ambition had driven them to a
thoughtless view of birth which led them to intervene obstetrically
in even uncomplicated deliveries. Yet the passage contains a hint
of the possibility of normality in childbirth. It just depends, according
to DeLee, on how normalcy is defined. In DeLee's other work one
finds that, in fact, some births are normal, even to his well-trained
eyes. In the preface to the first edition of his textbook, DeLee said
he was convinced that a minority of births were normal.[3] This small
admission is more than just a slip, though, for later in the same book
DeLee offers this advice and reproach:

> The duty of the accoucheur is to observe the efforts of
> nature, not to aid, until she has proven herself unequal to the
> task. Only when nature fails is art to enter. Nothing is so
> reprehensible as meddlesome midwifery.[4]

And then in the preface to the fourth edition of the text published
in 1924 DeLee makes a statement which is bound to surprise those
who cast him as the leader of the enemy forces:

> A strongly conservative attitude has been kept throughout the
> book. Something must be done to stem the tide of obstetric
> operating now prevalent, with its resultant maternal and fetal
> mortality. While the expert obstetrician in his specialistically
> [sic] manned maternity can obtain more nearly ideal results
> from his work by extending, somewhat, the indications for
> interference, at the present time it is the general practitioner
> who conducts the largest number of births, either in the home
> or in the frequently poorly equipped, small hospital. He must
> be given advice and methods applicable to the milieu in which
> he works, and *non-interference with the processes of nature,
> with their careful supervision, i.e., watchful and armed
> expectancy, had been proved to give the best results.*[5]

Superficially, this is hypocritical. The proponent of prophylactic forceps and routine episiotomy could not be siding with advocates of nature, could he? The reader has two ways to understand DeLee's views. DeLee might be an irrational person given to tidal swings of judgment, or he could be a rational person who earned his respect by understanding his profession and who wrote to respond to the profession's needs. Viewed from the latter perspective DeLee's seeming shifts of opinion reflect a dilemma with which obstetrics had to grapple in the early part of this century: birth was pathological and it was not; men should intervene in nature's processes and they should not.

This dilemma ran throughout the profession, and appeared in the writings of DeLee's strongest critics. J. Whitridge Williams, an earlier surveyor of the state of his profession, disagreed completely with DeLee's proposals for routine care. He implicitly challenged the profession to compare systematically DeLee's interventionist strategies with his own more conservative approach:

> In many instances I have been greatly surprised to find that [women one year after delivery] are in far better shape than one has any right to anticipate. . . . I am quite convinced that if Dr. DeLee's practices should become general, and the women were examined in a similar manner that they would be found to be worse off than the majority I see.[6]

But it had been Williams who had written in his textbook, published ten years before DeLee's, the following passage which only the most sensitive reader could have distinguished from the work of the more hawkish DeLee:

> From a biological point of view pregnancy and labor represent the highest functions of the female productive system, and *a priori,* should be considered as normal processes. But when we recall the manifold changes which occur in the maternal organism, it is apparent that the border-line between health and disease is less distinctly marked than at other times, and derangements, so slight as to be of but little consequence under ordinary circumstances, may readily give rise to pathological conditions which seriously threaten the life of the mother or the child, or both.[7]

Williams did not consider childbirth "decidedly pathologic" but the threat of each delivery crossing that fine line from normalcy demands DeLee's "watchful and armed expectancy" nonetheless. The two

eminent obstetricians of the day, who took opposite positions on
what constituted appropriate care, had started from similar views
of birth as potentially pathological.

There were other "strange bedfellows" problems in the early days
of the profession. For example, DeLee endorsed Rudolph Holmes's
contention: "The basic error has crept into the obstetric field that
pregnancy and labor are pathological entities, that childbearing is
a disease."[8] Yet on the question of what effects obstetrical practice
had on mortality, DeLee argued that his practices saved lives, while
Holmes embraced a wholly different position:

> The fact that modern maternity hospitals, where is centered
> the obstetric skill and knowledge of our profession, have been
> unable to decrease the dangers of birth to mother and child
> over the figures in the early part of the nineteenth century is
> *prima facie* evidence that modern obstetric surgery is
> ineffectual in combating those dangers.[9]

Birth was pathological, Holmes and DeLee agreed, and obstetrical
intervention helped, according to DeLee, or it did not, according to
Holmes. The profession was in disarray and the exasperation
showed. The discourse was stripped of its shell of scientific propriety, and a language of *rights* replaced a language of scientific legitimacy.[10] At one point, DeLee even cast obstetric intervention as a
matter of manly courage instead of medical appropriateness. In response to criticism of his "shoehorn maneuver" to extract a placenta
manually, he admonished his colleagues by saying simply, "I am not
afraid to put my hand into the uterus."[11]

Is there a vantage point from which to make sense of this disarray?
If we view the debates and controversies as merely arguments over
the inherent nature of childbirth or over appropriate care and professional practices, the early profession looks like a playground of
rather quarrelsome children. However, if these debates are seen as
one manifestation of the organizational problems faced by American
obstetrics—problems of the profession's own creation, for which it
was struggling internally to find solutions—one can make sense of
the many logics that seemed to coexist in the early days of the field.

The American profession had no basis for organizing itself as a
distinct group with a clearly defined province of its own. In fact, the
profession had achieved its present status by systematically eliminating even the possibility of finding an organizing principle.

Obstetricians had established their profession by blurring the boundary which might separate the material of obstetrics, per se, from the material of the midwife, of the general practitioner, or of anybody else. The problem, then, was what to do with the nonobstetrician who delivered babies, the faceless entity often referred to in the early professional literature as the "average physician."[12] The debates about childbirth and about obstetrical practices were really debates about what to do with the average physician, whether to work him into the profession or keep him out of it. A person's position in this debate depended on whether he wanted the profession to separate itself from the rest of medicine or whether he thought it should accommodate the needs of nonspecialists.

DeLee, the separatist, used the "average man" as a scapegoat in dismissing some of the problems with his preferred procedures, a tactic that would be used by others in the future. He did this to distance himself from the general practitioner and to set up his argument for the elevation of the profession. He urged that "we must not bring the ideals of obstetrics down to the level of the general, the occasional practitioner—we must bring the general practitioner of obstetrics up to the level of that of the specialist."[13] He argued for a division between the generalist and the specialist, and his real interest was in increasing the sophistication of his art. He wanted to be left alone and wished to leave all those without high aspirations for the profession behind, "trust[ing] each man to do according to his limitations."[14] Charles Gordon, a proponent of the "birth as nonpathological" school of thought, had different feelings about the organization of the field. He felt that obstetrics was going forward too quickly. He wanted to incorporate the average man into the field by teaching him fundamentals. He suggested that "hospitals might well open their doors for the practice of obstetrics to all those near them who will agree to follow the rules," and he suggested that the answer to the profession's problems would be found "not in the training of more specialists, . . . but in the continuous education of the average man."[15] We see the correspondence between doctors' positions on professional topics of the time and their ideas about the social future of the field. Those who wanted to avoid categorizations of birth as normal and abnormal tended to want to accommodate the needs of the average physician, as Gordon did. Those, like DeLee, who wanted to form a separate profession of obstetrics worked to formulate a conceptual basis for their separation, argued for the pathological dignity of birth, and favored binary categorizations.

B. P. Watson held an intermediate position on the question of the pathogenicity of childbirth and an intermediate position on the organization of obstetrics. He exhorted teachers to "impress upon their students the essential normality of the vast majority of cases." Not all cases were abnormal, a situation which would be consistent with DeLee's call for a superprofession, nor was birth strictly normal, a situation which would call for training in fundamentals. Rather, most births were normal, but some were not. Watson's corresponding organizational proposal was that hospitals employ "competent interns or nurses" to watch for signs of abnormality while the obstetrician "proceeds with the rest of his day's work," an organizational structure intermediate between the proposals of DeLee and Gordon. Watson's plan extended to home confinements as well, where he would use a system of "trained obstetric nurses" in order to "give the busy practitioner conditions approaching those enjoyed by the hospital obstetrician and . . . enable him to maintain the standard of obstetrics at a higher general level than has hitherto been possible."[16]

It appears, then, that the confusions, the superficial hypocrisies, of the formative years of the profession of obstetrics can best be understood as manifestations of a more fundamental problem, namely, whether obstetrics was to become a specialty distant from medicine to which the regular physician could aspire or whether it was to become a discipline which would incorporate the general practitioner and be sensitive to his needs.

In 1930 the social problems of the American profession were resolved in a way consistent with DeLee's interests by the establishment of the American Board of Obstetrics and Gynecology. This body developed criteria by which to judge the qualifications of obstetrical specialists and thereby put an end to the debates that had occurred over the preceding ten years.

As the profession achieved its specialty status within the broader profession, the medical gaze narrowed until the obstetrical "case" was effectively distilled from the person. Obstetrical material was carefully circumscribed and located within the confined space of the uterus and pelvis. Taking care of a patient meant focusing on the narrowly obstetrical aspects of her existence. A series of papers critical of aggressive, operative obstetrics that came close to calling on obstetricians to look on their patients as women and not simply "cases" received this reply: "I hold that a patient should be treated as judgment dictates; that we should act as practitioners of medicine instead of those who cater to the wishes of their patients."[17] Women who were part of research studies were described in journal articles as the "material" of the research, a practice that continues to this day. Obstetrics made women faceless vehicles of obstetrical material. They had no important part to play in childbirth: "The part which the patient takes in labor is largely a passive one, consisting chiefly of breathing the anesthetic as directed."[18] To the American obstetrician, women were simply carriers of the case, the "passage" and the "passenger" as the texts referred to the woman and her baby.

Things were different in Britain. Debates over the nature of childbirth and the structure of the profession did not occur nor was the woman so removed from childbirth. Instead of trying to decide whether births were pathological or not, the medical profession there considered births as either normal or abnormal. They existed on one side of the conceptual boundary or the other and they were treated according to their categorization. A fine line divided the categories, to be sure, but so did definitions:

> The condition of pregnancy, physiological though it may be theoretically, has a very narrow dividing line separating it from the pathological. . . .[19]

> By a *normal labor* is meant a case in which the fetus presents by the vertex, and which terminates naturally, without artificial aid and without complications. Presentation is not the only criterion of *normal labor,* for even when the presentation is normal, complications may arise which carry the case into the category of *abnormal labor.* It follows that abnormal labor is somewhat difficult to define.[20]

Not only was there a definition dividing "normal" from "abnormal," different kinds of attendants had different, clearly delineated responsibilities on either side of the dividing line. In the first stage of labor, for example, "there is little for the medical attendant to do . . . after the diagnosis has been satisfactorily made; a skilled nurse is quite as well able to attend to the patient's wants and watch the course of labor as a qualified medical practitioner."[21] Nonspecialists had their place as did specialists. No debates arose from organizational problems of the profession because the profession had a clear organizational structure, strongly related to the ideology of normality and abnormality. Books by the specialists were written "not for the use of specialists, but as a guide to that practical and adequate knowledge of midwifery which is essential to the student . . . and to the practitioner whose early years are so often largely occupied with obstetric work."[22] With a strong boundary protecting his field and his material the obstetrician could afford to consider the needs of other physicians and midwives.

British obstetrics also accorded women a larger role in childbirth. Perhaps, though, it would be more appropriate to say that obstetrics was organized so that it could pay attention to more aspects of the woman than simply the narrowly obstetrical ones. Home confinements were attended by midwives whose job it was to select for hospital confinement those women who crossed the line of normalcy. She selected, of course, according to the criteria of professional obstetrics, but those criteria encompassed more than the strictly obstetrical aspects of the case. The midwife's attention extended to the person, her beliefs, her concerns, and beyond her to the concerns of her relatives and to the environment in which she found herself. Midwives were instructed to select some women for hospital delivery for social reasons as well as for strictly medical reasons. The expansion of the medical gaze through the midwife was different from the approach to home deliveries recommended by DeLee. He had said, "when the parturient cannot be taken to the hospital operating room, the operating room must be taken to the parturient."[23] In Britain the operating room remained behind the boundary provided by the hospital. There the obstetrical specialist was available to handle abnormal deliveries should they be brought to his attention. In America the obstetrician had to accommodate those women who were unable to bring their case, filled with its pathological dignity, to the obstetrician's place of work. In Britain, the hospital was the place where abnormal births were taken as the need arose.

To summarize, the residual normalcy of childbirth, that which remained in the wake of obstetrics' partially unsuccessful attempts to conceptualize birth as pathological, was handled differently in Britain and America, and that difference can be attributed to a difference in the strength of the boundaries that the two professions had been able to erect around themselves. American obstetrics was organizationally unable to handle "normal" births. There was no clear demarcation of responsibilities between average physicians and specialists and no clear distinction between normal and abnormal births. The weak boundary with which American obstetrics entered its professional life gave rise to curious debates which were fundamentally arguments about the structure of the profession. In contrast, British obstetrics had no such problems since it entered the twentieth century with a strong professional boundary. In the following sections we see how the different boundaries gave rise to different obstetrical practices and conditioned the strategies of change available to meet challenges to professional practices.

Obstetrical Practices
Birth Position

To the first obstetricians, women seemed like savages; they had to bring some discipline to childbirth in order to do their work. With regard to posture during delivery, obstetricians confronted extant knowledge about so-called primitive people who reportedly adopted many different birth positions, all according to instinct and circumstance.[24] Obstetricians' search for the ideal birth position through available ethnographies and through observation of women left to their own devices during delivery was unsuccessful, and they were left with the disconcerting fact that nature had not provided a standard birth posture which they could discover scientifically, copy, and call their own. Bringing discipline to birth meant eliminating the challenge instinct posed for the conduct of obstetrical work. The temporal ordering of birth into stages, which obstetrics had inherited from the nineteenth century, was augmented by imposing on women birth postures designed to separate the woman from her obstetrically important parts and to make the "passages" easily available to the obstetrical operator. Because the organization of obstetrical work was different in Britain and America, different strategies for effecting discipline and order developed and different practices became standard practice.

The savage confronted obstetrics from the available literature. For example, in *Labor among Primitive Peoples* George Englemann reviewed the research on "natural" positions for labor published up through 1883 and then compiled a catalog of the positions usually assumed by laboring women in over a hundred cultures. His review of the few ethnographic reports available at the time and of the experiences of "unfortunate and inexperienced girls" observed during unassisted labor led him to say:

> It soon became evident, and impressed itself forcibly on my mind, that the *recumbent* position in labor is rarely assumed among these people who live naturally and are, as yet, governed by their instincts and have escaped the influence of civilization and of modern obstetrics. It certainly appeared as if the ordinary obstetric position of today [with the woman lying on her back] must be an unnatural one.[25]

After his study of labor among women of "nations of the past" and of "the savage races," he said:

> The care with which the parturient women of uncivilized people avoid the dorsal decubus, the modern obstetric position, at the termination of labor, is sufficient evidence that it is a most undesirable position for ordinary cases of confinement; and I am convinced that the thinking obstetrician will soon confirm the statement not unfrequently made by the ignorant but observing savage, . . . that the recumbent position retards labor and is inimical to easy, safe, and rapid delivery.[26]

The textbooks of the 1930s made it clear that the aim of obstetrics and thinking obstetricians was to tame this savage. Schumann's 1936 text says that a woman will try to assume a squatting position during the second, or expulsive, stage of labor "in an instinctive attempt to increase the diameter of the pelvic outlet and to enable the abdominal muscles to exert their utmost contractile force." But in properly managed labor, the obstetrician will eliminate instinct and effect an order which simulates the natural order: "the squatting position may be simulated to some extent in bed, by an exaggerated lithotomy position, the legs held in place by attendants."[27] Williams thought that a woman instinctively sought a recumbent position due to the pains of the last part of the first stage of labor, *but* "if she is still moving about the room or sitting up, she should go to bed immediately upon the rupture of the membranes and the beginning of bearing-down pains"[28] (the beginning of the second stage of labor).

The prescriptive stance on birth position developed concomitantly with the profession. Previously there had been a bias in the texts to permit women to assume the position most comfortable for them. The physician was advised to "accustom himself to conduct labor with equal facility" regardless of the position selected by women.[29]

The early science of midwifery even suggested that positions popular among obstetricians were irrational:

> The usual posture of the parturient woman is either on the back or on the side, but it must be admitted that neither realizes what may be reasonably expected from a rational position. The posture of the parturient woman is to be so arranged that first the direction of the expulsive powers act as perpendicularly as possible to the plane of the pelvis through which the fetal head is to be pressed, . . . for thus only the amount of friction will be the least, and, therefore, very little force will be lost, and secondly, the gravity of the child itself will not be prevented from aiding.[30]

The profession overlooked these kinds of arguments, even though they were cast in the language of the new science, and opted instead for schemes which were specific, detailed, and prescriptive, if less well reasoned scientifically. William Dewees's approach, published in 1825, exemplifies the kind of writing to which the profession turned in deciding on its early practices:

> The woman will be placed for labor upon her left side, at the foot of the bed in such a manner as will enable her to fix her feet firmly against the bed post; her hips within ten or twelve inches of the head of the bed; her knees bent, her body well flexed upon the thighs; this position will bring the head and shoulders near the center of the bed, which must be raised to a comfortable height by pillows. The part of the bed on which the patient is now placed must, like the part on which she is permanently to rest after delivery, be secured by folded blankets placed over the under sheet.[31]

This was the approach selected by obstetrics from among available alternatives to bring order to its work: detailed and rigid specification. Justification would come later, as it became necessary.

As the profession developed in America, one birth position diffused throughout the profession and became standard practice. The lithotomy position, a variant of the dorsal position, permitted the obstetrician to "stand before" the woman and watch for the potential pathology of delivery, and it permitted timely intervention should anything go wrong. Adopting this single position was one manifestation of the American profession's disregard for categorizing births as normal or abnormal.

Interestingly, what differences of opinion over birth position did
exist followed differences of opinion concerning the resolution of
the profession's organizational problems. That is, there was a correspondence between ideas about the social organization of the
profession and ideas concerning the profession's practices. Williams, who wrote for the medical profession at large and did not
have designs for a superprofession of obstetrics, recommended one
customary position, the recumbent, for all. His ideology of equality
was reflected in his preferred practices as well as in his social plans
for obstetrics. His text simply acknowledged that the lateral position,
with the woman lying on her side, was preferred in England and
elsewhere.[32] DeLee on the other hand recommended that specialists
use different positions from those favored by other physicians:

> The patient may be either on the side or on the back. It is
> well for the accoucheur to learn both methods, since each has
> its advantages, and the principles of operation, with a little
> practice, may be practiced equally well in either position.
> Owing to the possibility of better control of the fetal heart-tones
> the author usually delivers the patient on the back. In out-
> patient delivery services, . . . the lateral posture is preferred.[33]

The pictures accompanying the text show delivery in the lateral
position, but the implication is clear enough: once the profession is
large enough to provide a specialist like DeLee for everyone, the
patient would be on her back. As the profession changed, DeLee's
text changed also, so that in the seventh edition in 1940, the pictures
of lateral delivery are preceded by a picture which shows a woman
in the lithotomy position, draped for surgical cleanliness, attended
by two masked and gowned figures; the picture carries the caption
"All ready for delivery—maternity practice." Four years later, in
the first edition of DeLee's text authored by J. P. Greenhill, lateral
delivery is not shown. The lithotomy position had replaced lateral
delivery completely.[34] Later, in the thirteenth edition, there is no
room for doubt about standard care. A woman delivers, the reader
is told, "lying on her back with her knees raised and abducted" to
which is added, "an unruly patient may need anesthesia."[35] Opportunities for doing proper obstetrics had changed, "maternity practice" had replaced outpatient practice almost entirely, and so
recommendations for practice changed. The savage had been tamed,

either by proper management with the patient's cooperation or by anesthesia if necessary.

Once the lithotomy position was established as standard obstetrical practice, various devices—beds and attachments to beds— appeared to accommodate the needs of obstetricians. The way these devices are described in professional journals reveals the interests which gave rise to the practice. The purpose of obstetrical appliances was total control of the patient. One text said, "restraint that will prevent any shifting of the patient's relative position by her own muscle-action is very desirable."[36] Beds complied:

> Shoulder braces, readily adjusted and well padded with spongy rubber, prevent the patient from moving her hips away from the edge of the bed. The patient thus lies, throughout the second stage, in a perfectly natural, comfortable, and nonfatiguing position *which she cannot change, even when only incompletely narcotized.*[37]

Obstetricians justified immobilizing the patient on her back by their concern for aseptic technique. Williams claimed that the lithotomy position facilitated asepsis and praised the bed described above because it kept the aseptic drapes from being moved by the patient. At this stage, though, claims about asepsis were nothing more than speculative, unfounded justifications for the practice since no one had tested the claims and, as DeLee had said, outpatient beds where many women delivered were "filthy."

The recumbent position and its associated technology made obstetrical intervention in birth easier. The lithotomy position created a clearer operative field than other positions. Not only was the obstetrician's job simplified by the recumbent position, but beds could be built which made the nurses' lives easier as well. For example, one bed solved the nurses' problem of moving anesthetized patients by putting the mattress on rollers so that

> instead of pulling and hauling a partially anesthetized or struggling patient to the foot of the bed all that is necessary is to have her buttocks at or below the center of the mattress, she may then be anesthetized and any nurse using the crank at the foot of the bed, may bring the patient easily down for stirrups and delivery.[38]

Practices and instrumentation changed somewhat in response to threats of various sorts to obstetrical practices. In the mid-1960s one letter recommended a particular delivery bed because "personnel in the delivery area are becoming more scarce. Using a special type of labor-and-delivery bed, fewer persons are needed to attend the parturient."[39] As outside groups organized in opposition to certain practices, instrumentation and rhetoric changed so that interests embodied in the practices would not be undermined. At the height of the early phase of the natural childbirth movement in the United States, one obstetrician tried to revise the profession's concept of "normal physiologic delivery" to include delivery in the sitting or squatting position. He proposed the use of a bed that could be rotated through 90 degrees but which would, nonetheless, restrict a woman's ability to assume the position she preferred.[40]

Noting temporal correspondences between the occurrence of challenges to professional practices and proposals for changes in practices might suggest that doctors conspiratorially create new knowledge and practices as circumstances demand in order to retain their social position. Knowledge, clearly, is a resource often used for just such a purpose, but the fact that there are rules for creating knowledge which generally must be obeyed[41] reduces the plausibility of a conspiratorial model, which suggests knowledge is concocted to meet challenges as they arise. A more reasonable model is one which rests on the notion that a profession functions as a repository of "residual knowledge"—proposals, ideas, data, and so on—from which the profession can draw when politically necessary. The case of American obstetrics' recent tentative moves toward acceptance of alternative birth positions in the face of serious challenges of the women's movement in the late 1960s and early 1970s illustrates this nicely. Papers which showed that contractions are stronger and less frequent (more efficient, in obstetricians' terms) in the lateral position than in the dorsal position appeared in the 1950s and 1960s, but they had little effect on general obstetrical practice at that time.[42] These findings and data became part of the residual, unused, even unrecognized, knowledge of the profession. In the 1970s, when women began insisting on alternative types of deliveries and backing up their insistence by turning in greater numbers to alternative medical practitioners for assistance in childbirth, the profession moved toward accommodation rather than confrontation. Statements like this one appeared in the professional literature: "The effects of the left lateral position by pregnant women on uterine contractility and blood flow are well known. . . . The lateral position should be considered in all labors."[43] The profession's accommodation was not a compromise since change was implemented on the obstetrician's terms. The left lateral position should now be considered for all labors not because women insisted on options or because it was more "humane," but because the lateral position was known to be a scientifically acceptable, perhaps even better, position for delivery. Change occurred, and the effects of the threat were attenuated, by turning some of the profession's residual knowledge into timely knowledge.

Preferred birth postures differed in Britain. British obstetricians permitted two, the left lateral and the dorsal. The circumstances under which one or the other was considered appropriate followed and reinforced the strongly demarcated division of labor in the profession: left lateral was to be used by midwives and others attending normal deliveries, dorsal was to be used by the specialist attending deliveries that required operative intervention.

The English preference for the lateral position has a long history. Even though William Smellie recommended that a woman should "consult her own ease" with regard to birth position, he made it clear that he preferred the "London method" of delivery with the woman lying on her side. Little has changed over the several centuries since Smellie trained the initial corps of English obstetricians. Now virtually all British texts recommend the left lateral position for uncomplicated deliveries.[44] Even authors who deem it convenient to have a woman lie on her back throughout most of the second stage of labor still recommend that delivery be accomplished in the lateral position.[45] The dorsal position became associated with abnormal births, and thus with obstetrical specialists, after the profession established its strong demarcation from other groups delivering babies. Since the hospital, the domain of the specialist, is associated with abnormal births and the home is associated with normal deliveries, it is not surprising that some authors recommended different positions based on the place of delivery.[46] It is also not surprising that, as hospital confinements have increased in Britain, preference for the dorsal position has increased also.

As the use of the dorsal position increased, professional discussion of the birth positions in Britain turned from the merits of the dorsal and lateral position to the merits of various sorts of dorsal positions. An interesting exchange over birth posture occurred in the *British*

Medical Journal from September through December, 1955. It opened
with a letter recommending a straight-leg lithotomy position which
claimed that nature, properly observed, shows this to be the best
method.[47] But obstetricians were not the only ones who had recommendations based on appeals to nature. Advocates of natural
childbirth had established themselves as an interested party, and the
way they expressed their interests in this debate is instructive.
Grantly Dick-Read did not argue that a woman should "consult her
own ease," as one might expect of a natural childbirth advocate.
Instead he expressed a preference for a position which facilitated
cooperation between the woman and her birth attendant. He recommended a different kind of dorsal position, one with the back
elevated because "it allows a woman to see and hear her attendant."[48] No longer did nature present a threat of disorder to the obstetrician. Nature had been tamed so well by obstetrics and the need
for order had been so thoroughly accepted that even advocates of
"natural childbirth" were prescriptive when it came to something
as simple as what position a woman should assume for delivery.

Obstetricians have used other procedures to bring order to birth.
Studies of these procedures demonstrate other boundary phenomena
which occurred in the history of obstetrics.

Episiotomy

Episiotomy, an incision in the perineum from the rear of the vaginal
opening toward the anus or to one side or the other, was a technique
institutionalized on the basis of a timely metaphor and one which
achieved legitimacy through a language of interests that could have
developed only in a male-dominated profession like obstetrics. In
Britain episiotomy was characterized as an operative intervention
for use in problematic deliveries. Presently, it is a procedure which
enjoys wide use but which still carries a restrictive characterization.
It remains a specialist's practice on the abnormal side of the symbolic
and organizational normal/abnormal boundary. In America the procedure became almost symbolic of the united, somewhat elevated,
but still loosely demarcated profession of obstetrics. The profession's leaders advocated that episiotomy become a routine part of
every delivery. It diffused throughout the medical profession without
respect for categorizations like normal and abnormal, and when it

attracted criticism various strategies were employed to ignore or attenuate the strength of arguments against the practice.

The idea of incising the perineum to enlarge the birth outlet is credited to Sir Fielding Ould, who recorded the practice in 1742 while he was Second Master of the Rotunda Hospital. The first episiotomy in America was recorded in 1851. By 1895 at least one physician, F. A. Stahl, had claimed that an episiotomy was in the best interest of mother and child.[49] Actually, episiotomies were done more in response to obstetricians' concerns about repairing perineal tears than in the interests of women. (Of course, fewer perineal tears were thought to be in line with women's interests, but no one ever tried to determine if, in fact, they were.) An episiotomy replaced lacerations with clean, more easily sutured incisions, but it was not in any sense the only, the most natural, or even the most appropriate response to concerns about perineal tears available at the time. Indeed, the literature showed that episiotomies caused many problems and it even contained suggestions for avoiding perineal tears without operative intervention. Schroeder's 1873 text reported a 60 percent higher incidence of perineal tears among women delivered in a recumbent position over those delivered in a lateral position. The implication was that if there was genuine concern for preventing perineal tears women should be delivered on their sides. But Schroeder's data were ignored in favor of surgical intervention. Such intervention prevailed over careful attention and slow, noninstrumental deliveries, in part, because episiotomy was introduced into obstetrics through metaphorical reasoning which presented the procedure as a preventive measure for problems that were of more general, public concern.

Talk of routine use of episiotomy began in 1915 when Brooke Anspach recommended its use in all forceps operations and claimed that it would reduce infant mortality and maternal morbidity.[50] Three years later Ralph Pomeroy made the appeal that struck a responsive chord. He called the fetal head a "battering ram" which "shatter[s] a resisting outlet," and he asked rhetorically, "Why not open the gates and close them after the procession has passed?"[51] The idea of the baby as battering ram focused attention on the violence that birth supposedly did to the fetal skull even under normal circumstances. Around the turn of the century common sense and sociomedical theory had it that "brain damage," which the metaphor and the literature suggested might result from such a violent encounter, led not to a vegetative existence, as we think today, but to a life of crime. Thus, through the use of a metaphor obstetrical practices were tied directly to the much broader social and academic concern with the biological bases of crime. Obstetricians were one step ahead of the psychometricians, who could only measure predisposition to criminality with their newly imported IQ tests. Obstetricians could *see* the predisposition to criminality occur on their delivery tables as the baby's head encountered the perineum. Furthermore they could do something about it. They could intervene to prevent criminality. So the episiotomy entered the profession's armamentarium without tests of the assertions about reductions in mortality and morbidity because of a fortunate conjunction of a particular view of the birth process with broader public concern over general social ills.

The profession brought legitimacy to the procedure by using a language of interests that would be well received by the male-dominated profession and by women's husbands as well. Obstetricians, with Joseph DeLee leading the way, decided that an episiotomy should be done not only because it spared the child from a life of crime but also because it served a woman's sexual interests, at least as those interests were construed by obstetricians. DeLee believed that a woman should be as "anatomically perfect" after delivery as she was before and that since birth was a process where the fetal "head has been pounding and grinding the muscle like a piece of steak is pounded by a mallet" an episiotomy was the only way to preserve the vaginal entrance and restore "virginal conditions."[52] Obstetricians never asked women whether the degree of restoration which obstetricians claimed they achieved was important to them or not. In fact the language used by Nicholson Eastman in his polemic for one form of episiotomy over another shows that obstetricians had so effectively distilled the obstetrical "case" from the woman that she was not even party to the discourse on the restoration of her sexual anatomy. Eastman summed up his case for a median episiotomy (an incision directed toward the anus instead of sideways) in a sentence that equated three benefits of the procedure: (1) savings on electricity for postoperative pain-reducing light treatments, (2) savings on time "because we do not have to listen to complaints about the stitches," and (3) the fact that "at the six weeks return visit, a virginal introitus *presents itself*."[53] That the woman is pleased or not is of no concern; she is simply the conveyor of that which is of real interest, the introitus which presents itself to the examiner. By 1959, it was claimed that a properly repaired episiotomy restored "conjugal as well as anatomical normalcy" and obstetricians who neglected the potential sexual sequelae of some deliveries were termed "thoughtless" and "callous in the extreme."[54] Doctors' conceptions of the interests of women, which they attributed to their patients but never documented as having originated with them, thus were used to bolster and sustain the case for episiotomy.

Science was invoked to justify episiotomies, but it was never accorded a definitive or even primary role in the decision to retain or discard the practice. DeLee claimed that "although statistics are meager, they seem to show that instrumental delivery is safer than prolonged, hard, unassisted labor."[55] Statistics, though, were not a strong base for decision-making at this stage in the profession; even DeLee said, "Statistics in general are very insecure building stones on which to base judgment."[56] Practice was a matter of clinical judgment or, as Williams put it when he finally acknowledged in the sixth edition of his text that many people were doing episiotomies, "it may be said that its employment is largely a matter of taste."[57]

When comparative studies started to appear, they presented problems for the profession, though the problems were certainly not insurmountable given the flexibility afforded the American profession by its blurred professional boundary. The first study to compare the effects of episiotomy to delivery without incision appeared in 1935.[58] In that paper Fred Nugent reported on some 200 cases, of which 130 received episiotomy because the obstetrician felt that a severe tear was inevitable. So, this was not a randomized trial, but the results, and more important, the response to the results, are interesting. Nugent found that the group with episiotomies had a 50 percent higher incidence of maternal morbidity than the group without. His first reaction was to try to find differences between the groups—differences in complicated operative procedures, infection, and duration of labor—to explain this difference in morbidity. He could not. He was forced to conclude that there was "a substantial increase in morbidity attributable to episiotomy." He did not stop there, though. He turned the reader's attention to other kinds of morbid conditions, including anterior vaginal wall lacerations, which occurred in only one out of every twenty deliveries, and to long-term problems in nonepisiotomized women. A vaginal wall laceration was a particularly useful pathology to support an anticipatory operation because it was one that had been termed "invisible" only eight years earlier, in 1927,[59] and that, in Nugent's eyes, was "difficult to recognize." By turning attention to the potential long-term effect of a pathology of low incidence that is difficult to recognize, Nugent and the profession were able to ignore the critical results of this study and come to the conclusion that the appropriate obstetrical posture should be, "When in doubt, cut," as Pomeroy had said earlier.

During the following two decades a number of complications of episiotomies were reported in the literature and people began to attack it as a procedure performed primarily for the convenience of the physician. Yet the profession made no move to assess the efficacy or safety of the operation. In fact, episiotomy was such an accepted practice that the only self-styled "critical" analyses to appear were comparisons of different kinds of episiotomies; no one systematically compared the effects of having an episiotomy with the effects of not having one. The profession just assumed that episiotomies were better for women.

As late as 1973, investigators would be able to follow Nugent's analytical lead and find support for episiotomies in studies where none existed. Using data from the massive Collaborative Perinatal Study, Niswander and Gordon[60] found no statistically significant differences in perinatal mortality or mental and motor test-scores at eight months and four years of age between a group of children delivered instrumentally and a group delivered without a high degree of intervention. Yet their reasoning followed a serpentine course to a conclusion supporting instrumental delivery. In spite of the fact that they had found no differences between the "intervention" group and the group of women who delivered spontaneously, they began their conclusion by saying,

> Our data might be interpreted as suggesting that a
> spontaneously delivered child might incur a greater risk of
> neonatal death and a greater risk of abnormality on the 8 month
> and 4 year developmental and psychometric evaluations than a
> baby delivered by low forceps.[61]

Then they added the caveat, "However, shortcomings in our data must be considered before we can reach such a conclusion." But then they recovered by saying, "Yet, the very consistency of the data in individual groupings, even when the cohorts are small and the differences not significant, is impressive."[62] Logic of this sort was necessary as recently as 1973 to preserve the procedure against implicit attacks generated by the profession's own study of its work.

When problems that episiotomy is designed to prevent occur even after the operation has been done, the "average man" argument is still invoked to defend the practice. Lacerations into the anus or rectum are not blamed on the failure of the procedure; instead, attention is turned to the skill of the operator. One study explained differences in severity of complications by pointing to a mild association between years in the profession and the incidence of complications. Despite the fact that many complications still occur in the hands of skilled physicians, such analyses deflect attention to the need for improved training programs and away from the possibility that the problems might be with the procedure itself. Problems with the procedure become "more theoretical than real."[63] Problems occur, but they are not real because, theoretically, they can be eliminated by tinkering with the milieu in which the procedure is employed. This is an argument available only to a poorly demarcated profession such as American obstetrics. If the profession were more strongly demarcated, the "average man" would be a matter of paternalistic interest instead of a person available as a scapegoat.

In Britain, episiotomy was characterized from the earliest days of the profession as an operative procedure to be used in abnormal deliveries. There was, therefore, no room for the kinds of criticism and subsequent defense that occurred in America. By characterizing episiotomy as a procedure restricted to decidedly pathological cases, obstetrics reduced the likelihood of criticism. Making an incision under these circumstances was prima facie evidence that something abnormal threatened the safety of the mother or child and, therefore, no defense of the procedure by the profession was necessary.

The difference in professional characterizations of episiotomy can be seen in textbooks. DeLee had relegated his detailed description of episiotomy and perineal repair to the section of his text headed "Pathology of Pregnancy," but he described the procedure, illustrated it, and recommended its frequent use in the section on the management of normal labor. Episiotomy did not straddle the normal/abnormal boundary in British texts. Instead, texts which urged that students have a definite method of procedure for delivery opted for careful manual delivery instead of instrumental operative delivery as the method of choice:

> Care in the prevention of rupture of the perineum is well repaid. There is less subsequent visiting required, less risk of perineal infection and of later prolapse or incontinence. Patients usually appreciate the fact that there are "no stitches."[64]

It is worth mentioning that the reasons given to support attentive manual delivery are curiously similar to reasons given in America for operative intervention in birth.

Very slowly, episiotomy crept across the boundary into normal deliveries but the transition occurred cautiously and has never been completed. First, midwives were permitted to perform an episiotomy but they were not allowed to suture their incisions. Texts stressed that an episiotomy was a surgical procedure which "should not be undertaken except for good reason." [65] The use of this specialist's procedure increased with the rise in hospital confinements until a major text of the 1960s conceded that episiotomy "is more frequently used for abnormal than for normal deliveries, but it has its place in the management of labor that is otherwise spontaneous."[66] As the procedure became more widely used, criticism not unlike that which had appeared in America began to develop, but public attention in Britain had turned to another obstetrical procedure. Protests over the increased use of episiotomies were muffled by the outrage over alarming increases in the artificial induction of labor.

Induction of Labor

The history of the induction of labor is the history of a search for a technology of control and for the control of a technology. Artificially inducing or augmenting labor carried recognized risks from its earliest days. Yet it was associated with obstetrical abnormality and was, therefore, a relatively protected procedure. It resided on the abnormal side of the normal/abnormal boundary and, while criticized, it enjoyed a status which allowed the procedure to be refined and amended rather than abandoned. The problems with induction became not so much condemnations of the procedure as challenges for the specialists whose tool it was. Slowly, technical solutions to difficulties were found, hazards of the procedure were reduced, and the induction of labor spread throughout obstetric practice.

Induction became accepted practice and turned otherwise normal deliveries into abnormal ones. Responses to this extension of the obstetrical franchise differed in Britain and America, and those differences were functions of the difference in the boundaries each profession had been able to erect around itself.

The induction of labor, like other obstetrical practices, had a simple, reasonable beginning. If the uterus, the machine designed to propel a baby through the bony passages of the pelvis and past other female parts, did not do its job at the appropriate time, then according to the prevailing medical logic it would be appropriate to do something, anything, to help it along. Physicians knew as early as 1738, perhaps earlier, that rupturing the amniotic membranes induced labor and got the uterus started on its task. Stripping membranes from the uterine wall around the cervix also induced labor, though no one knew why. During the nineteenth century various things—sponges, carbonic acid gas, rubber bougies, bags, and animal bladders filled with fluid—were inserted into women's uteri in order to overcome "uterine inertia." Women were subjected to alternating hot and cold baths, hot and cold vaginal douches, large doses of quinine and castor oil, and various methods for mechanically dilating the cervix, all because to the obstetrician's eye these methods worked. They seemed to take over where nature had proven herself inadequate.

Also in the nineteenth century labor was induced pharmacologically by the use of ergot, a rye fungus that had profound effects on the pregnant human uterus. Ergot was used primarily in the third, or placental, stage of labor to cause the uterus to clamp down on the vessels leading to the placenta in order to prevent postpartum hemorrhage. Because of the unpredictable and often uncontrollable contractions which ergot caused, texts recommended it not be used unless delivery could be effected "at any given moment." Still one finds that ergot *was* used, often with stripping of the membranes, to initiate or augment labor.[67]

Near the century's end, physicians started noting the physiological effects of extracts of various body organs and thereby prepared the path that would lead them past the difficulties experienced with ergot. An extract of the pituitary gland drew medicine's attention as early as 1895, and in 1909 W. Blair Bell published a paper recommending its use in cases of uterine atony. His evidence was of the most medically convincing sort; he saw firsthand what happened in response to pituitary extract:

In two cases of Cesarean section I have had the opportunity
of observing the naked-eye effect of a single injection; it is
immediate and convincing. The uterus contracts into a blanched
"ball," and only relaxes subsequently to a moderate degree.[68]

Other methods for producing labor worked somehow and therefore
met the test of clinical judgment. But pituitary extract did not just
work; physicians had Bell's visual observation which confirmed the
existence of a quick causal chain between obstetrical intervention
and mechanical effect. This accorded pituitary extract such notoriety
that it was virtually certain to achieve a significant place in the
obstetrician's armamentarium.

Induction, through chemical means or otherwise, did not develop
a wide following immediately. In fact, the practice was severely
criticized. During the early years of the profession, many hazards
of induction were reported. Uterine insertions were condemned because of the risks of infection or of hemorrhage caused by acciden-
tally separating the placenta prematurely. Quinine and castor oil
were termed dangerous. Cases of uterine tetany—uncontrolled sustained contraction—were reported in the first major series of inductions in 1913. Even the concern that was being attacked by the use
of episiotomies, perineal lacerations, was thought to result from the
use of pituitary extract.[69] Finally, there was always the danger that
induction could lead to a premature child since no reliable method
existed for determining gestational age or fetal viability. How could
such a practice survive this kind of critical assault?

One aspect of a profession is its capacity to contain and protect
practices that constitute its work. Obstetrics, in its early days, had
this capacity and exercised it with regard to induction. Control was
the heart of the matter, but not simply control of the patient. The
main problem with induction was that the procedure itself was at
times uncontrollable. As the profession brought the procedure under
control, indications for induction broadened and it became the means
by which obstetrics advanced further into the normal region than
it ever had been before.

The profession's advance into normal births is best seen through
changes in textbooks' treatments of induction. The first editions of
both DeLee's and Williams' texts agreed on a conservative approach
to induction. Williams, in 1903, condemned the use of ergot except
in the third stage of labor and suggested the artificial rupturing of

membranes only when a woman had been in the second stage for "some time."[70] DeLee's 1913 text listed several conditions under which induction was permissible, but all were clearly pathological conditions. Induction itself did not receive separate treatment in DeLee's early editions; instead it was sprinkled throughout the various pathologies and was presented as one possible, though not particularly attractive, therapy in some instances.[71] During the early 1920s no new ground was broken in the pharmacological induction of labor except that, perhaps, obstetricians decided that one should use smaller doses than previously recommended. Then, in 1927, Hofbauer and Hoerner recommended that pituitary extract be administered by inserting a sponge soaked with the drug into the nasal passages. They claimed their tests on eighty normal pregnant women during the last month of pregnancy and at term "[testified] to the *control we now possess over the action of pituitary extract* when used both for the induction of labor and for accelerating labor already in progress."[72] Textbooks responded to this advance. The sixth edition of Williams's book in 1930, recommended induction of premature labor in cases where problems might be expected to arise and in cases where a child might be postmature and too large for safe delivery. There remained a note of caution, though, because assessment of postmaturity was still a matter of personal judgment, an unsolved technical problem which prevented wholesale extension of induction beyond the limits of the potentially pathological.[73] In DeLee's 1933 text, in response to increased control over the procedure, indications for induction were collected from throughout the text and presented in one section. DeLee made it clear, however, that he still preferred episiotomy and forceps over induction for the second stage of labor.[74]

The 1940s saw two more technical advances in the control of induction. By diluting pituitary extract in saline and administering it intravenously, drop by drop, the obstetrician could control "the character and amplitude of contractions."[75] Also, agents other than anesthesia were used to control tetany. As a result, labor looked more physiological to the clinical eye, it proceeded more quickly, that is, it was more efficient, and it was better controlled. The texts took their cue. J. P. Greenhill, the new editor of DeLee's text, added a new chapter on induction at the end of the 1943 edition of this classic book. Following the unhesitating style of DeLee, the text boldly declared, "There is hardly any condition affecting the preg-

nant woman that may not be an indication for emptying the uterus."
Of induction by rupturing membranes, the text said, "when . . .
properly carried out . . . for legitimate indications, labor is generally
shorter than normal, operative intervention is not increased, the
cervix is not damaged more often than normally, morbidity is not
increased, and fetal mortality is no higher than usual."[76] Under its
new editor the 1950 edition of Williams's text proclaimed that,
because of induction, "the 'problem of postmaturity' is non-existent."[77]
Clearly, induction was becoming a much more attractive, acceptable
procedure.

Technical problems with the administration of uterine stimulants
were completely overcome by 1960. The synthesis of artificial pituitary extract in 1955 permitted greater quality control over drug
dosage, and the invention of a pump in 1960 permitted control of
the rate of administration. Bishop's score, an analytical device for
assessing the "ripeness" of the cervix and therefore the likelihood
of a successful induction, increased the certainty of an orderly induction and placed greater control in the obstetrician's hands. No
longer was there any need for a pathology or even a potential pathology to be present. Each case could be assessed for its suitability
for induction and the procedure could be employed under carefully
structured, highly controlled circumstances. With these advances
the legitimate indications for induction increased beyond what might
be called strictly medical indications. Williams's own first six editions of his text and the subsequent three under H. J. Stander had
all contained strong condemnations of inductions "solely for the
convenience of the patient or her physician" even though "knowledge that gestation will terminate on a definite date" had, as early
as 1920, been termed a "mental and financial relief to the patient
and a marked convenience to the doctor."[78] But in the 1950s, correlative with technical and analytical advances, things began to
change. The 1950 edition of Williams's text under its third editor,
Nicholson Eastman, dropped the condemnation of those who practiced premature induction, and the chapter on induction in DeLee's
text moved from the end of the book to the end of the section on
management of normal labor. No longer was induction a new tool
whose use one would learn if he read to the end of this enormous
volume; it was a procedure available to all for the management of
all labors. At the decade's end the convenience of obstetricians and
patients was made a legitimate indication for induction. In the paper

now widely cited as containing *the* indications for induction, Fields, Green, and Franklin said that labor was induced electively (without other medical indications) and appropriately in one-seventh of their patients for the following reasons:

(1) to prevent uncontrolled delivery prior to or immediately upon arrival at the hospital,
(2) for the peace of mind of the patient who had experienced such a delivery previously,
(3) to prevent anesthetic accidents during delivery,
(4) to assure constant physician attendance,
(5) to maintain orderly hospital occupancy for the comfort of the patient,
(6) to allow patients sufficient time to organize family responsibilities.[79]

The texts followed quickly. The 1961 version of *Williams Obstetrics* granted that "the elective induction of labor . . . may be justifiable under special circumstances"[80]; somewhat more cautiously DeLee's 1965 text said, "there is growing realization that inductions may be undertaken on an elective basis provided certain ideal conditions exist and relative contraindications are absent."[81] But there were still serious problems with induction, including prematurity of the infant, infection, and prolapse of the umbilical cord, a condition in which the umbilical cord falls between the fetal head and the birth canal, shutting off maternal-fetal blood exchange.

In the 1970s one of these problems, prematurity, was essentially solved and a method of detecting one other, prolapse of the cord, was found. Using ultrasonic imagery, physicians could monitor fetal growth through pregnancy and estimate gestational age. Using this method, physicians did not have to depend on a woman's report of her menstrual period dates and could estimate fetal age reliably on their own. Also, amniocentesis—aspiration of amniotic fluid through a needle passed into the amniotic sac through a woman's abdomen and analysis of components of the fluid—permitted predelivery assessment of fetal lung maturity, one of the primary prerequisites for a healthy neonate. With these techniques doctors could avoid inductions that would result in a premature infant. Electronic monitoring of fetal heart-rate and uterine contractions was assumed to give an indication of fetal distress including distress caused by a prolapsed umbilical cord.[82] In response to the advances the texts changed once more. Instead of the advantages of induction being "*more than offset* by the hazards," as they were according to a 1961 text, the "conveniences are *somewhat* offset by the hazards," and instead of there being a "growing realization" that inductions could be done electively, "experience [showed] that inductions may be undertaken electively *without apparent risk*"as long as certain conditions were met.[83] "The popularity of *elective induction . . .* resulted from its advantages to both patient and physician in terms of convenience."[84] But it was made possible in the first place by the ability of the profession to contain the procedure and protect it from internally generated criticism so that the problems it presented initially could be solved.

Technical developments in Britain paralleled those in America. Indications for induction expanded, but the British were more reluctant to admit "convenience" as a legitimate reason for an invasive procedure than were their American counterparts. They were constrained from admitting that inductions were done, or even might be done, for convenience by the strength of their professional boundary. Procedures which were invasive had to be cloaked in a rhetoric of medico-surgical propriety and kept on the specialist's "abnormal" side of the boundary. Something done for convenience could hardly be admitted to such a category.[85]

Yet in the late 1960s and early 1970s, induction rates skyrocketed in Britain. During the ten-year period beginning in 1965, inductions rose by a factor of two and one-half, from 15 percent to 41 percent of all births. Different reasons for this rise have been offered. One person has argued that the increase was the result of obstetrical traditions of intervention and control.[86] Doctors argued that mortality rates falling during a period of increased inductions supported their changes in practice. The public, through the media, argued that inductions had increased because of convenience.[87] Each of these positions makes sense from the point of view of those who hold it, but each has its limitations, given the history of the procedure and its place within the profession at the time. "Tradition" is much too simple, for it fails to explain why the practice was not more widely used for the sixty or so years it was available but lay relatively dormant. Likewise, the public's cry of "convenience," while probably an accurate description of one reason for the increase in inductions, also fails to account for the latency period of the procedure. The profession's own argument fails to admit other causal factors in the decline in mortality. Induction is best understood as a procedure which, from the point of view of the obstetrician, had certain advantages, including convenience, and certain disadvantages. Missing from previous explanations of the increase in inductions is a recognition of the importance of the profession's capacity to keep the procedure from critical scrutiny until technical solutions to the disadvantages of the practice could be found. A strong boundary around a profession with a self-ascribed mandate, not just a "tradition," of control helps explain not only the occurrence but also the timing and the suddenness of the increase in inductions in Britain.

The character of the boundary around British obstetrics also helps to explain the strong public reaction to increases in induction and the profession's response to the public's outcry. When there is a strong demarcation between normal and abnormal births it is much easier to notice when more and more women are being treated *as if* they were abnormal. Strong demarcation leads to clearer categorization. More women in Britain were being delivered by obstetricians with their plethora of procedures, and fewer were being attended by midwives. The movement of the normal/abnormal boundary to catch more cases, to place more women strictly in the obstetrician's domain, was publicly visible, ironically, *because* of the strength of the professional boundary. A profession trying to enlarge its domain is a common occurrence, but in the case of inductions the obstetrical profession in Britain faced a serious problem, namely, indications for induction, the justification for moving the boundary farther into the normal region, were not strictly medical indications. By not basing its practices on strictly medical indications British obstetrics was literally overstepping its boundary. Some people tried to convert "convenience" into a strictly medical indication by asserting that planned deliveries were safer because they could be done when hospital staffing was optimum, but research quickly showed that increased inductions did not increase the number of "daylight deliveries" or create a situation in which staffing could be rationalized. So, in the case of induction, the strong boundary, which was pushed far into the arena of previously normal births by indications that could not be made to seem strictly medical, left the profession exposed and vulnerable.

In this volatile context an epidemiologist, Iain Chalmers, teamed up with A. C. Turnbull, an obstetrician who originally had been influential in the proliferation of invasive procedures like induction, to study the effectiveness of inductions. They took advantage of a natural experiment in progress at a major medical center in Wales where two relatively independent obstetrical services delivered babies with two very different styles of practice. One team used more elective inductions and cesarean sections, more antenatal admissions, more radiography, more ultrasonic investigations, and more amniocenteses than the other team. In short, one team was more invasive, one might say more obstetrical, than the other. Outcomes of nearly 20,000 deliveries showed that while patients of the less invasive team suffered more perineal tears and had more prolonged labors, there was no difference in fetal outcomes. That is, there was no measurable difference in the incidence of fetal distress, in the conditions of babies just after birth, or in mortality. Even when they confined their analysis to the 12,338 "normal" births (determined post facto by a long list of stringent criteria) they found similar results: no difference in fetal outcomes.[88] In response to such evidence developed in such a volatile context, practices on the obstetricians' abnormal side of the boundary had to change, and to a large extent they did. As induction rates dropped in major obstetrical units throughout Britain, mortality rates did not increase and the shared wisdom of British obstetrics turned toward a more conservative position on induction.

In America, critics of induction were less vociferous and less well organized than their counterparts in Britain, and their concerns were less well focused. The difference was not a result of psychological or social differences between the groups of critics; it was a function of the weak boundary around the American profession. True, more women were being induced, but were they "abnormal" cases? Perhaps, but maybe not. The categories were not clear, if they existed at all, and consequently it was difficult to tell whether an increase in inductions signaled a different view of women who would be considered normal in other circumstances. Convenience of a woman and her family and perhaps even convenience of the doctor were legitimate indications for induction—or were they? Where induction sat with regard to normal/abnormal distinctions, or what place it occupied on the American physician's continuum of interventions, was simply not clear. Therefore the procedure was not as vulnerable as it was in Britain.

Critiques of induction did develop in America, though. They tended to originate in the women's movement and find their way into hospitals and doctors' offices through childbirth education classes. Obstetricians responded but their responses were much softer, much less direct, than those in England. The responses were generally rhetorical attempts to reconceptualize or reconsider practices, not to change them. For example:

> Any discussion of induction of labor reflexively prompts subdivision into elective and indicated (therapeutic) types. Though such a classification may be convenient, it is basically spurious. The fundamental decision to be made in any given pregnancy is: should the pregnancy be permitted to continue or should it be terminated. . . . Thus, all inductions of labor are in essence elective. Stated otherwise, if there is any indication for induction it cannot be considered elective induction.[89]

Obstetricians seemed to be saying: "All inductions are elective but they are not"; "elective inductions are medically appropriate because they are not elective inductions." At least, the distinction between elective and indicated inductions should be considered "spurious." The profession which had established itself in part by breaking down categorizations was once again asking that categories be ignored and boundaries weakened if not obliterated. Consider also this:

> Artificial rupture of membranes is often employed to shorten labor, provide data regarding fetal well-being . . . , or provide access to the baby for monitoring. . . . However, artificial rupture of membranes is of dubious benefit to the infant in the normal birth process. Patient concerns regarding its use should influence our practice.[90]

The use of a practice of "dubious benefit" should not be stopped, but should be negotiated with the patient. These are the kinds of responses available to a profession with a weak boundary, a boundary which cushions the effects of criticism. They are very different from those responses available to a profession which has encased itself in a stronger boundary as British obstetrics had.

The story of the induction of labor is not over. Further research and better technology are seen as the future saviors of the procedure. Recently, induction with prostaglandins has received considerable attention. The present position of induction in obstetrics is such that studies of prostaglandins compare their effectiveness and efficiency to other methods of induction. They do not question the wisdom of induction itself.[91] The hope for a more "physiological approach" to induction remains: "It may be possible in the future to unravel the delicate inter-relationships which exist between mother and fetus that precede spontaneous labor so that the most physiological approach may be used."[92]

This is getting ahead of social developments in the profession, though. As the next chapter shows, the profession began to change its approach to the notion of control some years back. Instead of searching out and containing potential pathology, obstetrics turned its attention to developing systems of monitoring and surveillance of *all* births. Monitoring and surveillance deal with the problem of residual normalcy by ignoring it. Under this new regime no distinctions between normal and abnormal exist. Instead of births being categorized for the sake of obstetrical invervention, interventions like induction of labor became part of integrated systems of control arrayed around a new conceptualization of pregnancy and childbirth that took form in the late 1940s and early 1950s.

Part Two

Re-forming the Profession

The profession of obstetrics experienced an important discontinuity in its mode of social control over women, their pregnancies, and childbirth generally, just after World War II. This shift was similar to that described for the profession of psychiatry by David Armstrong[1] and followed the lines of the general shift in modalities of social control described by Michel Foucault in *Discipline and Punish*. Foucault described the two sides of the transformation in this way:

> At one extreme, the discipline-blockade, the enclosed institution, established on the edges of society, turned inwards toward negative functions: arresting evil, breaking communications, suspending time. At the other extreme, with panopticism, is the discipline-mechanism: a functional mechanism that must improve the exercise of power by making it lighter, more rapid, more effective, a design of subtle coercion for a society to come.[2]

For its designer, Jeremy Bentham, the panopticon was a new kind of prison. For Foucault, the panopticon is a machine of power. It does not express power ostentatiously as a prince does, nor does it create a relationship of dominance through a reign of terror. The panopticon creates a structure of power through its design. By means of minimal but calculated architectural constraints it creates the capacity to see objects dispersed in a wide, heterogeneous field and

effects a new form of control through the creation of fields of visibility. After World War II obstetrics no longer controlled childbirth
by isolating it within a small, circumscribed space within the body
and by isolating the body within the confines of the hospital. Instead,
obstetrics located childbirth in a wider social order and subjected
it to the power of a structure that creates birth in a field of visibility.

With medicine informed by a mechanical metaphor, pregnancy
had meaning only within the confined space of the body and was
understood only by the severely localizing, informed gaze of the
physician. Once the ecological metaphor replaced the mechanical
one, pregnancy and birth took on meaning only in terms of their
relationships to other aspects of a system in which they were only
one process. A member of the faculty of the Albert Einstein College
of Medicine described the ecological approach this way:

> . . . ecological medicine is concerned with disease and health
> processes in terms of systems of values of several components
> of the living organisms.
> Ecological medicine is more than comprehensive medicine or
> a psychological medicine because its tasks [are] recognizing,
> evaluating, preventing, and treating all the physical,
> psychological, socioeconomic, and cultural variables which are
> an integral part of the disease process in their order of relative
> importance.[3]

Under its new logic, medicine must look to wider fields in order to
understand health and illness, attributing meaning to bodily processes only as they occur in relation to other processes occurring
in the cosmos. The ecological approach to medicine forces the physician to consider much more than he had ever considered before
when looking at childbirth.

In the ecological metaphor, the body is not a machine, but is "an
open system of communication . . . interacting with the exoteric
cosmos and its ecological processes."[4] The informed gaze which
circumscribes disease, locates it as an event at the end of a series
of physiological forces and events, and intervenes in the series to
effect a cure is outmoded and ineffective in dealing ecologically with
disease and health. Physiological processes must be located by a
normalizing gaze that has several components. Processes must first
be analyzed so that the effects on the process of everything at all
levels of the system are known and the trajectory of the process is

mapped out. After the "normal" trajectory of a process is known and probability distributions of deviations from the "norm" are constructed, each individual must be monitored, subjected to surveillance, and located precisely in terms of deviations on those probabilistic normalizing distributions.[5] Finally, any deviations for an optimal, "normal" course must be normalized. Management schemes must be constructed for each individual in order to insure that a process stays on its "normal" trajectory. Just as in Bentham's panopticon, which Foucault exploited as the symbol of the new order of social control, subjects must be separated, individualized, subjected to constant and total visibility, and then offered technologies of normalization to guarantee an optimal experience, not necessarily for the individual, but for the system as a whole or, more precisely, for the individual considered in relationship to other components of the system. Treatment schemes become lighter, more individualized, more precise, more rapid, one might even say more "humane," but management schemes become infinitely more effective means of control as well.

To appreciate fully the importance of the ecological metaphor it will be useful to examine how one set of authors thinks it affects day-to-day medical care. In 1978 McGraw-Hill published a major new text on pediatrics. The opening chapter, by Henry M. Seidel and Robert A. Hoekelman, was called "Ecology of Patient Care."[6] In a short fifteen pages Seidel and Hoekelman outline an understanding of medicine that would have been heretical thirty-five years earlier. They begin with the understanding of the effects of medical intervention which an ecological approach forces on the physician:

> Too often, we who provide care suffer the conceit that our interventions are the major determinants of the well-being of people. It is more likely that we play a lesser role and that other determinants of behavior, emotions, and physical health are the variables which dominate.[7]

The physician cannot and must not assume that his or her work is responsible for good health, but that does not undermine the importance of the physician. The orientation of the physician must simply change from intervention to monitoring and recording. Physicians must monitor everything about an individual and the environment:

The interplay of social and emotional factors may obscure the physical elements, and the patient may present too early to allow for differentiation of the diagnosis on the basis of the clinical course. Above all, in primary care the patient is seen repeatedly and with an intimacy that is not the privilege of the consultant. Thus, the observation, measurement, and recording of change over time [are] particularly important in pediatrics. Also, it is necessary to understand the incidence and prevalence of problems in the population served, be they physical, social, or emotional. It pays to know what's "going around."[8]

Absolutely everything must be made visible to medicine, be subject to observation, and recorded. This is the task of the modern physician; it is the principal task of the new order of social control I call "monitoring."

Fundamental medical concepts must change to accommodate the ecological approach to health and illness. Medicine's understanding of "patient" changes. Previously, the patient was the vehicle which brought the disease, or what was of interest to the physician (e.g., the virginal introitus), to the physician. Now the patient is the whole person and more. "The lesson of ecology is lost if we tend only the child rather than children and children rather than family and the family rather than the community."[9] The physician must now take many things, as well as many other people, into consideration when deciding care for the individual. "There must be active concern with the social, political, and economic processes which affect the health care system within which the patient seeks care and cure."[10] "We must understand as thoroughly as possible the *context* of the problems brought to us."[11] The "patient" becomes the individual cum family and perhaps even the family in the social system. The physician must change his or her approach to treatment: "To the traditional model of repair and restoration must be added the model of accommodation, facilitation, and enablement."[12]

In fact, what it is that must be treated is quite unclear under the ecological metaphor, for there is no longer any decidedly abnormal behavior or event nor any decidedly normal behavior or event. Behavior and events may be inappropriate or deviate considerably from "normal" trajectories, but deviations themselves are not "abnormal"; they are just closer or farther from the "norm" on normalizing distributions. Even "neurotic need, if its satisfactions serve societal ends, may not be understood as neurotic."[13] Medicine does not seek to "cure abnormal behavior" anymore, but it facilitates adaptation and coping when an individual's course or a family's course or a community's course differs from the professionally known "normal" course of a given process. "We do want to move the patients we serve toward, or maintain them at, some *mutually* agreed and acceptable levels of behavior and function."[14] However, the physician does not decide what those levels are but instead enters into negotiations with the ecologically expanded version of the patient to determine them.

The ultimate goal, for which the physician has assumed responsibility, is social order, an order in which the physician serves the key role of negotiator, arbitrator, and facilitator. The goal of theory is to create order, to bring about harmony, but in an ecological metaphor the nature of theory changes. When the body is a machine, the task of medical theory and medical practice is to get the machine to function harmoniously. The machine that breaks down or the machine that might potentially break down is the object of medical attention. In an ecological metaphor the medical space expands and the physician must reorient his work to effect or maintain harmony in the larger space, the ecology. The *space* in which "machines" operate, not just the machines themselves, must be ordered now.

Ironically, however, an ecological metaphor demands that the physician pay more attention to the individual at precisely the time that the physician's ultimate goal becomes harmony in the ecology. In an ecological field each case has its unique features, its own precise location on normalizing distributions. Everything about the individual must be known and recorded and management schemes must be tailored to fit the needs of the individual. Having to pay attention to the individual qua individual and having to be simultaneously concerned with the larger problem of social order creates a problem for the doctor. As Seidel and Hoekelman put it, "We need to define ourselves as individuals and find our fates" at the same time; "health care is feasible only if it is based on a sense of order."[15] How is this tension created by ecological medicine's dual orientation of individual and social order to be resolved? What is to be the basis of a social order in which each individual must, to a greater extent than ever before, be treated as such?

The answer, according to modern medicine, is that the model for order is to be found inside the individual. Individuality is much more than skin deep, but it is not infinitely deep. Individuality stops at our common sociobiological core, and it is there that models for the larger social order begin to appear. When E. O. Wilson termed sociobiology "the new synthesis," he was speaking of the basis provided by sociobiology for a common understanding of the seemingly diverse theories of many academic disciplines.[16] In fact, though, sociobiology is the basis for a synthesis of the individual–social order dichotomy which is made so much more profound by the demands of an ecological approach. Theory, as Jürgen Habermas points out in his appendix to *Knowledge and Human Interests,* is a word that derives from the ancient practice of looking to the rhythms of the cosmos for a model of order on earth. One gazed upon the cosmos and ordered one's actions through mimesis (imitation) to be in tune with the harmonic rhythms of the heavens.[17] The problem with an ecological approach is that it leaves the heavens out. The ecology is the cosmos, and there is no heaven left on which to gaze. One must look in a different direction, and not surprisingly modern theorists look inward. Seidel and Hoekelman are cautious about ascribing what order there is in the world to our genetic base, and they only suggest "that human behavior is probably as finely ordered as organic molecular structure,"[18] thereby stopping short of prescribing an order based on the messages from our genes (E. O. Wilson's "morality of the gene"). They leave little doubt, though, that a model for order must be found and that it will probably be found within.

In a curious turn of rhetoric, this inward biological orientation has become the "radical alternative" of the day. Alice Rossi, in a paper discussed at length in chapter 5 below, presents a self-styled radical vision of society which she describes as "a society more attuned to the natural environment, in touch with, and respectful of the rhythms of our body processes."[19] Selma Fraiberg, whose socibiologically based work is also discussed in chapter 5, aligns herself likewise with the "radical" cause of striving for an order informed by our inner, sociobiological selves.[20] We have "microcosmicized" Habermas's understanding of theory,[21] directing our attention to the cosmos within to find the model for ordering the human world. In the ecological metaphor the individual gains prominence only to be subjected to normalizing distributions which are supposed to respect not the individual but the common sociobiological processes which the scientist alone can make known. Theory based on an ecological metaphor effects the same indignities on indivduals and silences them just as effectively as theory based on a mechanical metaphor did, even though ecological theory looks in a different direction for its model of order.

The ecological metaphor is as demanding of medicine as it is of the individuals who are medicine's clients, and the metaphor is ultimately frustrating to medicine. The organization of care must be reformulated. Health-care professionals must be reorganized into *teams* of which the physician is not necessarily the leader, and "the relationship among health professionals on a team offering health care is as sensitive as their relationship with the patient."[22] The only way order and harmony can be achieved is by properly structuring the relationship of everything to everything else in the ecology. That includes the relationships of the "patient" to his-her-its environment, relationships among members of the team, and relationships of the team to the "patient." Yet, even after constant study and multiple reorderings of the ecology, the determination of whether or not health care is effective is difficult:

> Overall, health care . . . has not been demonstrated to be a positive force in changing illness rates and outcomes for more sophisticated populations. Nor has it been refuted. The lack of clear evidence in this regard can be attributed to the difficulties inherent in trying to isolate the influence of each of the components of the ecology of health care.[23]

To complicate matters further, ecologies have a habit of changing, of being dynamic. So an assessment of the effectiveness of health care today might be invalid tomorrow. The ecological metaphor forces medicine to widen its scope of interest, reforms its most basic concepts, but threatens it with the impossibility of claiming that it is effective. However, as the following examination of obstetrics will show, the expansion of a profession caused by the ecological approach to health care provides the profession with new forms of power and new forms of security that are effective even in an ecological world that changes constantly.

We can now turn away from medicine generally and review the changes that occurred in obstetrics. The transformation of obstetrics that occurred after World War II was rapid and striking. Instead of concentrating on the confining aspects of hospital birth and directing its attention inwards to the pathology which the hospital contained or to the potential pathology contained in every gravid uterus, obstetrics began to concentrate on the positive aspects of hospital birth and to direct its gaze outwards into the community and forwards and backwards in a woman's life. The ecology of birth replaced birth itself as the subject matter of the profession. As discussed in chapter 4, obstetrics literally discovered the fetus around World War II. This discovery had certain immediate political consequences, but it had more important long-term consequences for the profession as a whole. The fetus was the point of intersection of many social processes, and the profession could involve itself in those processes by following them outward from the fetus. A new language of normalcy emerged. Pregnancy and childbirth were no longer treated as discrete events with beginnings and ends, events to be terminated before pathology showed itself. Pregnancy and childbirth were reconceptualized as a set of processes, an infinitely divisible series of intimately known events to be kept on their obstetrically known "natural" courses by simple, undramatic, individualized, corrective management schemes. Pregnancy and birth were only one set of processes experienced by a woman, a system of systems within systems, and everything had to be considered in assessing a woman's trajectory through pregnancy and birth and in designing management schemes to optimize each birth. Monitoring and surveillance of every aspect of birth and every aspect of the environment surrounding birth replaced classic, dramatic interventions in pregnancy. A new order of obstetrical control appeared.

Foucault does not state precisely why the transformation from the heavy-handed power of the prince, characterized by the "discipline-blockade," to the lighter, more efficient power of the panopticon occurred. He says,

> [Discursive practices] possess specific modes of transformation. These transformations cannot be reduced to precise and individual discoveries; and yet we cannot characterize them as a general change of mentality, collective attitudes, or a state of mind. The transformation of a discursive practice is linked to a whole range of usually complex modifications that can occur outside of its domain (in the forms of production, in social relationships, in political institutions), inside it (in its techniques for determining its object, in the adjustment and refinement of its concepts, in its accumulation of facts), or to the side of it (in other discursive practices).[24]

All of these kinds of modifications occurred around the time of the second transformation of obstetrics, just as the natural childbirth movement began to gather momentum. The profession of obstetrics had been able to gain for itself a degree of autonomy, one might even say sovereignty, over childbirth. But the sovereignty of a profession is always a contingent sovereignty, dependent in part on continuing support from the state and on the willingness of clients to remain clients, accepting the work of the profession as offered. The natural childbirth movement threatened the contingent sovereignty of obstetrics by telling women that they had alternatives to the models of pregnancy held by obstetricians and to the ways obstetricians managed pregnancy and birth. At the same time, particularly in Britain, the government threatened to amend the franchise of medicine. Both social bases of obstetrics, its franchise and its "material," were on the verge of being withdrawn. Also, based partly on wartime advances in technology, the tools of obstetrics improved and the profession gained greater access to the fetus. These were the kinds of changes occurring in obstetrics' environment.

Obstetrics was certainly vulnerable to any threats to its sovereignty that might materialize. Two characteristics of the profession lay at the heart of its vulnerability: its scientism and its ethically neutral facade.

Obstetrics was, like all of medicine, scientistic and not scientific. That is, its practices were based only in part on science even though the profession presented itself before and during its professional period as a scientific discipline. The science of medicine was thickly overlayed with clinical judgment, the art of medical practice. So, for example, J. Whitridge Williams could write of a randomized clinical experiment designed to test the safety of predelivery cleansing of the vaginal and pubic regions (a practice he had strongly endorsed in his early editions):

> Observations . . . showed that the incidence of febrile puerperia [postpartum infection] was 16.3 and 12.4 percent in the [women who were cleansed and prepared as usual and in those who were unprepared], respectively, and indicated that if there was any difference it was slightly in favor of nonpreparation. *I have not yet had the courage to advocate complete nonpreparation.*[25]

Well-conducted scientific investigations did not necessarily determine clinical practice. Experience and judgment weighed heavily in
the conduct of obstetrical care. To the outsider, however, the profession presented itself as scientific. The "objective" stance of medicine based on its scientific character was one of regular medicine's
selling points in its campaign to have state licensing laws enacted
during the 1890s, and the scientific character of medicine is the basis
for the model of the profession's development that the profession
itself holds. A profession which poses as scientific is vulnerable
because anyone can read the results of scientific experiments and
tell what their implications for practice are. Science leaves clear,
clean records and makes the work of a profession visible. How the
profession's own deployment of a structure of monitoring, with its
multilevel technologies of surveillance, exposed the profession and
brought it, as well as pregnancy and birth, under control is one of
the subjects of chapter 4.

Scientism, though, in its aping of the scientific method, can at
times work to the profession's advantage. Occasionally, the implications of scientific theories strike such resonant chords, within and
outside the profession, that the slightest hint of scientific support for
those theories—even if it comes from seriously flawed research—is
taken as the basis for action and policy. How obstetrics used pseudoscientific reasoning and data to expand its field of interest forward
in a woman's life from the point of delivery to the hitherto obstetrically closed areas of mother-infant interaction, family dynamics,
and social order generally is the topic of chapter 5.

The second aspect of the profession's character which led to its
vulnerability was its ethically neutral facade. Medicine in general
deals with choices for life and death and consequently operates in
an ethically charged field. Medicine does not present the choices it
makes as ethical ones, however. Internally, obstetrics is a moral
community, but to the outsider the actions of the profession appear
to be scientifically based clinical judgments. The profession's autonomy depends on its ability to maintain this duality, on its ability
to make ethical choices appear not to be ethical choices, on the
ability to contain the ethical content of its work within its professional boundary. When the outsider begins to examine the work of
the profession, as the deployment of monitoring permitted or perhaps
even encouraged, he sees that the actions of medicine have ramifications throughout the social system. Seeming "good" done for

the patient has "bad" effects elsewhere, in the patient's family or in the economy. The ethical aspects of obstetrical work seep across the boundary. Because of its posture of ethical neutrality the profession has no capacity to resolve what came to be, in the public's eye, ethical dilemmas, and it is therefore open to analysis by another discipline, ethics, which has claims to forms of prescriptive knowledge different from those used by medicine. Medicine and ethics sometimes disagree on answers to the fundamental question common to both disciplines, "What ought to be done?" Ethics presents a challenge to medicine, and therefore constitutes a problem for the profession. Yet ethics can offer medicine assistance in reducing the overall degree of scrutiny to which it is subject. How medicine and ethics simultaneously resolve the conflict between them, forge a partnership, and work together to reformulate the doctor-patient relationship, thereby constructing a new, wider protective boundary for the profession is the subject of chapter 6.

With obstetrics re-formed, assisted by ethics, and new, broader limits placed around it, the profession could once again turn its attention inward to problems its re-formation had caused. How to rationalize care and get women to agree to be partners with obstetricians in the preservation of obstetrical power over birth are taken up in chapter 7. This last chapter shows that women and obstetricians have almost identical interests with regard to birth. Obstetrics made women "joint adventurers" in the obstetrical project and in this way, with the cooperation of women, secured its hold on birth. Women joined the obstetrical project and helped bolster the control monitoring exerts over childbirth, albeit within a flexible system of obstetrical alternatives.

Part Two of this work is primarily about the rationalization of obstetrical care. It focuses heavily on developments in American obstetrics because that is where the greatest movement toward rationalization has occurred. Britain put in place a fairly stable organization for delivering care under the National Health Service. The British system introduced regionalization of care, an important step toward rationalizing perinatal health care, long before the idea became popular in America. With the strong boundary around the profession, relationships within the British system changed little after the system was established. For example, John Tomkinson, a member of the Central Midwives Board, described the role of the midwife in 1978 in terms almost identical with those used in chapter

2 above to describe the role of the midwife just after the turn of the century.[26] American obstetrics was a late starter but has since gone farther than British obstetrics in following the logic of monitoring. Perhaps because of its weak boundary, the profession has had to undergo a significant internal reorganization in response to the deployment of monitoring. Thus, the transformation of the profession occurred more rapidly in Britain than in America, but changes there stopped sooner than here largely because of differences in the postwar organization of British and American obstetrics. This explains why the British profession appears only briefly at the beginning of this part and then disappears from the discussion.

4 Monitoring and Surveillance
A New Order of Obstetrical Control

In modern obstetrics "monitoring" brings to mind the laboring woman plugged into an electronic fetal monitor that continuously records fetal heart rate and uterine contractions. The fetal monitor is the focus of the most contentious debate the profession has experienced since the introduction of the obstetrical forceps. Supporters of the monitor claim that it reduces infant mortality and morbidity. Critics in and out of the profession claim that the monitor adds to the economic costs of pregnancy and childbirth, that it increases the cesarean section rate and thus maternal morbidity and mortality, and that it reinforces the atmosphere of crisis surrounding birth, further "medicalizing" a normal and natural event. Carefully controlled experiments have cast doubt on the fetal monitor's capacity to detect fetal distress and improve the outcomes of pregnancy. Yet with all this controversy the monitoring movement in the profession is healthy and vigorous, with proponents arguing that all labors should be monitored.

How can this happen in modern medicine, a field which presents itself as a discipline based in large part on science? Obstetricians say that to focus attention on the fetal monitoring machine is to misunderstand the current direction of the profession. They claim that the fetal monitor is but a small part of their attempt to understand "fetal ecology," a new field of inquiry within the profession. Old technology provided only glimpses at the life of the fetus. New technological advances provide access to the fetus throughout most of pregnancy and allow obstetricians to understand better the developmental needs of the fetus from conception through labor and delivery. When a pregnancy is monitored with a wide range of surveillance techniques, potential problems can be detected early and often corrected by precise, carefully designed interventions, much simpler and "lighter" than those that would have been necessary had the problem gone undetected, followed its natural course, and been allowed to present as pathology of a high order. The profession says the result of an orientation which emphasizes earlier, simpler corrective interventions is a more normal and natural childbirth that can be enjoyed by the parents and that is beneficial for the baby.

As this chapter shows, technological advances are only a part of a more broad-based, penetrating "monitoring concept." The monitoring concept represents a change in the deployment of obstetrical power and a new mode of social control over childbirth which I will call simply "monitoring." Monitoring allows the profession to extend the obstetrical project out into the community and into every aspect of every woman's life. Power and control are magnified by making the object of control more visible and accessible, more "known" through multiple monitoring schemes. After the monitoring concept was in place, obstetrics did not need to confine itself to the abnormal or potentially pathological birth; every birth became subject to its gaze. Monitoring permitted the "lighter, more precise" intervention of a disciplinary power to replace the harsher, more dramatic interventions of a power which sought to confine the evil that pregnancy might present. Monitoring changed the focus of interest of the profession from the mother to the fetus and thereby justified a wider array of interventions while, at the same time, it allowed the profession to make the claim that births were more natural and "physiologic."

Monitoring is a new order of obstetrical control to which not only women and their pregnancies are subject but to which obstetrical personnel themselves are subject. Gone, under monitoring, are the boundaries that afforded the profession a degree of protective insulation. By the same means the profession used to extend its project beyond its previous limits it exposed itself to view and necessitated the implementation of a discipline for itself as well as for its subject matter, birth.

The Fetal Monitoring Controversy

The electronic fetal monitor has been a focus of controversy for the past ten years. Debates about its benefits and risks have occurred within obstetrics and outside of the profession's boundary. Many women, individually and collectively, have protested its use; the United States Senate has investigated its effectiveness, casting a critical eye toward its costs; at least two separate offices of the Department of Health, Education, and Welfare have issued reports on monitoring; the newly established National Center for Health Care Technology has given monitoring high priority in its program of evaluative studies; and debate among obstetricians continues despite the fact that the American College of Obstetricians and Gynecologists published a policy recommendation for the use of monitoring.

For all their electronic sophistication fetal monitors are conceptually simple devices. They embody straightforward extensions of concepts which have informed the practice of obstetrics since its embryonic stage in the mid-nineteenth century. Lannec claimed as early as 1819 that auscultation of the fetal heart—listening to fetal heart tones either directly or with the aid of a mechanical device—could detect fetal life and fetal distress.[1] Once the advantages of auscultation were established in principle, how to listen best became a technological problem for the profession, and what to listen for became a theoretical and empirical problem. The stethoscope and the fetoscope (a special stethoscope that amplifies fetal heart sounds) were early solutions to the technical problem of listening. Later, an ultrasonic device was designed which bombarded the fetus with sound waves and "listened" to the fetal heart by measuring the Doppler shift caused by the movement of the fetal heart wall. The electronic fetal monitor was developed by Caldeyro-Barcia and Edward Hon in the 1950s. Some monitors detect the electrical activity of the fetal heart indirectly at the mother's abdomen in much the same way that adult electrocardiography detects the electrical activity of an adult's heart at the chest wall. The difficulty with indirect measurement of the fetal heart rate is that electrodes sensitive enough to detect fetal hearts also pick up the mother's heart's activity, rendering the signal difficult to interpret. Hon, in 1957, described a method for filtering the maternal and fetal components of the signal from the mother's abdomen,[2] but methods of measuring the fetal heart rate directly, either by means of a clip on the part of the fetus first appearing in the cervix during birth or by means of a spiral electrode screwed into the baby's scalp after the head is engaged in the birth canal, obviated any need for electronically complex monitors. A single signal, either from a phonocardiogram (a microphone) or an ultrasonic device placed on the mother's abdomen or from an electrode attached directly to the fetus, can be used to drive a pen which writes on a moving sheet of paper to provide a continuous record of fetal heart activity throughout birth.

Advances in electronics have facilitated changes in fetal monitors. For example, microcircuitry and radiotelemetry of electronic signals[3] permitted the reduction in size of sensors so that a fetal heart detector could be coupled with a radiotransmitter and inserted in a woman's vagina or strapped to her leg. The laboring woman then could move freely from the fetal heart recording device, and reliable data could still be obtained. But regardless of the levels of technical sophistication achieved, the problem to which monitors respond—how to listen to the fetal heart—is the same as it was over a hundred years ago.

The mere act of listening is no longer problematic; the technical difficulties of auscultation have been solved. The theoretical problem—what to listen for—remains the question at the center of the fetal monitoring controversy. For the moment let us attend to just those data and fetal heart-rate patterns that are widely thought to be associated with poor fetal outcome and that have received extensive treatment in obstetrics texts and teaching media. Later, we can pick up the threads of controversy that run throughout this field.

When the uterus contracts during labor it exerts pressure on the fetus. Some say that the uterus *stresses* the fetus. Very early, obstetricians tried to define the point at which stress became *distress,* for it was assumed that distress was a signal for intervention. In the first edition of his text, in 1903, Williams said that fetal heart rates below a hundred beats per minute were ominous signs "incompatible with prolonged life of the fetus" and indicated the need for rapid delivery, "provided it can be accomplished without too great risk for the mother."[4] Williams recognized, though, that some fetal heart decelerations, even some falling below a hundred beats per minute, were benign. It was not and still is not unusual, for example, for the uterus to compress the fetal head slightly, exerting pressure on the vagus nerve which, in turn, slows the heart rate. Decelerations caused by this means are transient and recover at the end of a contraction. Once fetal monitors were equipped to measure uterine contractions simultaneously with fetal heart rates, a deceleration of this sort—one that began with the onset of a contraction, mirrored the contraction in intensity, and subsided at the end of a contraction—became known as an "early deceleration" because of its early onset. Early decelerations are still associated with "head compression" and are still thought to be benign.

Other patterns are not viewed so lightly. Using stethoscopes, some early obstetricians noticed that fetal heart decelerations that persisted beyond the end of a contraction or that were uncorrelated with uterine contractions seemed to be associated with fetal death or with the birth of severely compromised infants. With an early fetal heart monitor, Hon studied the heart patterns of a fetus of twenty-five weeks gestation presenting as a footling breech whose mother went into labor after the umbilical cord fell into the birth canal between the fetus and the uterine wall. Hon and his associates did not deem the chances of survival for the baby good so they treated this woman and child as a research case.[5] The fetal monitor detected "severe variable decelerations"—decelerations which varied in intensity and had no consistent temporal relationship with uterine contractions—when the umbilical cord was compressed either by the force of contractions, by a shift in the woman's position, or by hand. Hon's findings were supported in later research, and "variable decelerations" became associated with "cord compression" and are still taken as an indication for immediate action: discontinuation of uterine stimulants, administration of oxygen, and repositioning of the mother to relieve pressure on the umbilical cord.

The third form of fetal heart pattern commonly detected by fetal monitors and thought to be ominous is the "late deceleration." It begins near the middle of a contraction, mirrors the contraction in intensity, although the contraction and deceleration are out of phase, and subsides sometime after the contraction has ended. Most obstetricians feel that this pattern is caused by the uterine wall clamping down on the placental vessels which supply the fetus with oxygen and carry away the waste products of respiration. The uterus probably occludes the placental veins first, an event which causes the products of respiration to start building up in the fetus. Then the placental artery is occluded, shutting off the fetus' oxygen supply. The fetus suffers hypoxia—a lack of oxygen—and the fetal heart slows. After the contraction, the blood vessels are released, blood flow is reinitiated, the fetus recovers gradually from its hypoxic state, and the fetal heart rate increases. The delay in the onset of the effects of hypoxia and recovery from it cause the deceleration to be out of phase with the contraction. In a healthy placenta, vessels usually resist occlusion by the uterine wall, so late decelerations are associated with "utero-placental insufficiency" and often indicate the need for rapid delivery.

The three major types of fetal heart decelerations are summarized in figure 4.1, taken from an article by Hon. The electronic fetal-monitor tracings show uterine contractions measured by a saline-filled catheter placed inside the uterus to measure the pressure of contractions directly; above each tracing is shown the fetal heart rate. These tracings are somewhat idealized versions of the patterns which can be detected by most electronic monitors in use today. Other patterns, including a sinusoidal pattern of accelerations and decelerations, increased or decreased fetal heart baseline or "average" rate, and changing variability around the baseline or "average" ("beat-to-beat variability") have been investigated, but considerable controversy still surrounds their interpretation and they will not be discussed here.[6]

Physicians do not decide care strictly on the basis of monitor tracings. Decisions to intervene in labor are guided by the fetal monitor, but most physicians use other clinical data as well in the formulation of their management strategies. In addition to a woman's medical history, the clinical course of her present pregnancy, and the clinical data that can be collected through simple physical examination or direct visualization of the fetus with a fiber optical "amnioscope," further tests are often done in the face of ominous fetal heart patterns. For example, if late decelerations are indeed causing hypoxia, the fetus's acid-base balance will be upset by the buildup of acid in its blood caused by decreased respiration. A physician can assess the acid-base balance directly by nicking the part of the fetus visible through the cervix with a knife, drawing out some of the blood that appears, and measuring its pH, its acidity. Capillary blood pH, obtained through "fetal scalp blood sampling," as this procedure is called, seems to increase the predictive validity of ominous fetal heart patterns and reduces the incidence of interventions in pregnancies that would result in healthy babies if left to proceed on their own.

For being such a straightforward extension of very old obstetrical

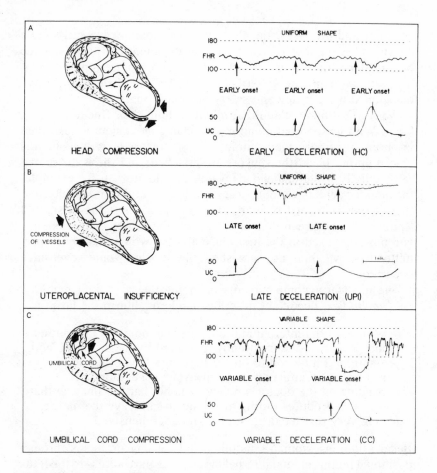

Figure 4.1. *A,* This FHR pattern of uniform shape, which refelects the shape of the associated intrauterine pressure curve, has its onset early in the contracting phase of the uterus and has been labeled "early deceleration." *B,* This FHR deceleration pattern, which is also of uniform shape and also reflects the shape of the associated intrauterine pressure curve, has its onset late in the contracting phase of the uterus and has been labeled "late deceleration." *C,* This FHR pattern of variable shape, which does not reflect the shape of the associated intrauterine pressure curve and whose onset occurs at varying times during the contracting phase of the uterus, has been labeled "variable deceleration." (From Edward H. Hon and Aida F. Khazin, "Observation on Fetal Heart Rate and Fetal Biochemistry. I. Base Deficit," *American Journal of Obstetrics and Gynecology* 105 [1969]: 723. Used by permission of the C. V. Mosby Co.)

concepts and practices, the electronic fetal monitor has attracted a considerable number of critics. Using the same body of evidence but speaking from different perspectives and representing different interests, women, the government, and certain obstetricians have questioned the efficacy and safety of monitoring.

Women justifiably claim that monitors limit their freedom during labor. With an external monitor a woman's movement is restricted in order to increase the accuracy of monitor tracings. A woman is placed on her back, the sensors are attached, and she is instructed to lie quietly while technicians watch the monitor. If, for example, the monitor detects variable decelerations, a "crisis" is signaled and the woman is turned on her side. This may avert the crisis and "prevent" a cesarean delivery, but, say the critics, if the monitor had not been used in the first place and the woman had been permitted to move about as she wished, the "crisis" would never have occurred.

The medical accompaniments of monitoring also limit mobility. As *Our Bodies, Ourselves* describes modern labor in the hospital,

> With both the internal and the external monitors the mother's blood pressure is intermittently measured by means of a blood pressure cuff attached to one of her arms. The other arm is very frequently attached to an intravenous solution unit, depending on the doctor's policy. It is not hard to imagine that all these procedures during heavy labor can leave the mother feeling very restricted, immobile and apprehensive.[7]

Besides limiting women's mobility and causing problems through positional requirements, internal monitors require access to the fetus which can only be gained through the membranes that contain the amniotic fluid. When physicians want to use a monitor, these membranes, if they have not ruptured spontaneously, must be ruptured artificially. The artificial rupturing of the amniotic sac is sometimes painful, sometimes causes the umbilical cord to prolapse into the birth canal as the amniotic fluid rushes out, and often requires further interventions in labor such as augmentation with uterine stimulants if labor does not proceed according to schedule. Women protest that "some of the fetal stress picked up by the monitor might itself be a product of the placement and operation of the monitor,"[8] and they receive support for their claims from some obstetricians.

Women also complain that the monitor transforms the birth experience into more of a medical event, something it need not and, some say, should not, be. Little can be said of this claim except that it seems eminently reasonable and that men can never hope to verify the claim independently.

The government has a different set of interests and a somewhat different set of concerns about monitoring. With women and obstetricians, the government is concerned about safety and effectiveness, but in this era of inflation and calls for "cost containment" in the health sector, the cost of fetal monitoring seems to be the government's underlying concern.

Without question, monitoring is big business. In 1968 Edward Hon, one of the inventors and early proponents of monitoring, set up the first company to manufacture fetal monitors, Corometrics. The company was influential in popularizing fetal monitoring through its educational programs, and Dr. Hon's published research was the basis for the early acceptance of monitoring by the profession. In 1975, American Home Products, a multinational conglomerate, bought Corometrics, and around the same time other giants in the electronics field, including Hewlitt Packard and Texas Instruments, entered the fetal monitoring business. In 1978 a single monitor cost between $3,000 and $6,000 and the total market in the United States was over $30 million. In Britain, with a much smaller market and somewhat tighter controls on spending for health care, one manufacturing firm sold over eight hundred monitors in one year for a total of more than 2 million pounds (about $4.4 million).[9]

The question for government, as it always is in the face of such large amounts, is whether monitors are worth it. Even with unequivocal data on effectiveness, which are not available yet, this would be impossible to answer because of the problems of attaching monetary figures to human experiences and of finding the appropriate comparison. These problems have not stopped people from doing "cost/benefit analyses" of monitors, however. For example, Drs. Edward Quilligan and Richard Paul,[10] both associates of Dr. Hon, estimated in 1975 that an obstetrical service of three thousand deliveries over five years would require an outlay of $106,500 for monitors and for the personnel to use and maintain them for the five-year period. They point out that this rather substantial expense means a cost to each patient of only $35.50 ($11 in expendable supplies and $24.50 in recovery costs), which they say "seems reasonable when a comparison is made with the estimated costs of procedures such as chest X-ray, electrocardiogram, SMA 18 analysis [automated blood chemistry analysis], and X-ray pelvimetry." To drive home their point they calculated the amount that might be saved by preventing fetal deaths and serious brain damage through the widespread use of monitors and found that a yearly expenditure of roughly $100 million on monitoring—enough, they estimated, to monitor all 3 million births each year—would prevent long-term expenditures of nearly $2 billion that would be required to take care of the damaged infants who would be born.

Other authors' estimates differ from that of Quilligan and Paul. In 1974, H. David Banta and Stephen B. Thacker, both physicians but who worked in the U. S. Congress' Office of Technology Assessment and the Center for Disease Control, estimated a yearly cost of $411 million for monitoring only the high-risk half of all births in the U.S. They estimated the direct cost of monitoring to be $80 million. In addition, they said, other costs would accrue, including $222 million for the extra cesarean section operations caused by using monitors, $5 million in fetal morbidity and mortality attributable to monitoring, and $58 million in maternal morbidity and mortality attributable to monitoring and the increase in operative deliveries. They compare their cost estimate to the $80 million spent annually on all public and private childhood immunization programs and find the required expenditures unjustifiably high. Furthermore, they dismiss estimates of expenditures prevented through the prevention of mental retardation by saying "without further study, the effect of EFM on the costs of mental retardation to the society cannot be estimated."[11]

The estimates of the National Institutes of Health's "consensus-developing" Task Force on Predictors of Fetal Distress, which issued its report in the same month that Banta and Thacker's findings were published, are cautiously worded and appropriately couched in admissions of having "inadequate information about the critical effects of monitoring on the health of mothers and babies."[12] They estimate direct increases in health costs of $92 to $192 million if all births were monitored. They estimate an increase in direct and indirect costs due to cesarean sections of $6 million and savings of up to $900 million in direct and indirect costs due to reductions in perinatal mortality and mental retardation, but they draw no conclusions from their figures. They present their cost/benefit analysis as merely interesting, not as something on which policy should necessarily be based.

What the ultimate impact of these disparate analyses will be remains to be seen since the government moves cautiously in the regulation of obstetrical practice. With regard to regulating fetal monitoring equipment, the government can certify the machinery itself, but only to the extent that it insures that a machine does what its manufacturers claim it does. Fetal monitor manufacturers claim only that their machines monitor and record fetal heart rate and uterine contractions, and so they do. The government has not given itself license to insist that monitors be shown to prevent death or mental retardation, as some physicians claim the monitors do. The government sets up task forces, but they have little direct impact on policy. The National Institutes of Health's task force termed auscultation an "acceptable" means of monitoring low-risk patients, but their recommendations contain no force for change except indirectly, through the courts, which will undoubtedly use the report in settling malpractice suits, and through women using the report to negotiate regimens of care with their own doctors.[13] Cost/benefit analyses could influence regional health planning through the federally mandated HSA structure established recently, but whether it will or not remains an empirical question.

At the heart of the fetal monitoring controversy and behind any cost/benefit analysis is the interpretation of studies purporting to establish the effectiveness and safety of monitoring. All critics—women, government, and obstetricians—have had access to the same data on fetal monitoring and have reached widely divergent conclusions concerning this new technology. A review of the controversy would be incomplete without a review of the studies and data available so far.

The questions about fetal monitors are simple. Are they beneficial? That is, do they decrease deaths which occur during the birth process (intrapartum deaths) or deaths in the first twenty-eight days of life (neonatal deaths), or do they decrease neonatal morbidity, a vague term meaning incapacity, ill health, trauma, or localized specific problems such as minor infections? Are they perhaps harmful? Might they *increase* neonatal morbidity or mortality? Might they increase maternal morbidity and mortality by increasing the number of cesarean section operations or by increasing the incidence of infections? Beyond these basic questions are more complex ones: If monitors are beneficial in some respects and harmful in others, do the benefits outweigh the risks? Can we identify populations for which monitors are beneficial, or should everyone be monitored? These are the questions on which the case for monitoring necessarily rests, but getting answers has proven enormously difficult.

There are three basic types of studies of the fetal monitor: experimental, quasi-experimental, and retrospective record reviews. Experimental studies compare patients who were monitored during the birth process with those who were not monitored but who gave birth during the same period of time and under similar circumstances as the monitored group. Experimental studies can be done with randomized assignment to monitored and control groups or with assignment based on specified criteria. Nonrandomized experimental studies suffer selection biases, and results from them are usually considered less reliable and valid than results from randomized designs. Quasi-experimental studies compare patients who delivered during a period when monitoring was not available with patients who delivered after the introduction of monitoring. Quasi-experimental designs suffer biases introduced by the passage of time, for example, changes in patient population or changes in obstetrical practices other than the introduction of monitoring. Generally, in medicine, results from these quasi-experimental studies are considered less reliable than results from randomized experimental studies. Retrospective record reviews do not involve purposeful selection of comparison groups at all. They involve the systematic but retrospective study of patients who were monitored, for whatever reasons, and those who were not. Record reviews are limited to data available in hospital records, which may or may not have been recorded with some idea of what constitutes "important" data, but it is often felt that large samples, appropriately analyzed, can provide useful results.

Table 4.1[14] summarizes all the randomized controlled trials and nonrandomized experimental analyses of fetal monitoring available through mid-1979. It also includes a sample of quasi-experimental studies and one large retrospective analysis in which the data were recorded in a uniform, reliable manner and subjected to rigorous, appropriate statistical analyses. The following review is restricted to a few representative or important studies.

Lee and Baggish's report on Mount Sinai Hospital, Hartford, Connecticut, is typical of studies published after the early rush to monitoring. A thorough review of their study and its results will serve as a guide to the issues involved in the monitoring controversy. After January 1972, all patients admitted to Mount Sinai Hospital for delivery were monitored except for those having planned, elective cesarean deliveries and those who experienced an intrauterine death before the onset of labor. Their reasoning for monitoring everyone was straightforward enough: "most indications for monitoring arose during the course of labor. In order to achieve maximal surveillance during this critical period of pregnancy, it would seem that every labor should be electronically monitored when circumstances permit."[15] All 3,529 deliveries during the period from 1972 to 1974 were monitored externally initially and then internally if membranes ruptured spontaneously or "if the external monitor [did] not show a satisfactory tracing." The experiences of this group of women and babies were compared with the experiences of the 4,323 deliveries that occurred in the preceding three-year period, 1969 to 1971. The critical variable in most obstetrical studies is perinatal mortality, babies born dead weighing 500 grams or more or born after twenty weeks of gestation, plus those babies born alive who die in the neonatal period (the first twenty-eight days of life). In this study there were 104 perinatal deaths in the premonitoring period and 52 after monitoring was introduced. The pre- and post-monitoring perinatal death rates of 24 per thousand births and 14.7 per thousand births, respectively, are significantly different in a statistical sense. Obstetricians often correct rates like these to exclude "unsalvageable" fetuses, those with congenital anomalies and other conditions incompatible with life. The remainder are theoretically "preventable" deaths. Table 4.1 shows intrapartum and neonatal death rates based primarily on figures corrected in this manner. The corrected neonatal death rates in Lee and Baggish's study were 13.1 per thousand for the unmonitored group and 6.0 for the monitored group, a "reduction" of 50 percent. Fetuses which die during birth are termed intrapartum deaths. In the Lee and Baggish study there were fifteen babies that died during birth in the premonitoring period and only one intrapartum death after monitors were introduced. They suggest that even the one intrapartum death in the monitoring period could have been prevented had an internal monitor been used earlier in labor. Thus, the unmonitored group had an intrapartum death rate of 3.5 per thousand live births and the monitored group had a rate of 0.3.

Table 4.1 Summary of Studies of Fetal Monitoring

First Author and Date[1]	Number of Patients[2]		Year of Intervention[3]
	Unmonitored	Monitored	
			Randomized
Haverkamp, 1976[4]	241 (high risk)	242 (high risk)	1973
Haverkamp, 1979[5]	232 (high risk)	463 (high risk)	1975
Renou, 1976[6]	175 (high risk)	169 (high risk)	1974
Kelso, 1978	253 (low risk)	251 (low risk)	1976
			Nonrandomized
Chan, 1973[7]	5,427	1,162	1968
Kelly, 1973[8]	17,000 (low risk)	150 (90% high risk)	N.A.
Paul, 1977[9]	36,602 (low risk)	14,038 (high risk)	1970
Tutera, 1975	6,179 (low risk)	608 (96% high risk)	1969
Amato, 1977[10]	2,994 (37% high risk)	422 (46% high risk)	
			Quasi-experimental and
Edington, 1975[10]	991	1,024	1974
Koh, 1975[11]	1,161	1,080	1973
Shenker, 1975[12]	11,599 (11% EFM)	1,950 (80% EFM)	1973
Lee, 1976[13]	4,323	3,529	1972
Neutra, 1978[14]	7,182	8,664	1969–75

NOTES

1. See chapter notes for full bibliographic information.

2. Number of patients in each group in experimental designs; number of births in each time period (before and after the introduction of monitoring for quasi-experimental designs).

3. First year of study for experimental designs; year monitoring initiated for quasi-experimental designs.

4. Excluded babies under 1,500 grams in weight.

5. Excluded babies under 2,000 grams or under 34 weeks gestation.

6. Discontinued randomized trial.

7. Excluded babies 1,500 grams and less; rates corrected for congenital anomalies.

Most studies of fetal monitoring report changes in babies' "Apgar scores" in addition to changes in mortality. A newborn's Apgar score is assessed at one minute and five minutes after birth and is based on the child's appearance, its pulse rate, its respiration, and its overall condition and behavior. The score can vary from 0, for

Intrapartum Fetal Death Rate/1,000 Births		Neonatal Death Rate/1,000 Births		Cesarean-Section Rate	
Unmonitored	Monitored	Unmonitored	Monitored	Unmonitored	Monitored
Controlled Trials					
0	0	0	4.1(1)	6.6%	16.5%
0	0	0	6.5(3)	5.6%	{17% EFM {11% EFM + FSB
5.7(1)	0	0	5.9(1)	14%	20%
0	3.9(1)	0	4.4%	9.5%	
Experimental Designs					
3.1(17)	1.7(2)	2.7(15)	4.3(5)	—	—
0.9(15)	0	14.0	6.0	8.3%	18%
0.9(34)	0.4(6)	5.1(184)	5.5(72)	7.0%	16%
6.0(37)	1.6(1)	8.0	1.6(1)	4.8%	10.1%
4.0(12)	0.2(1)	8.2(24)	0.9(4)	6.1%	8.6%
Statistical Designs					
4.0(4)	0	13.3(13)	3.0(3)	8.9%	
3.4(4)	4.8(5)	5.1(4)	3.5(1)	6.4%	
1.2(14)	0.5(1)	9.7(25)	3.1(6)	4.8%	
3.5(15)	0.3(1)	13.1(56)	6.0(21)	7.3%	
	N.A.	5.5	3.2	N.A.	

8. Excluded babies 1,500 grams and less.

9. Excluded babies 1,500 grams and less; rates corrected for congenital anomalies and birth trauma.

10. Rates corrected for congenital anomalies.

11. Excluded babies under 1,000 grams; rates corrected for congenital anomalies.

12. Excluded babies 1,000 grams and less.

13. Excluded babies 500 grams and less and 20 weeks gestation and less; rates corrected for congenital anomalies.

14. Multivariate statistical analysis; rates shown are aggregates of all risks.

almost hopelessly compromised newborns, to 10, for extraordinarily healthy newborns, with 6 being considered a "low Apgar," an indication that an infant is depressed or compromised. The five-minute Apgar score is thought by some to be a very good predictor of long-term development prospects, but its value in predicting poor outcomes beyond the immediate neonatal period has been questioned. Lee and Baggish report a statistically significant drop in the percentage of babies born with low Apgars after monitoring began, a finding that suggests that monitoring may be beneficial.

It may be that perinatal outcomes are improved after monitoring is introduced, but are there harmful effects of monitoring as well? Lee and Baggish report a significant increase in the rate of cesarean sections over time, from 7.3 percent of all deliveries in the three years prior to monitoring to 10.4 percent of all deliveries during the monitoring period. More important than the basic cesarean-section rate, though, is the proportion of cesarean operations done for "fetal distress," the condition monitors are supposed to diagnose. Most authors report diagnosis-specific rates because cesarean-section rates have increased threefold over the past ten years and most of the increase is attributable to reasons other than fetal distress. In the Lee and Baggish study, though, cesarean sections for fetal distress increased from 5 percent of all sections to almost 20 percent of all sections, a finding that suggests monitors may be responsible for subjecting more women to the risks of cesarean delivery, a major surgical procedure. Whether such an increase is good or bad is a hotly debated issue. Lee and Baggish seem to think the broadening indications for cesarean delivery are good in light of the increased safety of the operation and increases in the capacity to control postoperative infections. But others point out that cesarean-section operations carry with them a maternal mortality rate of 0.5–2 women per 1,000 operations and argue that such a risk is high enough to justify a second look at the widespread implementation of fetal monitoring programs.[16]

Besides the risks incurred due to cesarean-section operations, monitoring devices themselves may cause perforation of the uterus (by the uterine pressure catheter or its insertion device), may increase the incidence of maternal postpartum infection, may cause fetal hemorrhages or infections, and may cause injuries at the site of electrode attachment. Lee and Baggish report no instances of fetal infection or uterine perforation and a maternal postpartum infection rate that remained constant at just over 4 percent.

Most quasi-experimental studies report improved perinatal outcome and substantial increases in cesarean-section rates after the introduction of monitoring, although Edington and his associates in Britain report a decrease in cesarean sections in the second year of a general monitoring program, a decrease they ascribed to more intelligent interpretation of monitor tracings. Overall, though, results of quasi-experimental studies are encouraging and lead one to have faith in monitors. But, because of the inherent design defects of quasi-experimental studies, one may be going too far if one claims with Lee and Baggish that, "the improved perinatal mortality witnessed in this study is due in part to a program of unselected monitoring."[17] The design of quasi-experimental studies prevents one from attributing any change to the use of monitors. One cannot attribute benefits or risks, with the exceptions of uterine perforations and scalp abscesses at electrode attachment sites; one can merely note change and speak in terms of temporal coincidence.

Experimental studies take one a step closer to attribution, but when patients are not randomly selected to receive monitoring, selection biases limit the utility of such studies. Nonetheless, nonrandomized experimental studies seem to have had a substantial impact on obstetrical practice.

At the University of Southern California's School of Medicine, Dr. Edward Quilligan constructed a high-technology delivery room in which all indicators of fetal and maternal well-being can be monitored and recorded by computer for later analysis.[18] From that institution, directed by Dr. Richard Paul, has come the largest study of fetal monitoring available to date. Paul, Huey, and Yeager's results are based on a series of 50,640 births which occurred in the five-year period from 1970 to 1974. Only women considered "at risk" were monitored. The percentage of women monitored increased from about 10 percent of all births in early 1970 to about one-third of all births from mid-1973 on. The increase was due not to an increase in high-risk patients but to the institution's increased capacity to monitor all high-risk cases. Fetal and neonatal mortality continued the decline during the monitoring period that began before monitoring was introduced. The striking finding in Paul's series, though, was the higher intrapartum fetal death rate in the unmonitored, but *low-risk,* group than in the monitored high-risk group. Low-risk women should inherently have lower perinatal mortality rates. Overall, intrapartum death rates were 1.3 per thousand among monitored, high-risk deliveries where the fetus was known to be alive before labor, and 3.3 per thousand among unmonitored, low-risk labors. Excluding babies weighing less than 1,500 grams (about 3.3 pounds) and those with congenital anomalies or severe birth trauma, the rates were 0.5 and 0.9, respectively, rates which are not significantly different. No difference in neonatal mortality was observed either. The authors argue that their results undermine the concern that monitors may shift deaths from the intrapartum period to the neonatal period. They also argue that their results demonstrate that "presumed 'normal' " patients contribute significantly to perinatal deaths, an indication, they believe, that all labors should be monitored.

As with other studies, Paul's shows a substantial difference in cesarean deliveries between monitored and unmonitored groups. Sixteen percent of monitored women and only 7 percent of unmonitored women had cesarean sections. The difference is even more remarkable if one eliminates repeat cesarean sections which are often done for fear of previous cesarean scars rupturing under the stress of labor. In Paul's study the incidence of primary, or first, cesarean sections in the unmonitored group was 3 percent, one-fifth the incidence in the monitored group.

Drawing any conclusions about the effects of monitoring on cesarean sections or on perinatal outcome from this study is difficult because of bias caused by selection. Yet the authors conclude: "The monitored fetus apparently enjoys an enhanced survival over its unmonitored counterpart." But they also add: "The desirability and need for a well-designed perinatal study with long-term follow-up to further evaluate the role of clinical monitoring is evident."[19] At least part of their wish, that for well-designed studies, was fulfilled in the mid to late 1970s with the publication of four randomized controlled trials.

Randomization reduces bias due to selection criteria, but it does not necessarily insure comparability of experimental and control groups. Having large numbers of people in experimental and control groups tends to reduce intergroup differences, but group comparability can be a problem even in a well-done, randomized trial. In fact, this was a major problem for some of the randomized controlled trials of monitoring.

Of the four randomized trials, two have been conducted by Dr. Albert Haverkamp at the University of Colorado. Both studies were of high-risk patients only. The first compared a group of 242 patients monitored electronically with a group of 241 patients monitored by auscultation. After agreeing to participate in the study, all patients had an internal monitor, including a fetal scalp electrode and an intrauterine catheter, connected *before* being randomized into monitored and auscultated groups. After a woman had been assigned to the experimental or control group, the monitor was either covered and the fetal heart auscultated by a trained nurse using a fetoscope (in the control group) or it was used in the management of labor and delivery (in the experimental group). Monitors were attached in both groups to insure that experimental and control patients were treated the same up to the point that data were obtained and to permit subsequent comparisons of recorded but unused fetal heart patterns from the auscultation group with those used to manage the monitored group. Realizing that a randomized trial of some sixteen to twenty thousand patients would be needed to assess the effects of monitoring on mortality, given the low incidence of mortality even among high-risk patients, Haverkamp and his associates measured many other outcomes thought to influence survival and subsequent infant development. Their outcome measures included analyses of blood taken from a section of umbilical cord clamped before the newborn took its first breath, Apgar scores at one minute and five minutes, immediate neonatal outcomes including need for resuscitation, the infant's hospital course, and any morbidity reported by the mother and documented at a six-week pediatric checkup.

Haverkamp's research documented no differences in any perinatal outcome measures. He did find substantial differences in the rates of cesarean deliveries, however. Of all deliveries in the monitored group 16.5 percent were by cesarean section while less than 7 percent of the auscultated group underwent an abdominal delivery. The cesarean-section rate for fetal distress was also significantly higher among monitored patients than among patients in the auscultated group (7.4 percent compared to 1.2 percent). This led to differences in the kind of anesthesia used, the monitored group having a higher incidence of general anesthesia, and accounted in part for a difference in postpartum maternal infections. But even after correcting for differences in cesarean sections, an unexplained difference in maternal infection rates still remained.

Unfortunately there is some indication that Haverkamp's experimental and control groups may have been somewhat different. Review of the fetal monitor tracings for the auscultated and monitored groups showed that monitored patients experienced a higher percentage of ominous fetal heart-rate patterns early in labor, although the differences in ominous patterns over the whole course of labor were not significantly different. This bias, which occurred in spite of randomization and which cannot be attributed to the monitor directly since both groups had monitors in place, has been used by Haverkamp's critics to discredit the entire study. While wholesale dismissal is unfair, it can be shown that the differences in cesarean-section rates can be accounted for by differences in the early fetal heart patterns of the two groups.[20] This finding undermines, to a degree, the damaging conclusions of Haverkamp's first study.

Haverkamp's second study, published in 1979, compared 232 auscultated patients to 463 electronically monitored patients, 230 of whom were in a group where the physician had the option of doing fetal scalp-blood sampling if this was indicated by the monitor patterns. All 695 patients were randomly assigned to one of the three groups. Haverkamp obtained results almost identical with those from his first study. No differences in neonatal outcome could be documented and cesarean-section rates were higher in the monitored groups than in the auscultated group. These results stand unchallenged at this point and are the most serious threat to the continued diffusion of the monitor throughout obstetrical practice.

The other two randomized trials, one conducted in Sheffield, England, and one in Melbourne, Australia, obtained somewhat different results. The English study of low-risk patients, conducted by Dr. Ian Kelso and associates, reported no differences in neonatal outcome and supported Haverkamp's findings in this regard. But in spite of increased cesarean deliveries in the monitored group, the authors were reluctant to attribute the difference to monitoring because the rates of cesarean sections for fetal distress were identical. Renou's study of high-risk women in Australia is the only randomized trial to report data favoring the monitor. No differences in Apgar scores occurred, but in virtually every other aspect of immediate neonatal welfare—the need for resuscitation, correction of acidosis, the incidence of minor neurological symptoms and major brain damage, levels of oxygen and carbon dioxide in the blood, and time spent in the nursery—the monitored group fared better than the control group. A stillbirth in the control group that the authors thought, in retrospect, could have been avoided if the monitor had been used, caused them to terminate the study. Renou reports a higher cesarean-section rate among the monitored group but, as in Kelso's study, he could not confidently attribute the difference to monitoring.

One other study has significantly influenced contemporary obstetrical thinking about monitoring. Neutra and his colleagues analyzed the records of 17,080 births which occurred from 1969 through 1975 at the Beth Israel Hospital. After excluding babies born before twenty-eight weeks of gestation and those who died of anomalies incompatible with life, they divided the remaining 15,846 babies into five risk categories based on eighteen different risk factors. Then they compared the death rates of monitored to unmonitored babies in each risk stratum. Their results are shown in table 4.2. Despite the fact that none of the differences within strata are significantly different (i.e., despite the fact that the null hypothesis of no difference between monitored and unmonitored groups *cannot* be rejected according to standard statistical criteria), the authors still conclude that their results "suggest that there may be benefit from monitoring in the high-risk groups"[21] and their conclusion has been accepted in at least one influential review of the monitoring literature.

Now, what is to be made of these results? Three randomized trials show no effect of monitoring on neonatal outcomes; one shows profound effects. Two randomized trials show that a woman who

Table 4.2 Effect of Fetal Monitoring on Neonatal Death
Rates in Five Risk Strata

Risk Stratum	Monitored	Number	Death Rate/ 1,000	Death-Rate Ratio[1]
Highest risk	No	79	303.8	1.6
	Yes	41	195.1	
High risk	No	62	80.7	2.1
	Yes	53	37.7	
Medium risk	No	338	20.7	1.4
	Yes	271	14.8	
Low risk	No	1,722	5.2	2.1
	Yes	1,225	2.5	
Lowest risk	No	6,463	0.5	0.4
	Yes	5,592	1.1	

1. Ratio of death rate in the nonmonitored group to the death rate of the monitored group. A death-rate ratio of 1 indicates equal death rates; a ratio of greater than 1 indicates a result favoring the monitored group.

Source: From Neutra et al., "Effect of Fetal Monitoring on Neonatal Death Rates," *New England Journal of Medicine* 299 (1978): 324–26. Used by permission.

is monitored incurs a substantially increased risk of having a cesarean delivery; two show no increases attributable to monitoring. Virtually all nonrandomized experimental studies show that monitored populations have lower mortality even if they were at higher risk initially than their nonmonitored counterparts. And the general experience of most developed countries has been that, as fetal monitors came into more general use, perinatal mortality and morbidity continued their rather remarkable declines started years before. Also, cesarean-section rates increased almost geometrically over the same period. There are, as might be expected, differences in professional opinions concerning the meaning of these results.

On one side are those opposed to monitoring. Banta and Thacker conclude their report on monitoring by saying:

> Careful review of the literature indicates little increased benefit from EFM [electronic fetal monitoring] compared to auscultation. This is not surprising, given the lack of precision of EFM for the diagnosis of fetal distress, and the general difficulty in separating normal fetal stress during labor from fetal distress. If EFM has benefit it appears to be for low birth weight infants, but no RCT [randomized controlled trial] of its use in this group has been carried out.
>
> The risk from EFM is substantial, especially but not wholly through the increased CSR [cesarean-section rate] that its use apparently engenders.[22]

Dr. R. Alan Baker, writing in *Obstetrics and Gynecology,* says that "the pendulum of obstetric intervention has swung too far" and wonders what effect increasingly "mechanized birth" will have on families.[23] An editorial in Great Britain, where economic pressures on health service are more severe than those experienced as yet by American medicine, claims that monitoring is useful in cases with increased risk, interpreted broadly, but that the economic and clinical implications of monitoring every woman in labor compel the conclusion that a very large randomized trial of monitoring is still necessary.[24]

On the other hand there are die-hard proponents of monitoring. Drs. John Hobbins, Roger Freeman, and John Queenan, all obstetricians of some note, reviewed Banta and Thacker's analysis of the data on monitoring and said:

[Auscultation] is not only of inferior sensitivity, but it imposes significant demands on the nursing staff. Here it becomes difficult to question the cost effectiveness of the monitor.

To argue that low-risk patients should not be monitored is a mistake. The decision should depend on the physician's discretion, patient's wishes, and on the availability of nurses.[25]

Even the "consensus-developing" Task Force on Predictors of Fetal Distress, which only urged that use of a monitor in high-risk patients be "strongly considered," said of low-risk patients:

Although the Task Force finds that the weight of present evidence does not show benefit of electronic fetal monitoring in low risk patients, it recognizes that under certain circumstances, mothers or physicians may choose to use electronic fetal monitoring in low risk patients.[26]

Obstetricians are always ready to implement broad-based policies if they have evidence which supports their actions. In the unminced words of the *British Medical Journal,* if monitors can improve perinatal mortality in low-risk women "then monitoring will be mandatory for all women in labor."[27] Presently the evidence does *not* support a move toward routine monitoring of all labors, and still the monitoring movement is vigorous. Some people estimate that 60 percent of all labors are monitored, some people still recommend that all women be monitored, and, as noted above, there is no movement in the profession to control the use of monitors even in circumstances where available data reveal no demonstrable benefit from them. How can one understand this curious lack of relationship between evidence and practice?

If one maintains the belief that there is a direct connection between scientific inquiry and medical practice, as the scientistic interpretation of medicine would have us believe, then developments around the modern fetal monitor cannot be understood. In fact, with regard to fetal monitoring the profession of obstetrics has sounded the retreat from clinical science and rallied once again around the standard of clinical sense, the acquisition of knowledge which directs clinical action on the basis of clinical experience—the unshared, private, day-to-day experiences of the doctor. NIH's Task Force put the profession's position succinctly: "Electronic fetal monitoring or any other technology should never be a substitute for clinical judgment.''[28] This is a significant change in posture for physicians who five years earlier seemed anxious to receive their directive knowledge from scientifically designed, randomized trials of monitoring. But as David Armstrong points out, reliance on science, epitomized by the randomized controlled trial, exposes medicine to evaluation by nonmedical people, including those groups on which medicine's autonomy and authority are dependent, patients and government. A shift away from scientism and renewed reliance on clinical sense represents a retreat to the protection of the unapproachable, privileged knowledge of medicine. It ''restore[s] the authority of the doctor and enable[s] him to resist the incursion of clinical science into clinical sense.''[29] Without question, a renewed emphasis on clinical judgment will protect the physician from destabilizing attacks on his social position from within or without the profession, but to explain the continuing privilege of the obstetrician in terms of the ebb and flow of clinical science and clinical sense is too facile. That the obstetrician can possibly retreat from scientism suggests that he has a more firmly grounded basis for his profession than clinical science or clinical sense, alone or in concert, can provide. It suggests that we must look beyond the scientific controversies to more subtle and yet more important mechanisms through which obstetrical power was expressed and through which the obstetrical vision was extended.

The electronic fetal monitor is, as close attention to the obstetrical literature reveals, only one rather minor aspect of a generally deployed ''monitoring concept'' through which obstetrics developed a network of surveillance over childbirth. The monitoring concept is an idea that developed through the 1940s, coincident with the rise of the ''natural childbirth'' movement, an idea that informs obstetrics generally and that underlies a fundamental change in the modality of control exercised by obstetrics over childbirth. The change is characterized not by ''medicalizing'' childbirth or construing it as an ever more pathological process in need of increasingly sophisticated intervention, as some would suggest,[30] but by a lightening of the heavy medicalizing hand of obstetrics and an extension of the analytic, programmatic, ''helping hand.'' Monitoring is a structure of control—of which the physician is but a single, somewhat remote component—that allowed the extension of the obstetrical vision to all births while simultaneously permitting the withdrawal of punitive, negative characterizations of birth, and of the practices such characterizations fostered, on which obstetrical control of birth had previously been based. One can understand the continued professional control of childbirth regardless of the outcome of the fetal monitoring controversy or other assaults on the contingent sovereignty of the profession of obstetrics.

Surveillance and Monitoring

Some thirty to forty years ago the organizing concept in obstetrics changed from "confinement" to "surveillance." Birth moved into the hospital but women were not confined there. The hospital became the center of a system obstetrical surveillance that extended throughout the community. Implementation of maximal surveillance over childbirth involved several components. The fetus became the obstetrician's second and ultimately primary patient. The regimentation of pregnancy—its rigid categorization and lockstep staging—was refined and smoothed out conceptually and a corresponding emphasis on continuity of care (and deemphasis of the division of labor surrounding birth) emerged. Surveillance extended into the community through epidemiological analyses. With the development of sophisticated monitoring technology, concepts like "fetal distress" and other terms that carry notions of pathology and abnormality lost their definition instead of becoming more refined as one might expect they would. Birth became more individualized but no less controlled. Indeed, the individualization of birth was a major component in the new, more effective order of obstetrical control, an order called "monitoring."

Monitoring is a Janus-faced structure with one face watching over women and their births, the other watching over physicians. Continuous surveillance requires a disciplined, trained staff. Through the increased analytical capacity of the profession and the individualization of birth that monitoring provided, disruptions of the order and harmony of childbirth became more visible and responsibility more readily attributable. Monitoring made results of obstetrical work open to scrutiny. Thus, while monitoring and surveillance exerted a new form of control over birth, they exerted control over physicians and nurses as well.

Only by using the notions of monitoring and surveillance in a generic sense and tracing out the mechanisms by which they altered the obstetrical project can we understand how obstetrics protects childbirth in the face of controversies like that surrounding the electronic fetal monitoring. In fact, we shall see how the obstetrical project feeds on such controversy.

Hospital Birth

The hospital was originally a place of confinement for pregnant women. The Wertzes' interpretation of why birth moved into the hospital in America is a plausible one,[31] and merits review. Early obstetricians wanted no part of home births since they believed that there were fewer normal births than in the past. Specialists paid less and less attention to behavioral and social aspects of pregnancy and disease generally as they learned more about biology. The hospital was the place where the biological aspects of pregnancy could be analyzed and treated with convenience and efficiency. Birth was segmented and regimented in the hospital. The obstetrical space was partitioned just as pregnancy was. Labor and delivery rooms were separated and a woman was, and in some places still is, transported from one to the other as she progressed through the stages of childbirth that had been neatly mapped out by obstetrics. Obstetrical practices like those described in the last chapter caused birth to become a predictable drama directed by the obstetrical specialist. Appropriate treatment of pregnant women eliminated the savage, the inherent threat to disorder. Obstetrics tamed childbirth, and the hospital became a place of busy, active harmony based on the confinement of women and the profession's dominion over their bodily processes.

The harmony of hospital births was not to last for long, though. Socially, women were becoming less confined. Bottle feeding and maternity clothes allowed pregnant women to emerge from their confinements. They could go out in public just like "normal people." As the Wertzes put it:

> Hospital delivery had become for many a time of alienation from the body, from family and friends, from the community, and even from life itself.
> Hospital birth became a regime against which many women began a critical struggle, questioning the need for such extensive manipulation, questioning the safety of the procedures, and demanding that birth be an experience that

permitted a sense of self-fulfillment. They set out to regain posession of their bodies and of the life they had lost.[32]

Women provided one incentive for the hospital to deemphasize confinement and change its approach to childbirth; tensions in the structure of the hospital and the professional conduct of birth provided another. Obstetrical specialists were only one component of the drama of birth in the hospital. Their interests were narrowly biological, confined to the mechanical aspects of birth. Their technical skills were the basis of their authority as well as the mechanism through which they exerted power over birth. On the other hand, the hospital staff constituted a potentially competitive basis of power and was therefore a threat to the fragile order of the obstetrical project. The staff's authority derived from its institutional mandate to provide emotional and social support to women. In practice staff members were not always supportive, as the protests which fueled the early days of the natural childbirth movement showed, but they did represent another function than that of the medical technicians— the obstetricians—in the division of labor in maternity hospitals. The tension this division created would be resolved by changes in obstetrics' approach to childbirth that would have their focus in the hospital and spread from there throughout the larger community.

The change that transformed the hospital from a place of confinement in childbirth to a center for a network of surveillance of pregnancy and birth can be traced more easily in Britain than in the United States because the transformation was a matter of national policy there and because structural problems were so much more severe in Britain than in the United States.[33] Recall that in Britain the division of labor was more strongly demarcated than in the United States. General practitioners, obstetrical specialists, and midwives were all involved in birth and each had their own distinct institutional base. The specialist had the hospital, the general practitioner had his practice but used the hospital's in-patient and out-patient facilities. And the midwife had her bases in the community, where she sometimes cooperated with general practitioners, and in the hospital, where she cared for "normal" women who opted for hospital confinement. After the National Health Service was established in 1946, these three groups were responsible to different authorities: GPs were responsible to local Executive Councils, hospitals were overseen by the national health authority, and local health authorities provided midwives and local clinics for antenatal and postnatal care. Birth was moved into hospitals in Britain beginning in the 1950s, not to confine pregnancy but to resolve the tensions in this structure by integrating services to form a network of surveillance centered in the hospital and extending outwards from there. The relatively independent types of practitioners were to be integrated into an obstetrical team which would make every birth visible to an integrated system of oversight which was at once centralized and diffuse.

One can trace the movement of birth into hospitals in Britain through three reports: a paper proposing a national maternity service prepared by the Royal College of Obstetricians and Gynecologists in 1944, the *Cranbrook Report* prepared for the Ministry of Health in 1959, and the *Peel Report,* a report on maternity-bed needs and the domiciliary midwifery service prepared in 1970 by a subcommittee of the Maternity and Midwifery Advisory Committee to the Ministry of Health.[34] These reports culminate with the recommendation that all births occur in hospitals, but the themes which inform all of the reports are the integration and continuity of care and the extension of an obstetrical vision from the hospital into the community and to all aspects of pregnancy. The reports were not concerned primarily with "confinement."

The Royal College claimed in 1944 that "the incidence of maternal mortality and morbidity is primarily a matter of obstetric personnel—of the individual skill of midwives, general practitioners, and consultants, with *the proviso that all must be supported by first-rate maternity institutions and equipment.*"[35] But the rest of the College's report made it clear that a good maternity service was one which was coordinated around the hospital, the institution which would *support* a national service of quality. The College said, "The integration of institutional, domiciliary, antenatal, and consultant services has had a notable effect on the maternal mortality of those boroughs that have planned on these lines."[36] Besides being available to all women, a good national maternity service would have the capacity to collect and use better statistics and improve the quality of record keeping so that research would be encouraged.[37] These are recommendations for the construction of a map of childbirth, for the identification and localization of childbirth, both inside the hospital through the use of medical records and outside of it through improved statistical collection schemes.

In order to map childbirth, "the country should be divided into large health regions each based wherever possible on a University medical center." The large regions were to consist of smaller divisions coordinated from the key, or primary, university hospital. "Clearly," the report says, "there must be central control, first to bring about and then to maintain a high standard throughout the country."[38] Along the radii of the map, personnel and support services would be arrayed, for a good service is characterized by "fuller coordination within the service of general practitioners and specialists, of health visitors and midwives, of pediatricians and obstetricians, of hospitals, clinics and domiciliary services, of local and central administration." A service so construed would penetrate the community and the entire temporal spectrum of pregnancy by making available "better care of the mother during pregnancy and of the infant in the early weeks of life" and "by making arrangements for childbirth that were more accessible, less inconvenient and costly, and safer."[39] While the College supported continuation of domiciliary midwifery services because hospital beds were limited, it summed up its recommendations by saying, "We regard [the] principle of integration as absolutely essential for efficiency."[40] The College wanted previous divisions in the delivery of care retained in form but integrated under a new, efficient obstetrical order which radiated out from the hospital to cover the entire country.

The *Cranbrook Report* was the first thorough review of maternity services provided by the National Health Service. At the time the committee reported in 1959 more than 65 percent of births in Britain took place in hospitals. The committee supported this trend, saying, "hospital confinement is essential for all women with medical or social need," and by the late fifties medical and social indications for hospital delivery had expanded considerably. The committee also recognized, though, the position advocated by the active home-birth movement of the time, saying, "We believe that the advantages of home confinement for the apparently normal case probably outweigh the very slight risk of unforeseen complications."[41] Many people who read the *Cranbrook Report* today miss the point that whether birth should occur in hospitals or in homes was of secondary importance to the committee. The Cranbrook committee's primary concern was the coordination and rationalization of care. The committee supported home births not because they were more humane or because women desired them but because care could be easily integrated around a home birth: "There was a feeling that continuity of care was more readily achieved when a confinement took place at home. The mother had the doctor of her choice, the family link with the general practitioner was strengthened and the domiciliary midwife . . . had a better understanding of the mother and her background than could a hospital midwife."[42] Home births were better because a woman's entire case could be known more easily and integrated more carefully into the obstetrical delivery system.

The committee's recommendations were not directed exclusively toward the control of birth itself; they were also aimed at those who exercised the control. Births should be well integrated into the system of care, but the system itself had to be a well integrated, smoothly functioning system which was not handicapped by the divisions of responsibility which had existed earlier. To this end, the committee issued recommendations on educational standards for practicing obstetricians, urged that obstetricians be required to attend a certain number of deliveries each year in order to be admitted to an "Obstetric List," and suggested that

> Some interchange of domiciliary and hospital staff would be desirable, if the practical difficulties could be overcome, particularly where the proportion of domiciliary confinements is below 30 percent or the actual number of deliveries is small. . . . There should be a firm link between the general practitioner obstetrician and the hospital so that he becomes part of the obstetric team.[43]

No longer was it sufficient for the "case," the woman and her pregnancy, to be integrated into the delivery of good care, but it was important that care providers be well integrated into the system as well and that they be subject to the developing system of surveillance.

A decade later more than 80 percent of all births in Britain occurred in hospitals, although significant regional variations in this figure existed. This caused difficulties for domiciliary midwives. It reduced the number of deliveries available to them, it made the midwives more expensive, and the expansion of the health-visitor services provided by local health authorities resulted in duplication of the postnatal care midwives provided. The *Peel Report,* issued in 1970, also found that one in four women who wished to have a home birth eventually required hospital care and that those who had to be admitted suffered high perinatal mortality rates. This indicated to the committee that women were not being properly screened before being allowed to have a home delivery. The committee said, "wishes for home confinement should be respected provided, of course, that there are no medical or social contra-indications."[44] Yet their own data showed that even "normal" women selected for home delivery by available criteria might require hospital care, so even "normality" became a potential contraindication for home delivery. In response the *Peel Report* recommended "that sufficient facilities should be provided to allow for 100% hospital delivery."[45]

But the *Peel Report* did not mark the culmination of the "confinement" of births in hospitals. Rather it represented the culmination of the deployment of a surveillance network and the destruction of such dichotomous categorizations as normal and abnormal, pathological and physiological. In the words of the committee, the principal goal was

> the best deployment of skilled staff. . . . The district hospital
> will be the obvious focus for all maternity services, hospital and
> domiciliary, in the area served by it. . . . Medical and
> midwifery care should be provided by consultants, general
> practitioners, and midwives working as teams.[46]

Obstetrics extended its project outwards from the hospital by de-emphasizing the division of labor around birth, integrating previously disparate components of the care system into teams, and centralizing the supervision of a dispersed system of care in the hospital. But to extend the obstetrical vision outside of the hospital the profession needed to know where it was going; it needed a map.

The Analytic Power of Maps

From the hospital, obstetricians saw the threat to obstetrical order: even those segregated into the normal population could suddenly become abnormal and require sudden reorientation of effort. The *Peel Report* showed this. Categorizations failed obstetricians because birth failed to respect categories. Birth did not respond well to treatment regimens based on binary divisions. The space outside of hospitals, which the reports on maternity services had vowed to respect in .the reorganization of care, became threatening to obstetrics.

The problem obstetrics faced when it looked beyond the hospital was the problem of an infected space, a region that held the constant threat of disorder. Foucault uses the image of the plague, the "disease which is transmitted when bodies are mixed together," to describe this kind of space. The plague could not be excised by command, by separation and binary division of the sick and well, normal and abnormal. Instead, the plague had to be met by discipline and the power of analysis: "multiple separations, individualizing distributions, an organization in depth of surveillance and control, an intensification and a ramification of power." Analysis individualizes and localizes everyone and everything, not by crude designations, assignments to groups, and geographic relocation, but by "the assignment to each individual of his 'true' name, his 'true' place, his 'true' body, his 'true' disease" so that it is possible "to see constantly and recognize immediately." Once the "true place" of everything is known and a system of surveillance for monitoring all movement is in place, one can assess the effects of changes, interventions, and programs, and "carry out experiments, to alter behavior, to train or correct individuals."[47] Analysis creates a map by which programmatic intervention can be effectively and efficiently deployed.

The hospital could serve as the basis for deploying obstetrical resources only if the structure of the problem, the obstetrical anatomy of whole communities, was known. For an effective system of surveillance to be deployed, the space to be ordered had to be analyzed first. The first step in this analysis had to be the epidemiological mapping of childbirth.

Great Britain has a long history of collecting social statistics. Yet, as the country moved toward formation of the National Health Service, the lack of data adequate to the specific task of designing a national maternity service became apparent. In 1946, therefore, a Joint Committee of the Royal College of Obstetricians and Gynecologists and the Population Investigation Committee, a Cambridge-based group with interests in social policy and demography, conducted two surveys of British maternity services. One survey questioned 14,000 women "in every type of administrative authority, in all geographical regions, and among all social groups" about their experiences before, during, and after childbirth. The committee was not particularly interested in the clinical aspects of birth; instead, it focused on the social and economic aspects of pregnancy and childbirth. A second survey assessed the extent and quality of services offered in selected areas of the country. Together these surveys would help answer the crucial questions of the day: "What services are available to women bearing children? How far are they used and what are the factors affecting their use? Do they help women to regard childbirth as a normal process? How far do they prevent premature birth and infant death and promote the health of mothers and infants? Finally, what do parents spend on pregnancy and childbirth?"[48] The report dealt with every aspect of childbirth from antenatal care, to the place of delivery, attendance during delivery, pain relief, the extent of prematurity, postnatal examinations, infant feeding, and the use of infant welfare clinics. The ultimate interests of the committee were mapping differences and the analysis of variations so that all aspects of pregnancy as it existed throughout the land, not just in hospitals, could be known to the obstetrical profession.

Knowing the fine structure of the obstetrical anatomy, all variations and the correlates of variation, permits the construction of a map which dictates the deployment of resources and efforts. An analysis of variations in antenatal supervision, for example, revealed certain facts that are expressed in the following statements, which should be examined more for their form than for their content.

—"Few women receive no antenatal care. Those who do not, though, are largely "multiparous wives of manual workers, married women with illegitimate children, and unmarried mothers." (Multiple separation.)

—"Women often received supervision from more than one source. Thirty-one percent of those who went to private doctors went to clinics or midwives as well." (Every movement is subject to surveillance.)

—"Expectant mothers receive an average of eight antenatal examinations, the first one coming at 22 weeks before delivery. Private midwives are approached two weeks before municipal midwives and 30.6 percent of their patients begin care in the first trimester while only 22.6 percent of municipal midwives' patients receive first trimester care." (Individualizing distributions.)

—"Probably the most successful scheme would be to have a number of peripherally located clinics for routine supervision and a central consultative service for abnormal cases." When a woman cannot attend clinics, "supervision may be given by home visits from a municipal midwife or through a general practitioner scheme." (Organization in depth of surveillance.)

These are not judgments. They are analytical statements. They speak of variation and correlation, not of good and bad, not even of efficient or inefficient. Once variations in a phenomenon are known and the map is constructed, programs can be deployed where the map indicates need. But then the process of analysis and inquiry must be sustained:

> The data collected have led to specific proposals for amplifying and improving the existing maternity services. At the same time one of the most important results is to show the need for periodic examination of the services. . . .
>
> There is an urgent need for the regular collection of statistics to act as a continuing check on the efficiency of the maternity services, to enable expenditure on maternity and child welfare to be allocated to the best advantage, and to ensure that the services themselves are adjusted to the changing needs of mothers and children.[49]

The task of analysis is not to stabilize a situation but to make its every movement and twist known immediately so that programmatic intervention can be redeployed as necessary. The government implemented these recommendations and presently conducts both crude, continuous analyses and specialized, intermittent ones of the perinatal situation in Britain.[50]

In the United States, epidemiological studies on a much smaller scale appeared at about the same time the whole of Britain was being mapped. Interest was directed at the hospital catchment area—the geographical area served by a single hospital. The purpose and strategy were the same, however:

> Some . . . morbidity can be prevented by the simple provision of maternal and child-health services where they are needed. It therefore becomes of prime importance to delineate the segments of a city, county or state population that are thus at risk and in need of such services. To do this a method whereby these population segments may be located geographically must be devised. . . . In planning of programs for the population at risk it is further necessary to know the characteristics of the population and of any subgroups that may exist within it. . . .[51]

Researchers showed that by simply tracing the boundaries of perinatal problems on maps, problem areas made themselves evident. For example, putting regional differences in birth rates, infant and perinatal mortality rates, and rates of obstetric complications on a map of Buffalo demonstrated that the primarily black, low-income area of the city was at higher risk than the remainder of the city. But statistical analyses penetrate farther than this superficial distinction:

> Differentials [within the core area of Buffalo] highlight the types of care most needed in each subgroup [white suburban dwellers, blacks, and whites "with black demographics"]. For example, whereas the high infant mortality found in all three subgroups demonstrates the need for more intensive home visiting by the public health nurse and more intensive casework with families, the high perinatal death rate and high percentage of obstetrical complications of pregnancy in the Negro wards demonstrate the emphasis that needs to be placed on prenatal and perinatal care for this group.[52]

These analyses point inexorably toward refinement of the concept of "risk" from an aggregate level down to the individual level and perhaps even beyond that to the level of bodily processes. The group, the individual, and the processes inside the individual are localized and subject to analysis and programmatic intervention:

> It is evident that the newborn outcome is controlled by events of multiple origins which take place even before conception. It can be seen that many of the factors can be attributed to genetic background and health as well as socioeconomical status of the mother during childhood and adolescence. These factors can be controlled in part by parents, the government, and state or private agencies. Society certainly has a responsibility to develop programs in the community that can achieve this goal.[53]

Monitoring extends to the minutiae of life, but it begins and ends at the social level, the level of the map of birth.

Obstetrics did not deploy programs of surveillance that could be viewed negatively by expectant mothers, the people who would be subjected to them. Obstetrics could invest its programs of surveillance with a positive image because it had found a new object on which to focus its attention. The profession brought pregnancy under surveillance for the fetus, a new entity on the obstetrical terrain. Obstetrics justified "the need for detailed surveillance" by saying it was "in the interests of the child."[54]

Discovery of the Fetus and the Meaning of Obstetrical Intervention

The fetus captured obstetricians' interest around 1940. After 1950 obstetricians began to treat the fetus as a second patient. The discovery of the fetus was important to the deployment of obstetrical surveillance.

Dating the isolation of the fetus precisely is somewhat difficult, but changes in obstetric texts are helpful. Obstetricians correctly say that outward signs of fetal viability, primarily fetal heart sounds, have always guided obstetrical management, but it was not until 1940 that the fetus became recognized as a separate entity in obstetricians' eyes. The first edition of *Williams Obstetrics* cautions the physician to watch for signs of intrauterine asphyxia "inasmuch as their recognition frequently affords the indication for operative delivery." In the 1941 edition this phrase was changed to read "inasmuch as fetal distress frequently affords the indication for operative delivery."[55] This was the first time the term "fetal distress" had been used in the many editions of this text, and it was a subtle but significant change. In the first instance signs which originate inside the mother direct obstetrical management. In the second instance signs which originate not in the mother but in the fetus, a new object in the field of the obstetrical gaze, direct obstetrical management. By 1976 the authors of *Williams Obstetrics* had added a new chapter on fetal health and had justified it by saying:

> Until about 25 years ago, the intrauterine sanctuary of the embryo and fetus was held to be inviolate. The mother was the patient to be cared for, whereas the fetus was but another, albeit transient, maternal organ. The philosophy prevailed that "good maternal care" would automatically provide what was best for the products of conception.
>
> During the past quarter century, however, . . . remarkably intimate knowledge of the human fetus and his immediate environment has accumulated. . . . As did maternal health earlier in this century, fetal health . . . has now come to be appreciated . . . as a clinical discipline with great potential for

influencing favorably the quality of human offspring. Indeed, the fetus can now be considered the "second patient."[56]

Having the fetus as a patient changed the orientation of obstetrics. The fetus gave the obstetrician reason to extend his surveillance throughout pregnancy and gave him a new point of intervention into problems of pregnancy.[57] Edward Quilligan described the change in this way:

> Traditionally, the obstetrician's concern tends to remain fixed on the mother, for she is the patient he can best observe and the one he knows best. But when he has access to [technologies for fetal monitoring and surveillance] he suddenly finds that he has another patient on his hands—the fetus—who may furnish signs of viability or distress as clinically significant as those provided by the mother and frequently as treatable. Moreover, it has becomeapparent that the mother can tolerate without deficit most of the situations that put the fetus into trouble, while the fetus cannot. A fresh look must be taken at the question: Who is the primary patient?[58]

The focus of obstetrics did not swing completely to the fetus, but certainly the last twenty to thirty years have witnessed a significant change in obstetricians' approach to pregnancy.

Improved technologies of fetal surveillance may have facilitated the discovery of the fetus, but I suspect that other factors may have created a situation in which such a discovery took on added importance. Certainly, the timing of the discovery of the fetus must be described as fortuitous, given a clear threat looming on obstetrics' horizon. From the 1940s onwards, women posed a significant threat to the autonomy of obstetrics. Obstetricians had always thought themselves acting in the best interests of women and had always thought of their interventions as "good." In the 1940s, women, with help from some obstetricians, succeeded in bringing a new and decidedly negative interpretation to childbirth in hospitals. Not everyone shared the new meanings of hospital birth, but it was widely publicized and certainly held the potential for damaging the degree of sovereignty which obstetrics enjoyed. In this context, obstetricians found in the fetus not just a new point for intervening in pregnancy but also a way to blunt the critical edge of women's concerns about the way obstetricians treated them. The fetus provided the obstetricians an entrée through which they could invest pregnancy with yet newer meanings that would give them once again positive reasons for medical control of the birth process.

The struggle between women and obstetricians over the meaning attached to hospital birth is a fascinating example of conflict and its strategic resolution at the conceptual level. For the obstetrician, the potential pathology of childbirth came full circle at an inopportune time. Just as the natural childbirth movement gained momentum, obstetricians found that even "normal" pregnancies often surprised the obstetrician with manifestations of sudden, disastrous pathology. One study even ventured to quantify the extent of surprising pathology, saying "it is apparent from data [on 749 women monitored regardless of risk classification] that almost one-third of so-called normal patients have complications during labor."[59] In one hospital in Ireland the staff stopped trying to assess fetal vulnerability by using signs evident in the mother "because most fetal deaths during labor occur in normal mothers."[60] If the profession had acted in what was then an obstetrically proper way in response to this pervasive abnormality of birth, i.e., by developing interventions aimed at the mother, the results could have been disastrous in the context of the natural childbirth movement. More maternal interventions and greater maternal confinement would have fueled the arguments of women at a time when the profession was trying to accommodate some of women's demands. Some obstetricians held out, urging women to "accept the evidence that actual delivery, even of the normal case, can be most safely accomplished by the prophylactic measures recommended by DeLee two generations ago,"[61] but because of the discovery of the fetus obstetrics did not have to rest its case on such antiquated ideas or engage in the struggle over the treatment of childbirth on the terms women wished to use. Obstetricians could leave their treatment of the mother-to-be out of the debate entirely, for now they had the fetus, which they could defend against all the bad consequences that they claimed might result if they accommodated the demands of women for a more natural birth experience for themselves. The obstetrician no longer had to defend his practices on the basis of whether or not they were good for the woman; he could claim the practices were good for the fetus. The terms of the argument changed, so that one obstetrician could write, "more emphasis should and is being directed toward improving and protecting the quality of each birth. Ideal perinatal care should provide the optimum circumstances for each fetus and infant to realize its full genetic potential.''[62] Obstetricians became fetal advocates[63] and women were left to mount their struggle against an adversary who had acquired a potent ally in the fetus.

The health of the baby, loaded with positive meanings for both mother and physician, justified continued active intervention in childbirth, and these positive reasons for intervention overshadowed the negative meanings women had attached to obstetricians' work. The authors of the 1976 *Williams Obstetrics* put it this way:

> The widespread adoption of effective means for population control and consideration of their impact upon the well-being of current and future generations of offspring have logically accelerated interest in modalities for preserving and improving the health of the fetus and newborn infant. . . . The health team providing care for the mother, fetus, and newborn infant currently must deal with an appreciably higher percentage of pregnancies in which the fetus is at increased risk of unfavorable outcome unless an appropriate program of surveillance and at times active intervention is mounted.[64]

Obstetrics not only credited programs of surveillance and monitoring with improved fetal outcome, but it also attributed to them other changes in care which would be viewed positively by both doctors and mothers. In a study of obstetricians' feelings about the effects of electronic fetal monitoring in 150 cases, obstetricians said monitoring permitted "more accurate assessment of labor" in over 70 percent of the cases, permitted better management of labor in three-fourths of their cases, averted a traumatic forceps delivery in 4 percent of the cases, reduced their anxiety in over 80 percent of the cases, "accurately accelerated [the decision for a cesarean delivery] objectively" in twenty-six cases, and averted cesarean sections in twenty-eight cases.[65] Another study of obstetrical records indicated that a monitoring program allowed obstetricians to avoid a cesarean operation "despite monitor patterns indicating fetal distress" in 107 cases in a series of 608 patients.[66]

Obstetricians argued that monitoring and surveillance made birth a less traumatic, less anxiety-producing event. The literature shows, furthermore, that the deployment of surveillance mechanisms has allowed obstetricians to resurrect the notion that pregnancy is an essentially normal and physiological process and to offer this ulti-mately positive view of childbirth to their patients. *Williams*

Obstetrics now urges physicians and staff "to make the point that labor and delivery are normal physiologic processes," and Quilligan suggests that by "screening all women in labor or approaching labor," the obstetrician can avoid creating an "atmosphere of crisis about the normal and happy event of birth."[67]

How has surveillance given impetus to this "renormalization" of birth? The key to unlocking the curious return to a language of normalcy is to recognize that the profession reconceptualized pregnancy and carefully developed the idea that "pregnancy is a process." If pregnancy is severely segmented, assessed only intermittently with regard to relatively clear notions of normal and abnormal, the obstetrician is faced with only a few specific points at which one must decide whether therapeutic intervention is necessary to correct abnormal situations. If, however, pregnancy is a process, infinitely divisible, analyzed in fine detail so that one knows what is "needed" at each incremental step in the course of a natural process, and then if one subjects each pregnancy to continuous surveillance and monitoring, one can interject just what is "needed," no more and no less, into a process that begins to stray from its "natural," obstetrically known, course. The increased knowledge of the process of pregnancy which surveillance provides, then, is used in conjunction with monitoring of individual pregnancies to develop ever more precise, corrective actions designed to normalize deviations from a natural course. This strategy replaces the assessment of gross signs and symptoms of abnormality that permitted segregation of abnormal populations from normal ones and selection from among only a few interventions designed to hasten the termination of pregnancy when it crossed the line from normal to abnormal. The conceptual refinement of pregnancy and of interventions in it dissolved the distinctions between normal and abnormal on which obstetrical work had been based and permitted an increased emphasis on the naturalness of the process while retaining obstetrics' right of intervention in it.

Refinement of Pregnancy

The transformation of pregnancy from a segmented to a processual phenomenon, from an entity characterized by a demarcation of normal from abnormal to one with a natural course and quantitative deviations from it, is evident in many parts of the obstetrical literature. This section reviews counterintuitive changes in concepts like "fetal distress," the refinement of the concept of "high risk' to the point where risk becomes a nebulous idea that loses its power to discriminate among pregnancies but that pervades the space of obstetrical work, the changes in reasons for doing cesarean deliveries, and changes in technology that allowed an obstetrical response to concerns about the naturalness of childbirth while at the same time keeping all aspects of birth under surveillance. These are all aspects of the new, "lighter, more rapid, more effective" deployment of obstetrical power.

One might think that with increasing technological sophistication the definition of a concept like "fetal distress" would become clearer and clearer as clinicians accumulated data and gained experience in their interpretation. In the early days of monitoring, the profession suggested that with increasing information gained from improved technology a "generally acceptable definition of fetal distress based upon the fetal heart rate" might be achieved.[68] With the advent of the fetal monitor just the opposite happened. The meaning of fetal distress became less and less clear as time went on. Recall that *Williams Obstetrics* first used the term in 1941, associated it with intrauterine asphyxia, and placed clear limits around the normal fetal heart rate which, if exceeded, indicated a need for immediate action. "The most characteristic sign [of fetal distress] is afforded by changes in the fetal pulse rate" and a lower limit of 100 beats per minute remained, from the first edition of the text, the point at which action became necessary.[69] In the late 1960s and early 1970s, after more than a decade's experience with electronic monitoring, the same text said this:

> There is no consensus regarding the precise definition of fetal distress. In referring to this syndrome, most obstetricians think in terms of labor, but efforts have recently been made to ascertain the status of the fetus before labor. Disturbances of fetal function might well be considered part of this syndrome of fetal distress. . . . Although methods have been developed that may generally differentiate seriously ill from normal fetuses, they are not yet sufficiently precise to be completely dependable in individual cases.[70]

The move to eliminate binary divisions of normal and abnormal was on. Five years later, in 1976, after the great increase in devotion to the fetal monitor and before the controversy and dissension caused by randomized trials of monitoring, *Williams Obstetrics* moved the discussion of "fetal distress" from the body of the text to a footnote which read:

> *High risk pregnancy* and *fetal distress* are two terms commonly used in pregnancy to incite or intensify special concern for the quality of the ultimate product of pregnancy, the newborn infant. Precise definition of fetal distress and of high-risk pregnancy is not simple and will continue to change as the science of perinatology provides new information. These terms have much in common with some other terms of nearly universal medical usage, for example, shock.[71]

Distress was no longer a qualitative state. Instead it was a "syndrome," the main importance of which was to "intensify concern." Distress lost its place in the management of pregnancy. Research designed to develop a statistical definition of distress that would have predictive utility failed and showed just how difficult it was to achieve a satisfactory, useful definition. One team of researchers did a statistical analysis of the relationship between fetal heart-rate patterns and fetal scalp-blood pH (a measure of hypoxia thought to lead to "distress") and concluded, "No single characteristic of the FHR [fetal heart rate] was found to be an accurate predictor of fetal scalp blood pH." Only by using a computer to construct very complicated and clinically unintelligible combinations of subsets of the aspects of fetal heart patterns could they increase the usefulness of heart-rate patterns.[72]

The term "fetal distress" has not fallen from use completely. In fact, fetal distress is deemed responsible for about one-eighth of the threefold increase in the cesarean-section rate over the past ten years, although everyone admits that quantifying the increase attributable to fetal distress is complex and controversial.[73] But the concept has changed from a clearly defined problem to a less well defined syndrome. Strictly observed limits of abnormality have disappeared and given way to the need for monitoring and surveillance of the range of minutiae that constitute labor.

Eliminating limits of normalcy opened the way for the monitoring of all births. "It just seemed reasonable," as so many authors put it, to extend monitoring to all patients. Obstetricians turned away from using the monitor to detect pathology and began to evaluate the utility of the electronic monitor for determining normalcy. Obstetrics even developed a "nonstress test" of fetal well-being which may replace the "stress test" designed to detect a compromised fetus. In contrast to the oxytocin challenge test, the so-called "stress test," in which the reaction of a fetus to artificially induced uterine contractions is monitored for signs of "distress," the "nonstress test" simply monitors a fetus for thirty minutes looking for signs of fetal heart acceleration, thought to be indicative of a healthy fetus. Investigators concluded "that the outcome of babies demonstrating reactive [healthy] heart patterns [in the nonstress monitoring] is at least as good as that of babies demonstrating negative [healthy] contraction stress tests." The nonstress test had the further advantages of being an "inexpensive, convenient, time-saving screening procedure which can be made available to a greater number of patients than the contraction stress test alone."[74] The nonstress test increased the temporal segment of pregnancy which obstetrics could appropriately subject to monitoring, as electronic monitors, which previously were used only during labor and delivery, found a niche in the antepartum period as well.

The profession used more than just the electronic monitor to extend its network of surveillance. Robert Goodlin, an obstetrician who has been in the middle of several intraprofessional controversies, recognized the diagnostic difficulties surrounding the electronic monitor but was attracted by the intuitive appeal of extending the idea of monitoring to the antepartum period. He proposed that obstetrics should consider "simpler surveillance techniques" in order to find the "sick fetus prior to the stress of labor." To that end he instructed pregnant mothers to "consider any change in fetal activity during the third trimester as ominous" and enlisted them as monitors of their own pregnancy. This simple change, he suggested, would bring potential problems to the attention of physicians so that the antepartum health of the fetus could be assessed accurately through further tests. His data showed that, through the use of the mother as monitor, antepartum surveillance could help determine which fetuses were healthy.[75] The trend is clear: monitoring to determine normalcy and quantitative deviations from it instead of monitoring to detect abnormality is being extended to all pregnancies because concepts like distress, an abnormal condition which monitoring was expected to define, have lost their compelling form.

"High risk" has gone the same route as "distress" as the footnote from *Williams Obstetrics* suggested. Originally the basis for the epidemiological map of whole communities across which programs could be deployed, "high risk" was quickly refined to apply to the individual at risk instead of the group at risk. It was not sufficient to localize and identify high-risk *groups* or neighborhoods; the high-risk individual had to be located within the group, and within the individual the fetus at risk was sought. Throughout the late 1960s, then, a host of articles proposing "high-risk indices" appeared in order to provide "some practical method of identifying the fetus at risk." Proponents touted risk scoring systems as simpler, quicker, less expensive methods of screening women than clinical tests. Their goal was to achieve greater efficiency of analysis and more rapid localization of deviant cases. One person even suggested that "the ultimate aim would be almost *instinctive* application of such a score or tally to every antenatal patient."[76] Even a scorecard or systematic record entry should not impede the rapidity of obstetricians' assessments. Each proponent had his own ideas about what led to risk, so the construction of each score differed, but risk scores in general served to extend the gaze of obstetricians farther back into the pregnancy, into a woman's history and her environment. As one article put it:

> Effective care of the female to accomplish optimal reproductive efficiency during the adult years should logically begin during childhood, pubescence, and adolescence, before medical difficulties, dietary indiscretions, endocrine dysfunctions, emotional maladjustments, and poor social habits are entrenched. Ideally, patients at risk whose reproductive capacity is judged to be suboptimal should be identified early in the course of routine periodic checkups, premarital examinations, and preconceptional evaluations to permit workup, specific treatment, and appropriate family planning in context with the health and emotional status of the individuals so designated. If this supervision and continuity of care are neglected, proper screening should commence with the initial prenatal visit.[77]

This same article offered a risk scoring system to be used for screening purposes that included evaluations of a woman's "emotional survey" (based on "fears, attitudes, hostilities, motivations and behavioral patterns, previous pregnancies without supervision, etc."), her "social and economic survey" (based on employment patterns, income, education, and housing), and her race and marital status in addition to her obstetric history, her nutritional status, age, and so forth. Risk scores thus became a vehicle for expanding the scope of obstetrical surveillance to all aspects of a woman's life.

Risk scores also reduced the clarity of the idea of "high risk" by transforming risk from a dichotomy into a continuum. (For example, the score mentioned above varied from 0 to 100.) There was no set lvel at which a woman became "high risk"; she was simply placed at her "true" position on the infinite spectrum of possibility. This change freed the obstetrician from having to decide whether to designate a case as high risk or not, as normal or abnormal. Risk scores forced the doctor to consider the many factors that might put a fetus at some risk and provided a range of options—a continuum of categories—for the assessment of overall risk. A physician was no longer bound by strict categorization and was directed instead to pay attention to the subtleties and nuances of the individual case.

But if one pays attention to all aspects of the individual case, the score itself becomes redundant. The "perfect" scoring system, which would encompass all aspects of a woman's life which might conceivably affect the fetus, which would acknowledge the multiplier effects of certain combinations of factors and circumstances, and which would dictate management changes in the individual case, would be too cumbersome and too inefficient to use in every case. It would add nothing to the information in the medical record and would be simply a mathematical duplication of the clinical judgment physicians were quite capable of making without the score. So just as quickly as they gained popularity in obstetrics, risk scores fell into disuse. Only occasionally is another risk score proposed, and usually that is only done in connection with the construction of a finer epidemiological map based on individual women's characteristics instead of group characteristics.[78]

By the beginning of the 1970s risk scores had served their purpose: they justified the extension of surveillance farther back into the early parts of pregnancy and into a woman's personal life and they refined the notion of risk to a point where speaking of risk as if it were a unidimensional scale became impossible. The obstetrician's attention was directed to the fine structure of each pregnancy.

Obstetricians turned their attention to the dynamic aspects of childbirth, refined their conceptions of parturition, and plotted "ideal" courses around which individual cases might vary. Emmanuel Friedman led the way with the early development of his

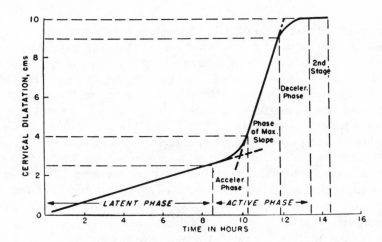

The mean labor curve, cervical dilatation versus time, based on the study of 500 primigravidas at term. The phases are defined in the text.

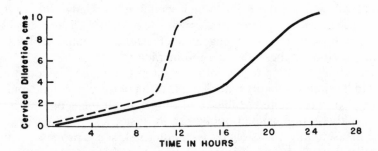

Clinical inertia, the mean curve of 46 primarily inert primigravidas. The sigmoid characteristics of the curve are apparent, despite the alteration in the time factor. The broken line represents the mean labor curve.

Figure 4.2. Examples of Friedman's "partographs" reflecting his calculus of pregnancy. The upper panel shows the continuous cervical dilation-time graph divided into subphases of labor. The lower panel represents one of the many problems that can arise in labor and be detected by the partograph. This is an example of "dystocia," "uterine inertia," or "failure to progress." (From Emmanuel A. Friedman, "Primigravid Labor: A Graphicostatistical Analysis," *Obstetrics and Gynecology* 6 [1955]: 569–89. © 1955 by the American College of Obstetricians and Gynecologists. Used by permission.)

"partograph," sometimes called the "Friedman curve" (see figure 4.2). He said:

> The dynamic nature of parturitional change had, in the past, rendered exceedingly difficult the detailed and critical analysis of its vagaries. The utilization of a method—involving graphic appraisal of cervical dilatation-time relationships—has made it possible to simplify this relatively complex clinical art.[79]

Friedman wanted to smooth all the discontinuities and "stages" out of parturition and, although he thought in terms of a calculus of labor and delivery, "for purposes of mathematical simplification" he settled for subdividing the former "first stage" of labor into "latent" and "active" stages with "acceleration" and "deceleration" phases bounding the active phase of cervical change. While admitting that cervical changes were specific to each patient and that there were "many variables associated with labor and its study," Friedman developed an "ideal" cervical dilatation curve, deviations from which indicated potential difficulty. Obstetricians could chart cervical dilatation on a "partograph" and use oxytotic drugs to keep labor progressing along its "natural" course. Statistically determined limits on normal progress in labor can be entered on the partograph to inform those with less technical skill—"the midwife working in the periphery or the junior doctor working in the hospital"[80]—when expert attention is necessary. In this way, the profession could deploy the "partographic control of labor"[81] across large geographical areas and reduce the need for women to be seen in specialized obstetrical centers before it was necessary to see them. Later devices which measured cervical dilatation would be connected in a feedback system to oxytocin infusion pumps to control uterine contractions automatically.

Even cesarean deliveries have changed to respect the dynamic nature of the labor process, and the cesarean operation, once an assuredly fatal intervention, has been incorporated into the new order of obstetrical control. When Williams wrote his text in 1903 he gave some figures on the relationship of the size of the fetus to the pelvic outlet which were *absolute* indications for cesarean deliveries and others which were *relative* indications for cesarean operations.[82] Subsequent editions changed, and then abandoned, these prescriptive limits and opted instead for long lists of indications justified by tables indicating the number of sections done for each reason in a reputable obstetrical center. The implication was that, the greater the number of operations done for a given reason, the more appropriate it was to consider a cesarean delivery should that particular problem present itself in your hospital. In the 1950 edition of *Williams Obstetrics* the dimensionality of abnormality changed; the main reason for a first-time cesarean operation, "dystocia" or failure of labor to progress effectively, was subdivided into many different reasons for dystocia. By 1980, when "dystocia" was blamed for one-third of the recent dramatic increase in cesarean sections, a changed understanding of the term existed. The change "corresponded to a shift from an anatomical consideration to a more functional approach to labor—that is, less pelvimetry and more labor graphs."[83] A few "absolute" indications for cesarean section remain, such as having had a previous cesarean operation, a baby presenting in the breech position, or of having a condition called placenta previa, where the placenta covers the cervix; but the wisdom of automatically effecting an operative delivery even in some of these cases is being debated. Many obstetricians will allow women with one cesarean delivery to attempt vaginal delivery during subsequent births. Some obstetricians are even proposing vaginal delivery of premature babies who present in a breech position.

Obstetrics is incorporating cesarean delivery into the structure of monitoring. What was once considered the ultimate in drastic obstetrical intervention in labor is now considered simply another component of childbirth delivery systems. Some authors claim that the functional view of pregnancy and the use of labor graphs permit "more prompt and *less traumatic* methods of management" and they include cesarean delivery under that rubric.[84] Women are told:

> Cesarean section was not always having a baby. For that matter it was not always having a mother. . . . Today, not only is having a section having a baby, but often, having a baby is having a section.[85]

Surveys of women who have cesarean births indicate that they feel alienated from the birth process. In response, obstetricians are encouraging greater participation by mothers in the decision-making that leads to cesarean delivery, allowing fathers to be present during the operation, using regional instead of general anesthesia so that early postpartum contact between mother and baby can be insured, and generally developing a "family centered approach to cesarean birth."[86] Cesarean sections are being done for more positive reasons focused on the fetus: "because of the widespread emphasis that is now directed toward prompt recognition of impairment of fetal well-being."[87] Some feel that the past decade's threefold increase in cesarean sections indicates that obstetrics is, in fact, "medicalizing" birth further and is not interested in lightening the medical hand. In truth, however, the meaning and experience of cesarean delivery— and on the medical side, the indications for and outcome of operative delivery—have changed and are capable of being incorporated into the structure of monitoring. Obstetricians are, in other words, smoothing out the disruptions that operative delivery used to cause and integrating it into the newly conceptualized process of labor and delivery.

Technology of Control

Once obstetrics had conceptualized pregnancy as a process, once it had done away with its discontinuities or expressed them in a calculus of accelerations and decelerations, and once obstetrics knew the course of the process of pregnancy in minute detail, pregnancy could become the subject of integrated systems of control that would not only monitor the process but would either institute corrective action or signal the need for it should the course of a given labor deviate too far from its "natural" course. In the words of one text, "the automatic control of labor by 'closing the loop' is theoretically possible."[88] Servocontrol mechanisms to normalize deviations rather than to direct interventions in pathologies insure that a modern pregnancy and childbirth will be "natural."

Monitoring, even in the narrow technological sense, has come to mean much more than just electronic monitoring of fetal heart rate and uterine contractions. Consider this array of available gadgetry.

For Monitoring Mother

Temperature. If maternal temperature is assessed only periodically or if an attendant fails to leave a thermometer in place long enough, detection of infection from amnionitis may be delayed. Thermocouples permit continuous monitoring of maternal temperature and can be attached to the maternal pad on present electronic monitors.

Blood pressure. Changes in blood pressure caused by medical intervention, including anesthesia, or by internal hemorrhage can be ominous. Existing systems can automatically measure and record blood pressure once every minute. Patient acceptance of more thorough monitoring will depend on the development of alternatives to the present cuff method of measurement, perhaps through the use of ultrasonic devices.

Heart rate. Can be measured using existing electronic fetal monitoring equipment or with a pad placed over the fingernail capillary bed.

Uterine activity. Can be measured directly or indirectly. Problems of false readings from intrauterine pressure catheters can be alleviated by devices which automatically flush the catheter before signaling that an ominous sign originated in the mother and not in the machine. That is, monitors can be made to monitor themselves as well as patients. Monitors can be connected in feedback systems to uterine stimulant infusion pumps so that uniform, regular, more "natural" contractions can be insured.

Cervical dilatation. Presently done by manual vaginal examination which increases risk of infection, or by rectal examination every hour. Friedman invented a mechanical device for continuous monitoring of dilatation in 1956. Recent improvements in Friedman's original design continuously monitor and record detailed dilatation versus time, including cervical response to each contraction.

For Monitoring Baby

Heart rate. Direct methods are better than indirect. Increased paper speed on recent machines permits improved assessment of beat-to-beat variations.

Fetal blood pH. Present methods require quick access to laboratory facilities, a separate vaginal examination for each sample, and a separate puncture for each sample. Researchers have invented a subcutaneous, continuous-reading pH electrode, the output of which could be displayed on another channel incorporated into existing monitors.

Oxygenation. Researchers in Germany invented an electrode to measure blood oxygenation transcutaneously, through the skin. It heats up a small area of skin and measures blood oxygen-levels noninvasively. This device has been used primarily in the neonatal nursery, but some obstetricians use it during the intrapartum period. Can be incorporated into existing monitors. A separate electrode can measure mother's blood oxygen as well.

Fetal respiratory movements. By the incorporation of cheap, continuous-beam ultrasonic devices into existing monitors, fetal chest-wall movement, an indication of well-being, can be monitored.

Each of these measuring devices could conceivably be integrated into control loops which would automatically keep labor on its natural course. One author has predicted, "There can be little doubt that in about 10 years time monitors will be capable of performing active functions involving microprocessors and programmable memories. We are entering the era of the 'smart' machine."[89]

Technology is not becoming more and more cumbersome as it becomes more sophisticated. Sophisticated electronics that keep the labor process on its "natural" course also allow physicians to respond, in their own way, to the concerns of women for a more "natural childbirth." Some authors, for example, have suggested that the fetal monitor annoys women,[90] and others have attributed changes—sometimes even drastic changes—in labor to the presence of the monitor.[91] Obstetrics has responded with telemetered fetal monitoring. Uterine pressure and fetal heart rate can be transmitted from a device worn on the patient's thigh or inserted in her vagina to a radio receiver/recorder several hundred yards away. Describing radiotelemetry of monitor data, a group of evaluators said:

> It allows for maximum patient mobility and comfort due to the absence of wires, straps and catheters coupling the patient to the machine. . . . One investigator believed there was less patient anxiety when radiotelemetry was used, due to the absence of the direct connection between the patient and the monitor as well as the potential for locating the monitor away from the patient.[92]

The space to which birth used to be confined literally opens up and the patient has, in the words of the doctors, maximum mobility. A Hewlitt-Packard spokesman praised telemetry saying, "This way the mother is mobile. . . . She can go down to the cafeteria if she wants and we'll still be able to keep track of her. One woman even got lost in the hospital but we still had her signal."[93]

Obstetricians think this lack of confinement is bringing back the "naturalness" of childbirth. One team of researchers said that not having a monitor in the room with a woman can be "an asset in the care of patients desiring 'natural' childbirth." Another team saw the positive reasons for the telemetered monitoring in a more humanistic, patient-centered light: "the naturalness of labor with the patient ambulant might be expected to increase the development of [the affectional bond between mother and infant]."[94]

No one need fear, however, what the *New York Times* called the "Orwellian scene of electronically controlled childbirth,"[95] a childbirth devoid of people. As one person said, "the first monitors of labor were midwives and doctors and . . . they are still irreplaceable."[96] Monitoring is a structure of control that has a significant technological component, but monitoring can be deployed through personnel as well as machines. As Haverkamp's first study showed, as long as nurses were specially trained to monitor birth closely, the absence of a machine made no difference in outcome. The authors remarked, "[We] have the impression that the reassuring atmosphere created by personal nurse interaction and the absence of the recording machine in auscultated patients contributed to the excellent infant outcome in [that group]."[97]

Controlling the Controllers

People remain monitors of childbirth, but reflexively they themselves are subject to the control of monitoring, the new order of obstetrical power. The analytic power of the panopticon is manifest throughout a space "in which the individuals are inserted in a fixed place, in which the slightest movements are supervised, in which all events are recorded." This description corresponds to the image of modern obstetrics deployed throughout the hospital and the community, too. Power is centralized, but "an uninterrupted work of writing links the center and the periphery" and "power is exercised without division, according to a continuous hierarchical figure." Just as the object of control—childbirth and women going through it— is re-created as a continuous process, analyzed in meticulous detail, and subjected to constant surveillance, so too is the staff, ostensibly responsible for effecting control, reconstructed as a well-integrated, continuously hierarchical, ubiquitous, fully knowledgeable entity. Discontinuities in the division of labor are smoothed out, specializations are dissolved, and obstetrical teams responsible for continuous oversight are created. But there is more. The controllers become subject to the power of the very structure through which they presume to exercise control:

> The Panopticon may even provide an apparatus for
> supervising its own mechanisms. . . . [The director] will be able

to judge [his employees] continuously, alter their behavior, impose upon them the methods he thinks best, and it will even be possible to observe the director himself. An inspector arriving unexpectedly . . . will be able to judge at a glance, without anything being concealed from him, how the entire establishment is functioning.

When every childbirth is individualized to such a fine degree, and the nuances of the course of every labor and delivery are recorded, the error, the unexpected death, or the injudicious use of high forceps becomes self-evident. Every threat to order, whether originating with the mother or with the obstetrical team, stands in high relief against a predictable background. The panopticon "enables everyone to come and observe any of the observers"; it becomes "a transparent building in which the exercise of power may be supervised by society as a whole" so that "there is no risk . . . that the increase of power created by the panoptic machine may degenerate into tyranny."[98] Monitoring fulfilled these functions of panoptic power, the reordering of the powerful and the subjugation of them to its power, and brought the transformation of obstetrical power full circle.

Jacques Roux and his colleagues said, "the increased supervision of labor provided by electronic fetal monitoring . . . *focuses the attention of the personnel* on the patient." Telling the mother to report changes in fetal activity *"gain[s] the attention of the clinic physician."*[99] Monitoring is a commanding, demanding structure. It directs attention where it was not directed before—to the finest details of pregnancy. It does more, however; monitoring changes the clinician's perception. Explaining the good outcomes of auscultated patients in his second study, Haverkamp said, "We are left with the impression that nurses auscultate with a *different perspective* since the advent of the electronic monitor, which has provided much more information about fetal heart rate patterns."[100]

No one is immune to the effects of monitoring. The "monitoring concept" is pervasive, bringing with it "changes in previous long-established routines, augmented education, and enhanced alertness among the medical, nursing, and paramedical personnel." It increases the size of the obstetrical record, adding "fetal monitoring tracings and written interpretations"[101] so that not only is the labor recorded and visible but the staff member doing the interpreting is, too. Everyone must be trained and properly organized:

Proper surveillance of the fetus during labor depends on adequate staffing and instruction of nurses, clinical clerks, interns, residents, and obstetricians in the techniques of fetal monitoring and interpretation of fetal heart rate patterns. The establishment of a fetal heart rate team, to include consultants with adequate experience in fetal monitoring, would improve fetal surveillance during labor. [A resuscitation team should be organized as well.] Moreover, fetal monitoring systems should not be confined to rooms of patients in the first stage of labor, but should be in the delivery room and in the cesarean section room.[102]

The monitoring concept is deployed along the lines of pregnancy reconceptualized as a process:

It is our contention . . . that unless an intensive care orientation pervades hospital obstetric practice from clinic to delivery room, many patients who need such care will fail to be identified or, if identified, may encounter a gap in the simultaneous availability of equipment and experienced personnel at the precise moment they are needed.

Intensive care, of course, is more than an orientation. It requires a concentration of equipment and testing procedures . . . that permits fetal-maternal status to be evaluated in much greater detail than is possible by traditional indices. . . .

Our intensive care approach . . . is in three phases—a special clinic unit, a special ante-partum unit, and a special intrapartum unit.[103]

Monitoring breaks down specialty divisions:

The optimal fulfillment of the concept will be achieved through a strong mix of obstetric and pediatric skills in both the antepartum and the intrapartum periods; the ideal would be for the pediatrician to know the fetus as well as the obstetricians do—or believe we do—before he has to deal with the newborn infant.[104]

The perinatal concept emerges, and a new specialty is created with its own journals, professional organizations, and board examinations. Its focus of attention is the fetus from the presumed point of viability, twenty weeks of gestation or so, through the neonatal period. In some training centers pediatricians are encouraged to go on obstetrical rounds and obstetricians to accompany pediatricians on their rounds.[105] At the University of Colorado Medical Center, a precipitous drop in perinatal mortality in the early 1970s could be explained only by a new policy which required that an attending perinatologist-neonatologist be in the delivery room during the birth of every high-risk infant. As with pregnancy itself, surveillance becomes a continuous, hierarchical process to which staff must conform.

With monitoring so thoroughly deployed, with the proper course of pregnancy recorded in journals and texts accessible to anyone who learns the language, and with each small part of every pregnancy documented and accessible in the medical record, obstetricians become just as visible to the inquiring eye as the process into which they have inquired. They become subjects of monitoring as well:

> Never before has the practice of medicine been subject to surveillance by consumer and government groups as at the present time. Both groups are questioning our practice procedures and demanding cost-benefit analysis and scientific justification before application of our technologic advances.[106]

The entire fetal monitoring controversy discussed at the beginning of this chapter is just one example of the way the new modality of control of childbirth—monitoring—has penetrated the protective boundary in which obstetrics had tried to seal itself. The sovereignty of the obstetrician is gone. He and his practices are subject to detailed scrutiny, a scrutiny that may bring controversy and refinement or even major change in some practices. It may cause more obstetricians to be subject to legal prosecution for negligence. But far from constituting a diminution of control or a "victory" for one group of critics, changes in practice are simply a demonstration that the new structure of control—monitoring—is working. Controversy, and the refinement of concepts, practices, and organization that it may effect, merely strengthens monitoring and magnifies its influence.

Obstetrics is no longer confined by boundaries built on notions of normality and abnormality or on the concept of pathological potential. Obstetrics is not even confined by traditional notions of pregnancy and childbirth as phenomena which occupy only a delimited part of a woman's life. Every aspect of every woman's life is subject to the obstetrical gaze because every aspect of every individual is potentially important, obstetrically speaking. The obstetrical vision looks at everything leading up to childbirth and, as the next chapter shows, it looks at everything after childbirth as well. Obstetrics does not have free reign to work its will at its own pleasure, however. Obstetrics is constrained by life, but it is constrained by a life so intimately known, so scrupulously investigated, so demanding of conformity, and so quick to notice threats to order that this life keeps the power of obstetrics in check.

5 Maternal-Infant Bonding
Monitoring and the Problem of Falling in Love with Your Child

Science, turned inward to the phenomena obstetricians claim as part of their domain, serves a corrective function by changing practices and refining the project so that the general authority of the profession is preserved while its fine structure is adjusted. Scientism, turned outward to phenomena related to the obstetrical project but not yet within its net, facilitates expansion of the profession's field of interest. The theory and research that developed around maternal-infant bonding were the beacons that illuminated obstetrics' expansion of its domain from the point of birth.

With scientism turned outward, professional domains expand quickly. A few experiments, based on rather old notions from the social sciences, appeared in the obstetrical literature and seemed to show that the process of "falling in love" with one's child just after birth followed regular patterns. Deviations from the natural course of the process seemed to lead to dramatically abnormal child development and to cause severe disruptions in family life. Patterns of development and deviations from natural processes are the stuff of which new obstetrical interventions are made. The profession seized bonding as a new aspect of its professional concern, and the theory served the profession well. Bonding helped the profession extend its interests beyond birth to the early postnatal period of adjustment; it facilitated a new

A longer version of this chapter appeared in *Feminist Studies* 6, no. 3. (Fall 1980): 547–70.

synthesis of mother and baby as a unit of interest, following the division of the unit that occurred with the earlier discovery of the fetus; and as bonding extended the obstetrical domain outside the hospital and beyond the family unit to other social institutions it picked up collaborators in the obstetrical project from other disciplines.

According to an independent midwife, "Bonding is that process [through] which the mother and the child come together and the child realizes that that's the mother it was born out of and the mother makes the outward realization that that is her child."[1] It is a process which, some argue, has both social and biological bases. Extant literature is unclear about the definition of bonding or the nature of the "attachment" process, but significant sectors of diverse groups—doctors, social workers, and feminists—have embraced the notion of bonding. There is widespread agreement that the effects of bonding, or more precisely of its absence, are profound and long-lasting.

Much of the research on bonding is methodologically flawed. Yet bonding theory has been accepted uncritically despite its demonstrable scientific problems. In this chapter I review the development of bonding theory, point out some of the methodological problems with bonding research, and suggest one mechanism through which a profession comes to accept methodologically flawed research as a basis for its work. I also show why it is necessary to consider the political context in which theory develops in order to understand fully a profession's activity.

The Research and Logic of the Maternal-Infant Bonding Literature

Evidence that suggests bonding occurs and that it has important consequences derives from two sources: ethological research and quasi-experimental and experimental human research.

Within the ethological tradition there are three major kinds of studies: inference from evidence of commonalities in birth practices across a wide variety of species, separation studies in which the effects of postnatal separation of mother and infant are examined, and adoption studies in which the researcher tries to get an animal to adopt some other animal's offspring after the newborn has been separated from members of its own species for varying lengths of time.

Species whose perinatal behavior has been studied intensively include cats, rats, goats, sheep, and various primates. Marshall Klaus and John Kennell's major summary of their own work, *Maternal-Infant Bonding,* and E. O. Wilson's *Sociobiology*[2] provide reviews of this literature. The results from these studies show that parental behavior toward offspring is species specific, but, it is argued, "different species have evolved comparable caretaking behaviors to meet similar needs of newborns." Regardless of the social behavior peculiar to each species, "individualized, enduring bonds develop between mother and infant."[3]

There is great variation in birth practices across species, and bonding researchers might be criticized for concentrating too much on commonalities instead of paying attention to this interspecific diversity. But bonding theorists would argue that their cross-species comparative research is suggestive, not definitive, evidence for the existence of bonding. Their case for the existence of "bonds" in animals rests on separation and adoption studies.

Separation studies begin by removing a newborn from its mother immediately after birth or by surgical delivery. Dependent variables in separation studies include "acceptance" of the young (nursing, retrieving young moved a short distance from the mother, etc.) and species specific maternal behaviors such as nest-building in rats. Different species have different reactions to separation. Goats whose babies are taken from them in the first five minutes of life will reject their young. Goats left with their young for five minutes after birth and then separated from them will reaccept their offspring after several hours. Rats, too, are thought to have a "critical period" (the time after birth when attachment is thought to occur), but it is longer and much less well defined than in goats. From these and other separation studies, attachment theorists conclude:

> Separation of a newborn or young animal from its mother therefore significantly alters maternal behavior. The sooner after birth the separation occurs, the stronger are the effects. For each species there seems to be a specific length of separation that can be endured. If separation extends beyond this sensitive period, the effects on mothering behavior during this breeding cycle are often drastic and irreversible.[4]

Adoption studies tend to confirm the existence of a sensitive period but add one qualification: the setting in which one tries to effect an adoption and the behavior of the infant both affect maternal response to the infant. This qualification suggests the importance of mother-infant interaction and the importance of the environment in "attachment."

Investigation of the physiological bases of attachment-behavior has paralleled observational studies. Spurred on by developments in endocrinology that demonstrate the impact of social stimuli on hormonal excretion and subsequent behavior,[5] investigators have tried to show how the presence or absence of a newborn affects the hormonal status of a new mother. The results of this work are summarized by Klaus and Kennell:

> Biological mechanisms are primarily responsible for a mother's receptivity to young at the time of birth but quickly subside afterward. Within the sensitive period, maternal behavior quickly disappears if young are not present to elicit and maintain it. . . . Because of her physiological state after parturition, a mother is sensitized to the behavior cues of her newborn and begins to respond to them. The infant, in turn, responds to maternal behavior, and patterns of interaction quickly develop that establish the bond between mother and infant, preventing her from abandoning him.[6]

One cannot experiment with human mothers and infants in the same way one experiments with animals, but one can study the effects of of various forms of separation. Quasi-experimental bonding research on humans involved babies separated from their parents by "accident," by war, or by death of parents. In fact, for "quasi-experimental evidence" one can often read "anecdotal evidence." That is, the evidence comes from studies which compare separated infants to *notions* of normal development instead of comparing them to a comparable group of nonseparated infants, as an experiment would require.

Researchers in the 1930s and 1940s studied children who were institutionalized, and claimed that deviant modes of mothering and nurturance led to long-term disturbances of personal-social relations, altered perceptual-motor functioning, and intellectual retardation.[7] Subsequent research questioned the long-term impact of institutionalization[8] and pointed out that the complexity of maternal-infant interaction made it difficult to isolate those variables related to observed developmental disorders. Furthermore, the detrimental

effects of institutionalization were found to be "apparently revers-
ible if the infant is placed in a home or given supplementary caretaker
attention and stimulation before he or she is past six months of
age."[9]

With hindsight it is appropriate to say that the findings of institutionalization studies and other anecdotal information on the deprivation of stimulation and attention were not extraordinarily
important in themselves. They are historically important because of
the impetus they gave to recent experimental research on bonding.

Ethical considerations prevent prolonged, indefinite separation of
mothers and infants for experimental purposes. So the independent
variables in human separation studies are timing and duration of
maternal-infant contact after birth. In the now classic study by
Klaus, Jerauld et al.,[10] a study typical of the genre, a group of twenty-
eight mothers was divided into an "extended contact group" and
a control group. Each member of the control group saw her baby
for a short time soon after birth, had brief contact again at six to
twelve hours after birth for identification purposes, and then visited
her child for twenty to thirty minutes every four hours for feedings.
This was standard hospital procedure for postpartum mother-infant
contact. Members of the extended contact group "were given their
nude babies . . . for one hour within the first three hours after birth,
and also five extra hours of contact each afternoon of the three days
after delivery."[11] Thus, the difference in contact totaled sixteen hours
over the first three postpartum days.

Dependent variables in separation studies of this kind are numerous. The studies reported in Klaus and Kennell's book take data
on dependent variables from three sources: interviews with mothers
when their babies are one month old, maternal behavior during physical examinations of babies at one month and one year of age, and
films of feeding at one month and one year. The studies report statistically significant differences in indices of maternal behavior at
home and during the physical exams. Also, it is claimed, analysis
of films taken during feedings shows that the extended contact group
engaged in *en face* behavior (alignment of mother's face with baby's
face) and fondling to a greater extent than did the control group.
Subsequent studies on subsets of the original twenty-eight subjects
showed differences in the mothers' linguistic behavior toward their
infants at two years of age and in the infants' language ability and
IQ at five years of age.[12] The conclusion from this extended series

of studies is, "just sixteen extra hours of contact within the first three days of life affect maternal behavior for one year and possibly longer, and they offer support for the hypothesis of a maternal sensitive period soon after birth."[13]

The work by Klaus and Kennell is representative of human experimental research on bonding. In such research, to put it simply, one manipulates maternal-infant contact and then searches for differences in maternal behavior or child development. Other studies have adopted variations on this theme using different schedules of maternal-infant contact and different dependent variables. But the conclusions are clear, at least to bonding proponents: "On the basis of [the] evidence, we strongly believe an essential principle of attachment is that there is a *sensitive* period in the first minutes and hours after an infant's birth which is optimal for parent-infant attachment."[14]

Methodological Critique

There are many problems with the research on bonding. In the introduction to an extensive review of the research on child care in the family, Alison Clarke-Stewart makes this sweeping, general, and accurate description of research on child development:

> The field is, in fact, one beset by methodological problems arising at all stages of the research endeavor: design, conception of variables, sampling, recording, compiling, analyzing, and interpreting data.[15]

In order to appreciate the full force of this criticism for the bonding literature, one must accept such research, for the moment, on the terms in which it is presented. Bonding research is offered as scientific research, so let us examine it from that perspective.

The first problem with the field is that there is no agreement on just what attachment or bonding is. There are definitions, of course. Klaus and Kennell say, "An 'attachment' can be defined as a unique relationship between two people that is specific and endures through time."[16] This is consistent with conceptions of attachment which existed before they started their research. Over the past few years, however, the vagueness of this definition has been questioned and alternatives to it have been proposed.[17] Some feel that attachment should be viewed simply as one aspect of mother-infant interaction.

As Miriam Rosenthal says, "Attachment is not a 'thing' . . . but rather a characteristic of some patterns of interaction between mother and infant."[18] Others have suggested that the child is an "active participant" in a "social network."[19]

Discovering a lack of conceptual consensus is not uncommon in social research, but in this case imprecision in the definition of concepts sets the basis for committing serious methodological errors. Lack of consensus permits a researcher to use multiple indicators of the concept under examination. Scientists generally search for correlative differences in several indicators—fondling, kissing, soothing, proximity-seeking behavior, *en face* behavior, attempts to breast-feed, laughing or singing to an infant, subjective feelings about separation, and so on—in the same study of attachment. Besides creating many measurement problems,[20] multiple indicators require multiple tests of statistical significance, a practice that biases results in favor of the researcher. The multiple indicator criticism is a common one in social research, which tends to deal with somewhat amorphous concepts, but it cannot be lightly brushed aside in this field because there seems to be a high degree of inconsistency in results and because replication of studies is relatively rare. Masters and Wellman conclude their critical review of the psychological literature on attachment by saying, "correlations which are significant in one sample often fail to reach significance in an independent sample and . . . the temporal stability, cross-situational consistency, and cross-behavioral consistency of attachment behaviors are not great."[21] They conclude that "correlational analysis of human infant attachment behaviors does not provide substantial support for the concept of attachment as a psychological state or central motive state."[22] A low degree of conceptual clarity and consistency of findings encourages one to develop new and improved measures of attachment instead of working with old ones. Therefore, few people attempt to check the reliability of reported results.

Beyond basic methodological errors there are other problems. Leifer et al., in a paper published in *Child Development*,[23] report many complicated tests of significance on many indicators of attachment. Some tests support a hypothesis to the effect that differences in behavior are caused by extended contact, some do not. Then, in a kind of scholarly postscript, they add:

> There are other differences between the groups that are not reflected in the observational data presented here *and are*

probably outcomes of their separation experience. For instance, within the sample of 26 separated and 23 contact mothers of prematures who participated in any phase of the study, two relinquished custody of their infants sometime after hospital discharge. Both of these mothers were in the separated group. Also, there have been six instances of divorce among the parents in this study, five of them in the separated group. . . . Finally, there were four mothers who attempted to breast-feed their infants. Two of these mothers were in the contact group and two in the separated group; one mother in each group was a primipara and the other a multipara who had successfully breast-fed at least one previous child. The only mother to succeed was the multiparous contact mother.[24]

They conclude:

These actions [divorce and relinquishing custody] represent severe disturbance of normal maternal and marital behavior. . . . The existence of these cases, while few in number, suggests that early separation of mother and infant may seriously disrupt normal maternal behavior.[25]

These researchers sought out data to bolster their theory when their original investigation was less than successful in producing such data.

Besides problems of conceptualization and measurement, there are problems with the design of separation studies. These are of two sorts: problems of obtaining comparable experimental and control groups and problems of experimental treatments being confounded with other variables.

Matching experimental groups with other mother-infant pairs who are not treated controls the effects of variables, other than the experimental treatment itself, which might influence attachment behavior. In studies reported to date, experimental and control groups are, in fact, quite comparable on variables which might influence results *prior* to the beginning of each study. The problem is that there is no assurance that groups *remain* comparable as a study proceeds. In bonding research, where important effects of early extended contact are supposed to propagate over many years it is important that experimental and control groups remain roughly comparable over time. Klaus et al.,[26] for example, randomly divided their subjects into control and experimental groups based on their day of delivery. They obtained identical experimental and control groups. But does knowing that the groups were matched to begin with permit the inference that differences at one month, one year, two years, and five years are attributable *only* to the experimental manipulation of sixteen extra hours of maternal-infant contact in the first three days of life? For such an inference to be made, the life course of experimental and control group members after delivery would have to be similar. To what kind of home environment did the mothers return? Was there continuing employment for the bread-winner(s)? Were there pregnancies during the five-year follow-up period? What impact did subsequent pregnancies and births have on households? Questions concerning post-discharge life course are especially crucial since attachment studies are often conducted on people drawn from the unmarried ranks of lower social strata where life courses are likely to change frequently and rapidly.[27] Simple randomization of a small number of subjects does not adequately eliminate the very plausible hypothesis that it is life-course events, not the experimental manipulations, which cause observed differences.

Another problem is that experimental manipulations in bonding research are often contaminated. Bonding researchers claim that extended contact between mother and infant is the only difference between experimental and control groups. This is not so. Experimental and control groups were treated differently by the doctors and nurses who facilitated contact between mothers and infants in one group and denied contact in another. It is likely that these health professionals influenced maternal behavior toward infants since they always affect patients' conception of their own health status and of their babies' health status as well. This observation is especially important since one indicator of attachment is maternal behavior during a physician's examination of the mother's infant. Mothers who have extended contact show a greater propensity to stand near the examining table and soothe their babies during the exam than do mothers in control groups. These mothers might presume that they need not surrender their children to health professionals and remain in the background during an exam since health profession-als—the nurses who brought the babies to the mothers for extra contact—had given them the tacit message that their babies were theirs, not medicine's. Similarly, *en face* or fondling and soothing behavior may be unintentionally or intentionally encouraged by staff members during the extended contact period.

Appropriate experiments that would allow one to attribute behavioral differences to separation or extended contact are impossible to design. That is, it is impossible to conduct the scientifically required "critical test" of bonding theory, for what would constitute such a test? If agreement on the meaning of attachment could be reached, experiments similar to those conducted by Harlow on monkeys would be required. One group of children would have to be reared normally and one group would have to be reared with surrogate mothers. Development would have to be monitored for many years, certainly through adolescence. To control for genetic endowment, it would be best if identical twins could be used, one from each pair going into the experimental group, one from each pair going into the control group. We must be so demanding in this case because, as attachment theorists tell us, there is a wide range of behaviors which can lead to a successful "bond":

> There are an infinite number of normal variations in patterns of mothering and *great diversity* in the mode of communication between baby and mother. Any of a *vast number* of variations in the pattern can be accommodated in the human baby's development and still ensure that a human bond will be achieved.[28]

Yet the literature leads us to believe that there is a period very early in life during which proper behavior is essential and during which improper behavior can have dire consequences. The test described above would meet the scientific obligations incumbent on attachment theorists, but it is unreasonable to demand that such a test be conducted. Consequently, it is impossible to determine the prolonged effects of early parent-infant contact.

Bonding theory very quickly found its way out of the laboratory and into medicine and social policy. Scholars and scientists developed the knowledge that was then used to foster some rather remarkable claims about human behavior. The effects of not bonding are thought to be clear and profound:

> In the case of a child who has been deprived of human partners in the formative years he may lack inhibitions of aggressive impulses or [experience] extraordinary problems in the regulation of his aggression.[29]

One can succumb to the "diseases of non-attachment" which may "give rise to a broad range of disordered personalities"[30]:

> In personal encounters with such an individual [one who suffers from the diseases of nonattachment] there is an almost perceptible feeling of intervening space, of remoteness, and of "no connection." . . . There is no joy, no grief, no guilt, and no remorse. . . . Many of these people strike us as singularly humorless. . . . A very large number of them have settled inconspicuously in the disordered landscape of a slum, or a carnie show, or underworld enterprises.[31]

That happens to the child who fails to bond.

The parent who remains unbonded comes under surveillance because of a propensity to child abuse. Several studies suggest that "separation is indeed one factor resulting in physical abuse of preterm infants."[32]

Bonding theory is only one contemporary manifestation of sociobiological reasoning. Sociobiological argumentation permits doctors and other policy-makers to claim legitimacy for their project by insisting that they are simply allowing the means-ends chains embedded in our genes to be realized. They are facilitating the realization of a truly "natural" order. This kind of argument thereby obscures the choices—the political choices—being made for all of us and it prevents scrutiny and discussion of those choices.

The Politics of Falling in Love with Your Child

The scientific method is an idealized set of rules for the creation of a particular kind of knowledge. If one follows the rules, the knowledge acquires a privileged status. Bonding theory, however, was accorded scientific privilege even though the method by which it was created merely imitated the scientific method. It was accepted by obstetricians and others because bonding theory is socially and politically useful. To understand this claim we must examine the context in which the theory arose.

Bonding theory has a broad appeal and is being used to reform various institutions with social practices of such long-standing that they have been objectified, reified, and have seemingly acquired a life of their own. The most immediate, and perhaps commonsensical, application of bonding theory has been in the reform of hospital practices involving childbirth and early postpartum care of mothers and infants. Outside hospitals, however, the theory provides both direct and indirect justifications for needed social reforms: direct by justifying social policies immediately affecting children, and indirect by resurrecting old justifications for certain social practices in a new scientific rhetoric.

Hospital Practices

Klaus and Kennell wish to change hospital obstetrical practices:

> All these clinical reports suggest that the events occurring during the first hours after birth have special significance for the mother. Nursery practices in the modern hospital in the United States do not generally acknowledge this, and, instead, separate mother and infant immediately after birth. . . . If there were convincing evidence of an early sensitive period in the human being, major changes in hospital care would be necessary.[33]

Why have an interest in changing hospital practice? Why have it at this particular time?

Bonding theory appeared just in time to facilitate change in hospital practice as the natural childbirth movement gained new vigor in the early 1970s. Natural childbirth, with its emphasis on ecstasy, psychosexual experience, safety, and a return to nature, caught the public interest in the 1940s.[34] The number of proponents grew steadily throughout the following three decades, so that

> By the 1970s the thrust for natural childbirth, which had been a loosely organized cultural movement among middle class women, aimed at enhancing their experience at birth, acquired a social and political cast; women of all classes began to organize, to educate one another, and to try to change or avoid the professional and institutional structures that exerted such dominance over birth.[35]

The profession did not respond to these calls for change when they first arose because, simply, it could not. Klaus and Kennell show[36] that hospital practices which the profession wished to change—early separation of mother and infant and little contact after birth—developed out of scientific concern over the introduction of infectious diseases into the newborn nursery. Practices that have their own scientific basis cannot simply be changed in a profession whose very existence is dependent on the autonomy which science, or at least a facade of scientism, accords it.[37] It was necessary to develop bonding theory and gain support for it in order to make changes in practice permissible.

Change might have been permissible because of the new research, but something which is permissible is not absolutely necessary. The actual impetus for change came not from research but from women who threatened obstetricians' livelihoods by taking their obstetrical business elsewhere. In a *Wall Street Journal* article on the rise of "birthing rooms" and the relaxation of hospital birth rituals and rules, David Stewart, executive director of the National Association of Parents and Professionals for Safe Alternatives in Childbirth, is quoted as saying, "Hospitals that don't set up a birthing room will go out of the baby business because of the competition. And there's no question that consumer pressure is bringing this about."[38] Women created an economic pressure for change.

If obstetrics had maintained a strictly medical view of pregnancy as a delimited event in a woman's life fraught with pathological potential, it would not have been able to use the research on bonding to change its hospital practices for at least two reasons. First, the profession would not have had license to pay attention to the family unit *after* birth. The obstetrician's job would have ended as the baby passed healthily out of the birth canal, when all the physiological processes of the baby had started on their natural courses, and when pregnancy and childbirth had come to an end. Second, women's demands that birth be treated as a more natural and more normal phenomenon would have threatened to its ideological core a profession of obstetrics based on notions of the pathology of pregnancy. But the monitoring concept had changed the profession's view of pregnancy and childbirth, making pregnancy into a process whose natural course was known and maintainable and which had no clear boundaries in a woman's life. The new view of pregnancy and birth allowed obstetrics to respond, in its own way, to women's demands and to incorporate extensions of bodily processes into the field of professional concern. Bonding theory made falling in love simply another phase in the pregnancy-birth process. Bonding theory outlined the normal and natural course of falling in love, and the horror stories which came from the bonding literature testified to the effects of deviations from that natural course. The theory suggested simple interventions that could correct a deviant process and set it on its proper trajectory, to the benefit of all. Fraiberg's "diseases of non-attachment" were the basis on which the physician's right of intervention in and control over birth were preserved while, at the same time, physicians could argue that they were responding to women's desires for more normal birth experiences: "By understanding the genesis of maternal and attachment behavior, perhaps we can better envision interventions that will foster change in those cases where such is desirable for the mother and infant."[39]

Interventions did not have to be medically dramatic, though. They could be extremely simple and noninvasive. Child abuse, for example, might be reduced just by encouraging parents to interact with their babies within the first twelve hours of life.[40] The doctor's job was no longer simply to deliver a laboring mother, it now included "Helping Mothers to Love Their Babies," as a leader in the *British Medical Journal* put it.[41] The obstetrician's job expanded and changed so that he could still intervene in birth, but the changes that bonding theory facilitated included precisely the kind of changes women demanded in their call for more natural childbirth: earlier, closer contact with their babies, contact on demand in the early postpartum period, less alienation for medical reasons. Obstetrical practices could change because of bonding theory, but the changes preserved the relationship that traditionally existed between physicians and patients.

Social Policy

The "diseases of nonattachment" are also used as the basis for criticism and eventual reform of social policies involving children. Lack of bonding in early infancy contributes to many social problems according to Fraiberg:

> These bondless men, women and children constitute one of the largest aberrant populations in the world today, contributing far beyond their numbers to social disease and disorder. These are people who are unable to fulfill the most ordinary human obligations in work, in friendship, in marriage, and in childrearing. . . . Where there are no human attachments there can be no conscience. As a consequence, the hollow men and women contribute very largely to the criminal population. It is this group, too, that produces a particular kind of criminal, whose crimes, whether they be petty or atrocious, are always

characterized by indifference. The potential for violence and destructive acts is far greater among these bondless men and women; the absence of human bonds leaves a free, "unbound" aggression to pursue its erratic course.[42]

From this point of view it is easy to propose changes in the judiciary system, in child-care practices, and in social welfare policy. Courts are asked to recognize the drastic implications of "unbinding" children through custody decisions. Just as obstetricians are encouraged to be a child advocate in the delivery room, there are calls that children be assigned advocates in court, since "the supporting staff of social workers and psychologists have neither specialized professional training nor the vocational commitment to children which qualifies them as advisors to the court."[43] "Child Care Industries, Inc."—day care—is issued a "blanket indictment" for providing "anonymous sitters for small children." And it is claimed that public welfare policy regarding children compels choices only among bad alternatives.

Bonding theory gives social reformers license to propose changes in these social institutions, to eradicate the "diseases of nonattachment," but criticism and proposals for reform are only one side of the phenomenon. Bonding theory also provides the institutions with relief that is sorely needed. The judiciary is presently under attack for alleged subjectivism and for creating loopholes which any good lawyer can use advantageously. A scientific theory for dispassionate judgment of all cases can be used by courts to create a facade of rationality, objectivity, and fairness based on science. Bonding theory can be used by the courts to assure the public that action taken is in the scientifically demonstrated "best interests of the child."

Bonding theory, like much theory developed in obstetrics, has all the characteristics of a pseudoscience, "a sustained process of false persuasion transacted by simulation or distortion of scientific inquiry and hypothesis testing."[44] A view of bonding theory as a pseudoscience helps explain its appeal to social reformers and the paucity of criticism directed toward the theory. A pseudoscience garners no popular criticism because it "serves as a kind of wish fulfillment, enabling people to discover what they would like to believe."[45] With bonding, people are discovering that a judiciary that "Divides the Living Child" (one of Fraiberg's chapter titles) between parents in custody suits can be reformed so that the institution is preserved while its more disagreeable aspects are eliminated. Bonding fulfills the desires of those who wish we could do without "Child Care Industries, Inc." but who are reluctant to speak against an institution which presumably frees people from the social requirement that children be attended constantly by one parent or the other. And it does all this in the name of science. Pseudoscience garners no criticism from science because "scientists generally do not like polemics, and when conflict occurs they usually try to minimize its importance."[46]

Using exactly the same kinds of theories, the same kinds of reasoning, and the same approach to intervention that obstetrics uses in pregnancy and childbirth, social scientists have set out to reform social institutions. The obstetrical project is being extended by another discipline to areas outside the hospital. The legitimacy of one discipline's work, that of obstetrics, justifies the other, social science, whose work then feeds back and augments the first discipline's power in its field of concern. Social scientists become indirect collaborators in the obstetrical project, not just by developing theory and research for obstetrical consumption, but by applying it to institutional reform in other fields. Bonding theory is being used in direct ways to reform social institutions which desperately need reform, but bonding theory is being used indirectly, in a more diffuse way, as well, and it is to this more subtle application of the theory that I now turn.

Social Order

In 1916 a paper in the *American Journal of Sociology* described how major social institutions and aspects of social life—law, art, public opinion, education, and other "devices"—were used to get women to bear and raise children. Leta Hollingsworth argued that the "social guardians" manipulated social life to increase the birth rate in order to "secure order, and insure that individuals will act in such a way as to promote the interests of the group, *as those interests are conceived by those who form the radiant points of social control.*"[47] In early twentieth-century America, it was in the national interest to produce children, particularly children from families of means. Women did bear and raise children despite the fact that doing so was "painful, dangerous to life, and involve[d] years of exacting labor and self-sacrifice" and despite the fact that according to the research of the day "there [was] no evidence to show that a maternal instinct exist[ed] in women of such all-consuming strength and fervor as to impel them voluntarily to seek the pain, danger, and exacting labor involved in maintaining a high birth rate."[48] Professor Hollingsworth, in a style appropriate in the sociology of her day, concluded:

> The time is coming, and is indeed almost at hand, when all the most intelligent women of the community, who are the most desirable child-bearers, will become conscious of the methods of social control. The type of normality will be questioned; the laws will be repealed and changed; enlightenment will prevail; belief will be seen to rest upon dogmas; illusions will fade away and give place to clearness of view; the bugaboos will lose their power to frighten. How will "the social guardians" induce women to bear a surplus population when all these cheap, effective methods no longer work?[49]

Over sixty years later we see bonding theory, a social-psychological-biological theory, a resurrected if somewhat modified and scientificized version of "maternal instinct," being used to keep women in their place, maintaining social order.

Social interests are different today but the strategies are similar. A high birthrate is no longer crucial, but continued subordination of women and other groups is. Bonding is a theory which lends legitimacy to the notion that women are the only appropriate attendants for children. It is an ideological justification for keeping women in the home with their children.

Bonding theory has a "constraining" side and a "liberating" side. Bonding's negative effect is to constrain women from participating fully in economic life should they want to have children. This is turned into a positive attribute, however, by pointing to the "liberation" women enjoy under bonding. Women are "liberated" to participate more fully in the *social* realm of life, that part of living Jacques Donzelot described as "the set of means which allow social life to escape material pressures and politico-moral uncertainties; the entire range of methods which make the members of a society relatively safe from the effects of economic fluctuations by providing a certain security."[50] Since the nineteenth century most social theories have associated the family with the cultural, the social, side of life, and have associated women with the family. Women have been created the conservators of culture, the curators of what Christopher Lasch called the "haven in a heartless world."[51] (Social theories differ on whether this placement of women is good or bad, but they all acknowledge the placement has occurred.) Bonding must be understood as one more theory in the social science tradition of justifying this association and rationalizing the interests from which the association originally flowed.

The social interests served by bonding research are revealed by the methodological biases of the work.[52] Consider, for example, some measures of attachment used in bonding research. At one month, Klaus et al.[53] asked mothers two questions about their behavior and took the sum of their scores as an indication of successful bonding. The first question was: "When baby cries, has been fed, diapers are dry, what do you do?" The respondent received no points if she "always let him cry it out," one point if she "tended to let him cry it out," two points if she "tended to pick him up," and the maximum three points if she "always pick[ed] him up." The second question was, "Have you gone out since infant born [sic]? How did you feel?" The respondent scored zero for going out and feeling good about it, one for going out and thinking about her child, two points for going out and worrying about her child, and three points for not going out or going out and thinking constantly about her child. The bias is clear. Mothers are better if they stay home and concern themselves entirely with their infants.

Also, the interests which lie behind the literature on bonding are indicated by the high degree of "father absence."[54] Rossi, for example, does not discuss the potential importance of nonbiological or nonfemale parents. And Klaus and Kennell focus to a very great degree on *maternal* infant bonding. Fraiberg is perhaps the most "liberal" in terms of recognizing the importance of *human* attachments, but her review is constrained by the "father absent" character of the literature on which her argument is based. "Father absence" is conspicuous in the face of the general finding that:

> It seems likely that in the first six months, at least, fathers and mothers have a parallel influence on their infant's behavior, the relative extent of their influence being determined by the amount and quality of interaction each has with the infant.[55]

Bonding theory is prejudiced against women interested in pursuing a life in which children are not the raison d'être of women or their exclusive focus of attention.

Bonding is an ideology which, like so many other ideologies that pose as social theories, turns social issues into individuals' problems. All of the social ills which concern bonding theorists are reconstructed by bonding theory as problems of women not bonding to their babies. Attention is directed away from fundamental social problems and toward the individual. Women are singled out by calling attention to the possible biological bases of bonding and through the argument that it is only women who possess the biological constitution for solving our social problems. Social order can be maintained only, it seems, by acquiescing to our biological heritage. This argument is being advanced despite the impossibility of making the attributions bonding theory makes and despite the rather firm location of sex-role behavior in history and society accomplished by the women's movement and feminist scholarship.

Obstetrics, in basing its expansion on a theory which has such widespread implications as bonding, stands only to gain. Bonding theory quickly finds roots in commonsensical notions about the social order. Thus, obstetrics, in extending its gaze beyond the birth of a child, is supported not only by its scientism but by its social appeal as well.

Conclusion

Bonding theory urges us to look inward to our biology for solutions to major social ills. Our prototype for order is to be the order apparent in the biological world. Rossi's "radical" proposal for society makes this clear. She wants, as I pointed out in the introduction to Part Two, "a society more attuned to the natural environment, in touch with, and respectful of the rhythm of our own body processes."[56] But to suggest that we orient ourselves to our biology is a political act. It is a decision to accept an ideology which provides an individualistic rationalization for social problems of crime and violence and for the social need to keep women by the hearth. Orientation to biology is disrespectful of the subjective expressions of interests by each individual concerning the way she feels about and experiences herself, her child, and her intimate relations generally. Adopting a biosocial view of the family presents a "significant retreat from the experimental mode" of social interaction.[57]

But this is exactly why obstetrics embraced bonding theory so readily. An experimental mode of social interaction would present a constant threat to the work of obstetricians. A profession which is subject to the control which monitoring exerts, which can change only through the plodding corrective changes of science, is dependent on a world which consists largely of "ideologically frozen relations of dependence."[58] Admitting women's subjectivity to the discourse about obstetrics would be disconcerting. A theory, the embodiment of objectivity, can be used as the basis for a response to the concerns of women without allowing the subjective, passionate component to surface and disrupt obstetrical work. Bonding is a theory which allowed obstetrics to change in order to keep the social relations, on which its work was based, the same in the face of calls for fundamental reform. The disorder which women threatened to bring to the profession was prevented by reworking the old order and adapting it to a new situation. In the next chapter we see how another discipline, ethics, joined with obstetrics to defend the profession against other threats of disorder.

6   Medicine, Ethics, and the Reformulation of the Doctor-Patient Relationship

The potential for detecting genetic problems in utero, the potential for screening populations in order to detect carriers of genetic problems, and the development of neonatal intensive care based on greatly improved knowledge of fetal and newborn physiology are all aspects of the culmination of the redeployment of a new order of obstetrical power. Monitoring and surveillance in the name of the fetus facilitated the expansion of the obstetrical project out into the community and back from childbirth into the details of a woman's life. Bonding theory extended the obstetrical gaze forward from childbirth through the period of nurturance and early child development. Bonding theory also permitted obstetrical penetration of other, nonmedical, social institutions involved in the care of children. The potential for detecting genetic diseases expands the obstetrical project back to the early weeks of pregnancy and intracellular structures while screening programs extend control to the period in a woman's life when she is only thinking about having a child. Advances in genetics equip medicine fully with the power to implement the rule of "no surprises." Mongoloid children may still be born, but their birth will not be a surprise to anyone for their unusual complement of chromosomes will have been discovered, their births discussed, and deliberate decisions about their existence made. In the imaginable extreme, any fetal defect will be known in advance and a defective child's birth will not be the shockingly disruptive and surprising event that it is now. Everything will be known, planned for, and well managed.

Intensive care for the critically ill neonate is the final component of the monitoring. Should a sick infant be born, intimate knowledge of fetal and newborn physiological processes permits numerous corrective interventions. Dramatic advances in knowledge and technology of newborn respiration, circulation, and nutrition can keep the sick neonate on its "natural" physiological course despite the presence of serious defects and diseases.

Medical genetics and neonatal intensive care are the two aspects of modern obstetrics which have attracted the most vigorous ethical debates. Some people claim that technological advances have made problems of informed consent, problems of agency (the question of who decides), and problems of determining criteria for deciding who is to benefit from limited medical resources so difficult and so acute that people without medical training—ethicists and others trained in moral reasoning—must be involved in medical decision-making. In fact, though, the "technology causes ethical problems" hypothesis is of little explanatory value. Medicine in general, and obstetrics in particular, has always faced and will always face difficult decisions involving matters of life and death. The question which the ethicist poses as the key question, "What should be done?" is the question on which the whole of medical practice turns, and the answer is not always clear-cut. "Value conflicts" occur and "ethical dilemmas" arise regardless of the technology available to obstetricians. The problem is not to explain the existence or the extent of ethical problems, as the "technology" hypothesis does, but to explain why, in the last ten years,[1] we have seen an explosion of open, public discussion of ethical problems. There has been a breakdown in the profession's capacity to contain the ethical dimensions of its work behind a professional boundary, and it is this social aspect of contemporary ethical debates that merits examination.

To understand this social phenomenon we must recall the nature of the doctor's work under the control of monitoring. The physician must, first, locate an individual precisely in terms of deviations on normalizing distributions. Then, the physician must employ normalizing technologies to manage deviations and monitor the effects of all interventions. Monitoring leaves a record of each individual's course vis-à-vis the normal, natural, optimal course of a process *and* a record of the work of the doctor who must restore various processes' trajectories. Monitoring leaves records that are open to scrutiny by anyone, and thus opens a rent in the professional boundary that outsiders can peer through. Ethics has examined the work of medicine and found that medicine's answers to the question, "What ought to be done?" are often debatable; and ethics is willing to debate them. Medicine never invited ethical inquiry, but given its scientistic, ethically neutral facade, medicine had no way to silence those who would mount such an inquiry from another disciplinary base. Medicine had no choice but to acknowledge ethics' view of what ought to be done. Consequently, medicine and ethics found themselves in conflict.

The history of the medicine-ethics dialogue through the 1970s is a history of compromise. Eventually medicine and ethics worked out a limited partnership in which ethics agreed to assist in the defense of the medical project and in which medicine made ethics a junior partner on the health-care team. The partnership, however, was based on medicine reformulating the doctor-patient relationship so that medicine could pay attention to much more than just the individual. Under the new arrangement, medicine could pay attention to the ecology of patient care.

Before reviewing the social dialogue that transpired, we should review the developments around which ethical debates have arisen.

Medical Genetics and Neonatal Intensive Care

The birth of modern genetics is normally dated to the work of Gregor Mendel in the late nineteenth century, even though Mendel's work was anticipated in large part by Pierre Louis Moreau de Maupertuis a hundred years earlier.[2] Mendel's contribution to genetics derived from his meticulous documentation of the results of cross-breeding and in-breeding different varieties of garden peas. He showed that the transmission of inherited "units," or "particles" as Maupertuis had called them, across generations could be described very accurately by simple statistical rules. He found, for example, that if he crossed yellow-seeded peas with green-seeded peas all the offspring were yellow-seeded. If he then bred the yellow-seeded offspring among themselves, almost exactly one-fourth of their offspring were green-seeded. One-third of the yellow-seeded plants in this second generation produced all yellow-seeded plants when in-bred, while the other two-thirds of the second generation behaved like the first generation of offspring, themselves producing one-fourth green-seeded plants. R. A. Fisher, the famous statistician, reviewed Mendel's research in 1936[3] and showed that Mendel must have been conducting carefully planned experiments to test a theory of genetic inheritance. Mendel's theory, now well known, was that both parents carried two "factors" for every trait and contributed one factor to each offspring. The two factors for each trait were "segregated" in the parent before transmission. Every trait in the offspring was the outward manifestation of a combination of "factors," one from the mother and one from the father. Some factors, according to the theory, are "dominant," others "recessive." So when an offspring inherits, strictly by chance, a dominant and a recessive factor, the offspring manifests the dominant trait, yellow-seededness in the example above, but carries a single, unmanifest, recessive factor. When, by chance, an offspring inherits two recessive factors it manifests the recessive trait, green-seededness in the example. Mendel's *law of segregation* of parental factors together with the concepts of dominance and recessiveness account completely for the statistical distributions of the plant types Mendel observed. (See figure 6.1.)

In 1903, Theodor Boveri and Walter S. Sutton suggested that the segregation of chromosomes (structures in the nucleus of all cells which separate by pairs during cell division) accounts for the law of segregation proposed by Mendel.[4] The study of chromosomes as the carriers of genetic information in plants and fruit flies flourished in the early twentieth century while the study of human genetics was driven along at the same time by concerns over mental deficiency, an interest in eugenics, and by an interest in the inheritance of anatomic and metabolic "errors" which are transmitted genetically.

Medical genetics can be divided into two fields according to the structural level—genetic or chromosomal—at which "errors" occur. An error at the genetic level causes an inborn error of metabolism. Over two thousand inborn errors of metabolism have been identified. Some genetic conditions are "X-linked." That is, they are carried on the sex-determining chromosomes. In an "X-linked recessive" condition such as color blindness, hemophilia, and some forms of muscular dystrophy, a female offspring only has the condition if both her X chromosomes, one from each parent, have the recessive trait

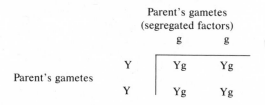

Parent's gametes
(segregated factors)

		g	g
Y		Yg	Yg
Y		Yg	Yg

Parent's gametes

Breeding of homozygotic (two factors of the same type) yellow-seeded plants with homozygotic green seeded plants produces all heterozygotic (two different factors, one dominant, one recessive in this case) yellow-seeded plants. Yellow is the dominant factor.

Parent's gametes

		Y	g
Y		YY	Yg
g		Yg	gg

Parent's gametes

In-breeding members of the new generation produces one-fourth homozygotic yellow-seeded plants which will themselves produce all yellow-seeded plants if bred among themselves, one fourth homozygotic green-seeded plants which will produce all green-seeded plants, and one-half yellow-seeded heterozygotes which will produce just as their parents do.

Figure 6.1.   One of Mendel's experiments.

gene. A male is afflicted with the condition if his single X chromosome inherited from his mother has the recessive trait gene. Thus, a father who has an X-linked condition will not pass on the trait to any of his sons, but all of his daughters will be unaffected carriers. Half of a carrier mother's sons will be affected with the trait, half will be normal; and half of her daughters will be unaffected carriers. (See figure 6.2. These concepts are important in the discussion of genetic screening programs below.) Errors can also occur at the chromosomal level. During cell division, chromosome pairs usually separate, one member of the pair going to one end of the cell and ultimately into one of the two new cells and the other going to the opposite end of the dividing cell and into the other product of cell division. Occasionally both members of a pair will migrate to the

| | Affected Father | |
	X*	Y
X	X*X carrier daughter	XY son
X	X*X carrier daughter	XY son

(Mother, rows labeled X and X)

The offspring of a normal mother and an affected father: No son will be affected because sons do not receive the father's X chromosome. All daughters will be carriers.

| | Father | |
	X	Y
X*	X*X carrier daughter	X*Y affected son
X	XX daughter	XY son

(Carrier mother, rows labeled X* and X)

The offspring of a carrier mother and an unaffected father: Half the male offspring will be affected, half will be normal. Half the daughters will be carriers, half will be normal.

Figure 6.2. Transmission of X-linked conditions such as color blindness, hemophilia, and some forms of muscular dystrophy.

same end of a dividing cell and stay together in the new cell. If this happens in the formation of the sperm or ovum, the offspring will receive one chromosome of a pair from one parent and a complete pair from the other parent. This gives the offspring a total of three chromosomes where there are usually only two. The offspring will be "trisomic" and, if the child survives, will suffer from one of a number of "trisomy syndromes." The best-known of these is Down's syndrome—mongolism—which results from having a third chromosome in the twenty-first pair of chromosomes as they are conventionally numbered. Other errors at the chromosomal level include "breaks" or "deletions" in an arm of a chromosome and "translocations" in which incompatible parts of two chromosomes are exchanged within a chromosome pair at cell division. These errors have various clinical manifestations.

Amniocentesis, a procedure for collecting a sample of amniotic fluid from the uterus, is the technical key to detecting genetic and chromosomal problems in the fetus. Fetal cells floating in the fluid can be cultured for chromosomal and biochemical studies and the fluid itself can be analyzed to detect certain chemical abnormalities. In the late 1950s, researchers tried transvaginal taps of the amniotic sac very early in pregnancy, but they often obtained little fluid and they caused a significant number of infections. In 1967, transabdominal aspiration of amniotic fluid and cell culture techniques led to the first diagnosis of a fetal chromosome problem. In 1968, the first intrauterine diagnosis of Down's syndrome was reported, as was the first diagnosis of an inborn error of metabolism. Today obstetricians can do an amniocentesis at twelve to eighteen weeks in pregnancy and have an analysis of the fetus's chromosome complement, including knowledge of its sex, plus the results of tests for over fifty inborn errors of metabolism, in four to eight weeks. In addition, most of the 125 centers now doing prenatal diagnosis can test amniotic fluid for increased alpha-fetoprotein, an indication that a fetus has a neural tube defect such as spina bifida.

One group of researchers estimated that 15,000 amniocenteses were done in the United States in 1978.[5] White, well-educated, affluent women are overrepresented in this group in relation to their proportion in the population, even though a number of programs to improve the availability of amniocentesis to "women at risk" who are disproportionately nonwhite, not well-educated, and poor, have been mounted in various areas. If all women considered medically eligible and appropriate for amniocentesis had the procedure, laboratories would perform 150,000 to 200,000 procedures and associated analyses each year.

Whether amniocentesis is safe or not is a vigorously debated issue at the moment. In October 1975, the National Institutes of Health released the results of a study of 1,040 women who had amniocenteses and 992 somewhat comparable women who did not have the procedure done. Physicians greeted the results enthusiastically because they showed no difference in the incidence of fetal loss or stillbirths in the two groups. Similarly, there was no difference in complications of delivery, congenital anomalies, or injuries attributable to the amniocentesis. Two percent of the women having an amniocentesis suffered immediate problems—vaginal bleeding and amniotic fluid leakage—as a direct result of the procedure. Although "individual tragedies" occurred, including three failures to detect a mongoloid child, the report ended by saying, "Hopefully, the results of this study will stimulate increased use of the procedure, for only if it is used can its potential be realized."[6] The decision to change the status of amniocentesis from a research procedure to an accepted part of clinical practice was supported by a subsequent Canadian study of 1,223 amniocenteses which found no difference between outcomes of women's pregnancies after amniocentesis and provincial vital statistics for all pregnancies in Canada.[7]

In 1978, a British Working Party chaired by Professor A. C. Turnbull released its findings on 2,428 pregnancies where midtrimester amniocentesis was done (there were the same number of control pregnancies). They found that amniocentesis probably increased fetal loss by 1.0 to 1.5 percent and increased "unexplained respiratory difficulties at birth and major orthopedic postural abnormalities" by the same amount. They concluded that the benefits of amniocentesis outweigh the hazards only in limited circumstances, such as when a previous baby had a genetic or chromosomal abnormality, when tests on the mother indicate she might be carrying a fetus with a neural tube defect, or when the mother is over 40 years old.[8] The design of the British study has been criticized[9], but its results have thrown the question of the safety of amniocentesis into doubt.

Results of prenatal diagnostic tests on amniotic fluid are accurate if done by competent technicians in laboratories that have good quality-control programs. The American collaborative study showed that the overall predictive accuracy of amniocentesis was 99.4 percent, although cell cultures from amniotic fluid failed to grow in one of every eight cases. When cells failed to grow, second taps were required to obtain usable results, and this delay caused longer waiting periods before the fetus' condition was known to physicians and parents, and thus delayed medical management decisions.

At the present time little can be done if amniocentesis detects a defective child. A few inborn errors of metabolism can be managed by diet or drugs and some defects can be corrected surgically, but except for fetal blood transfusions in the case of maternal-fetal blood group incompatibilities, no in utero therapy is available for genetic or chromosomal defects. The only "therapy" medicine can offer parents, once a defective child is detected, is abortion. One person described programs of genetic and chromosomal abnormality detection as aimed at prevention of the person rather than the disease, and she called them "the ultimate in preventive medicine."[10] Deciding whether to have an abortion is often a difficult decision for a woman, but it is complicated by several aspects of genetic disorder detection. For example, some doctors refuse to do amniocenteses unless the woman is willing to commit herself, before the test is done, to an abortion in case a defective fetus is found.[11] The NIH "consensus-developing" Task Force on Predictors of Hereditary Disease or Congenital Defects recommended against requiring prior commitment to abortion, but there is no mechanism for enforcing their recommendation. Also, the results of amniocenteses can be known only late in pregnancy, often after a mother feels fetal movement. Abortion after quickening is often more depressing than abortion accomplished earlier in pregnancy. The incidence of severe depression following elective abortion for genetic reasons is so great that "it may be more difficult to deal with than either an abortion of 'convenience' or a stillbirth at term,"[12] or perhaps even more difficult than bearing and rearing a defective child.[13] A third problem is that with some kinds of disorders women can be fairly confident that they are aborting a defective fetus. In other cases, as with X-linked disorders, a woman has to make a decision for or against abortion knowing that the chances of her fetus becoming an affected child are only fifty-fifty. While diagnosis may be fairly safe and very accurate, the alternatives following a positive finding are not ideal, even in the eyes of practitioners.

The impact of amniocentesis has not been thoroughly assessed. We do know the following, however. Each year more than 100,000 infants, 3 to 5 percent of all births, are born with a congenital malformation, a genetic disorder, or a chromosomal abnormality. About one-fifth of all infant deaths are due to these problems. More than 25 percent of hospital admissions of infants one to eighteen days of age are for conditions of genetic origin.[14] In the United States, the 15,000 amniocenteses done each year detect 665 "abnormal" fetuses, including male babies which have a 50 percent chance of having an X-linked disorder.[15] Those 665 fetuses include only about 150 of the 2,500 or more children born with Down's syndrome in the United States each year. The NIH task force concluded that if the availability of the technology could be increased and physicians and the public educated about the benefits of amniocentesis, "a significant reduction in the incidence of selected hereditary diseases and congenital defects might be realized."[16]

Cost-benefit analyses for diagnosis and abortion of mongoloid fetuses[17] and those with Tay-Sachs disease[18] have been done. Economists estimate the cost of detecting one mongoloid child through a well-designed program would be $35,000 (in 1974) and the savings due to preventing the birth would be $65,000 or more. Active, aggressive community screening for Tay-Sachs disease results in benefits outweighing costs by as much as ten-to-one, while simply having a screening service available in communities at risk still brings a benefit-cost ratio of more than two-to-one. But cost-benefit analysis is notorious for collapsing "the human factor" into economic terms and has done little to deter others from mounting competing analyses emphasizing different dimensions of the issue.

While amniocentesis offers the individual the opportunity to learn about her unborn child, genetic screening programs offer the opportunity to know the extent of hereditary disorders in populations and to identify individual carriers of genetic disorders. Several kinds of screening programs exist. Phenylketonuria (PKU) is an inborn error of metabolism that can be detected only by a postnatal screening program. Children with PKU are severely retarded and suffer convulsions. The progress of the disease usually can be retarded by restricting the dietary intake of the amino acid phenylalanine, although phenylalanine cannot be eliminated entirely from the diet since it is ubiquitous. In the 1960s and early 1970s, forty-three states passed laws requiring postnatal testing for PKU. Bessman and Swaezy[19] have shown how PKU legislation was the result of several interested parties mounting campaigns for the widespread adoption of screening legislation. Despite Bessman and Swaezy's and others' criticism of mandatory screening, some states regard screening as so important that they have passed legislation which enables the implementation of screening for any condition that might result in neonatal deficiency. Postnatal screening has clearly benefited from a bandwagon effect,[20] being driven along by a concern over retardation, the concern that has driven much of obstetrics from its earliest days.

Some chromosome abnormality screening programs exist, but systematic programs to screen for chromosome anomalies are primarily limited research efforts. In the mid-1970s, for example, considerable attention was directed to screening for XYY trisomies after it was noted that high percentages of institutionalized and incarcerated populations had the XYY triploid.[21] Chromosome screening of "at risk" populations as for trisomy 21 (mongolism) are not mandatory as yet and the degree of their organization across the country varies.

Carrier screening programs are the logical culmination of the screening movement. Carrier screening seeks not the person who is or might be afflicted with a disease but the person who might pass on a predisposing gene. Two carrier screening programs have attracted considerable attention: Tay-Sachs screening and sickle cell anemia screening.

Tay-Sachs is a horribly degenerative disease that kills affected children usually before they reach the age of five. It occurs primarily among Jews of eastern European origin. A simple, inexpensive test can detect the heterozygotic carrier and, based on probabilities of genetic combinations as discussed above, reproductive decisions can be made. Where Tay-Sachs screening programs have been deployed, community acceptance has been good and the utility of the programs has been unquestioned.

Sickle cell anemia is a disease which kills about half of its victims before they reach the age of twenty, but many people with the disease live much longer. About one in every twelve black Americans carries a recessive gene for the disease and about one in six hundred black babies is born with the disorder. The disease is *not,* however, limited to the black population, although the incidence among whites is about one one-hundredth of the incidence among blacks. Carriers can be detected, but unlike with Tay-Sachs disease, there is no way of improving one's estimate of the probability that a given fetus is affected. Couples may choose only to conceive or not. Screening programs clearly have effects on peoples' decisions about marriage,[22] and probably influence a couple's sexual activity.[23] And at one time the National Academy of Science joined others in recommending that blacks be screened prior to being allowed to enter military service.[24] Sickle cell screening has been met with cries of outrage and accusations of genocide. At the very least it can be said that efforts to implement widespread screening have been motivated by a liberal political desire to do something "good" but inexpensive for black Americans without regard for the cultural and even medical implications of such programs.[25]

In addition to providing information to individuals, screening programs are attractive to medical researchers. Only by mass screening programs can rare diseases be detected early enough so that medicine can study their "natural history" and perhaps devise therapeutic interventions.[26] Whether the law will permit mass screening programs for the many disorders that can be detected remains a question; that we have the capability to conduct large screening programs relatively inexpensively is no longer in doubt.[27]

Medical genetics, which is clearly an extension of the monitoring concept, traces the causality of disease processes back to their subcellular origins, extending the medical gaze into a woman's cells, into the cells of her unborn child, and back through her and her husband's family pedigrees. Interestingly, medical genetics offers a new synthesis of the normal and abnormal distinction which was destroyed by monitoring. Geneticists inform us that everyone carries three to five abnormal genes and that this is a completely "natural state of affairs."[28] So, under genetics, everyone is normal and everyone is abnormal, normality and abnormality are conjoined and old distinctions are entirely obliterated. At the level of social action, screening programs change the posture of the doctor toward disease. The doctor need not wait for the patient to seek help as traditional physicians did; physicians now actively seek out disease, and the rarer the condition for which screening is implemented the farther afield is the medical net cast.[29] The presumed voluntary character of the medical encounter is eroded by screening and the physician's orientation is changed from treating incapacitated individuals to active study of the ecology.

Reflexively, medical genetics exerts its own form of control over health professionals. Equal in importance to a "monitoring and surveillance program . . . to measure . . . technology utilization [in genetics], and to monitor the degree of reduction in birth incidence of infants with specific hereditary disorders and congenital defects" is a program of "quality control assessment of all laboratory facilities at regular intervals, and for the rapid dissemination of new and innovative procedures and knowledge." Equal in importance to programs to educate the public about genetics and the advantages of screening are programs to change the doctor's orientation from one which is illness-responsive to one which emphasizes prevention.[30] Genetics looks inwards to the medical encounter and advises physicians to learn the subtleties involved in being an effective genetic counselor or to turn their patients over to a well-qualified person.[31]

Medical genetics blurs divisions of labor even further by incorporating ancillary laboratory personnel, the geneticist, and genetic counselor into the "medical team." Some people suggest the need to develop a "team ethic" and to provide effective team models in medical school curricula dealing with genetics.[32] Even the sociologist is trying to become a member of the genetic team as he notes the possible social and psychological issues involved in screening and shows how he can help insure that "the benefits offered by screening [are] realized and any unintended consequences worked through" and why "all concerned must expect to adjust their views and expectations in response to biomedical innovation."[33] Even the patient becomes part of the team,[34] being called upon to make decisions that would have been made only by doctors in the past. (This is a topic taken up in detail below and in the following sections.) Genetics demands that training and accreditation programs for counselors be expanded and overseen by professional organizations such as the American Society of Human Genetics. Training programs for laboratory personnel are likely to be centralized under government control.[35] All of these are aspects of genetics' reflexive influence on medicine.

Finally, just as with monitoring generally, medical genetics is justifying its progress with positive reasons for its work. Advances are made in the name of extending health, not in the name of confining and combating disease. Genetic screening is identified with preventive medicine[36] and public health.[37] "Such programs rest on the rationale that an anticipation of disease is itself desirable because it allows identification of a population at high risk for later disability. . . . While screening may have begun as a mechanism for detecting, isolating, and treating the sick, it may in the future be directed toward the identification and preservation of health."[38] The control exerted by genetics is not heavy-handed. Screening programs do not restrict one's freedom of choice; they merely offer the possibility of making informed choices. Informed choice, knowing what it is possible to know—not control or restraint—is the rationale for extending the obstetrical gaze to intracellular structures and into the preconceptional period of a woman's life. The expansion of the obstetrical gaze, a new synthesis of the concepts of normal and abnormal, and reflexive controls on medicine, all for "good" reasons, make medical genetics an important part of the deployment of the monitoring concept and the extension of obstetrical control.

Advances in genetics improve screening capabilities and provide more information about certain diseases; newborn intensive care provides an array of therapeutic interventions in disease processes and a wide spectrum of supportive care. Any review of advances in perinatal care is bound to be inadequate and out of date by the time it is published, but consider the nature of some of the major developments in neonatology over the past two decades.

Respiration. Respiratory problems in the newborn period account for a great percentage of neonatal deaths. Physicians now have techniques for intervening in respiratory processes before as well as after birth.

Premature infants often suffer from atelectasis, an inability to expand the lungs easily. The problem is caused by a lack of surfactant, medical shorthand for "surface acting agent," a compound secreted by the lungs which acts like soap to reduce the surface tension of the water in the lungs. It is water in the lungs unaffected by surfactant that makes lung expansion difficult. Initially, physicians treated this disorder by a rather simple respiratorlike device that keeps "continuous positive airway pressure" (CPAP) in a newborn's lungs even while the infant expires air. If positive pressure is kept in a newborn's lungs, the infant does not have to work as hard as he or she would otherwise to expand the lungs for each breath. Thus, an infant's energy stores are not depleted as rapidly as when he or she has to work against the surface tension of the water in the lungs. With maturity the lungs' secretion of surfactant increases, the water tension decreases, and the child can breathe normally. More recently, neonatologists have found that they can induce surfactant production by the fetal lung with a drug, betamethasone, given to the mother prior to delivery. If a premature delivery is imminent and prenatal tests done on fluid taken by amniocentesis show that the fetal lungs are not producing enough surfactant to prevent atelectasis, delivery can be delayed pharmacologically and the mother given two injections of betamethasone twenty-four hours apart. An infant born after this therapy has its chances of suffering respiratory distress syndrome reduced by 90 percent.

(It is interesting to see how these interventions, particularly the betamethasone therapy, change the meaning of a term like "prematurity." Previously, prematurity was defined by gestational age; prematurity was time-dependent. Now, it is not the infant who is premature; it is the infant's lungs. Just as "normal" and "abnormal" lose their meanings and merge as the processes they described become better understood, prematurity loses its meaning as the biophysical "causes" of the specific problems of premature neonates are better understood.)

Understanding "normal respiratory processes" permits the design of aggressive corrective interventions in deviations from the normal, natural course of physiological processes. Similarly, understanding the course of pathological processes permits appropriate, more studied interventions in their course. For example, about 4 percent of all babies suck into their lungs meconium, the abrasive, tarlike substance that accumulates in the fetus's colon and is expelled in utero in about 8 percent of all births. Studying the normal course of meconium aspiration syndrome, physicians found that the meconium gradually works its way to the periphery of the lungs, creating an often fatal condition. Once this natural course of the disease process was known, it became evident that aggressive resuscitative efforts at birth might, in fact, cause the meconium to start its insidious diffusion throughout the lungs. Now, obstetricians withhold aggressive resuscitation and delay an infant's first breath until the meconium an infant has aspirated can be suctioned from the respiratory tract.

Nutrition. "A clearer understanding of the relation between nutrition and cellular growth has been brought about by . . . elegant animal studies and . . . clinical correlations in humans."[39] Feeding the sick newborn infant—maintaining it and more importantly, getting it to grow—is the field that has seen some of the most remarkable advances in the last fifteen years. In 1968, a surgeon found that a solution containing amino acids, vitamins, minerals, and sugars could completely support patients who could not eat.[40] Hyperalimentation, as this therapy is called, is remarkable but it does not supply the small infant with enough calories for proper growth over very long periods of time. This final problem in nutrition was solved by the development of intravenous lipid (fat) infusions. The United States government delayed clinical trials of intralipids for a long time even though they were part of medicine's therapeutic repertoire in Europe for some time. Now, total parenteral nutrition[41]—hyperalimentation together with intralipid infusion—is a standard part of care in intensive-care nurseries.

Metabolism. For those inborn errors of metabolism not detected in utero, there is "an awareness, relatively recently acquired, that many [of these errors] are manifest as distinct and recognizable biochemical abnormalities in a newborn infant who is *entirely normal clinically*. Thus, timely treatment can prevent clinical manifestation from ever occurring in a number of these disorders."[42] The concept of screening, so important in genetics, is incorporated into neonatal medicine and brings more and more infants under medical surveillance. Screening for biochemical disorders extends medicine's gaze to the intracellular aspects of pathological processes where predispositions to illness can be detected and perhaps corrected.

Surgery. Surgery for infants has made considerable advances over the past twenty years. Neural tube defects can be corrected, although correction requires many operations and rarely restores an infant to a high functional level. Plastic surgery can attenuate the impact of many congenital defects. Gastrointestinal surgery is commonplace now that nutrition can be maintained parenterally. Infant heart surgery to close an opening between major heart vessels that sometimes remains open after birth can now be done in the nursery instead of the operating room. Recently, there have appeared isolated reports of intrauterine surgery to correct fetal defects.

One must add a note about pediatric surgery. Surgery is often regarded as an unfortunate necessity, one that would be eliminated by adequate understanding of the process leading to a given disability. The ideal in medicine has always been to develop "physiologic" treatments, treatments which mimic the natural course of a process. Thus, medicine speaks of its desire to correct genetic anomalies in utero instead of relying on corrective surgery after birth. In the case of some neonatal heart defects, researchers have developed drug therapies to mimic or augment physiological processes that usually occur without intervention. Thus, today, some infant heart defects can be closed pharmacologically that only a few years ago had to be closed surgically. The dream of modern medicine is corrective intervention without unnecessary invasion—the implementation of power from a distance.

Advances in perinatology extend beyond birth the control embedded in monitoring. When an infant deviates from the natural course of events, therapies exist for putting the organism back on that course. Control is no longer exerted strictly through diagnosis, labeling, and dramatic intervention, however. Control is exerted through the sorting function of screening programs, through monitoring every aspect of birth, and through precise corrective therapy. These two extensions of monitoring, genetics and newborn intensive care, are the aspects of obstetrics around which the most intense ethical debates have developed. It is tempting to attribute increased ethical concern to technological advances, but, as the next sections show, understanding ethical debates as the result of a technological imperative is inappropriate.

Ethical Discourse

The dimensionality of ethical discourse is surprisingly small. Consideration of a single case provides an overview of those dimensions.

The now-famous "Johns Hopkins"[43] case involved a Down's syndrome child born with a duodenal atresia, an easily corrected obstruction between the stomach and the small intestine. The physicians informed the child's parents of the problems and sought their permission to operate on the gastrointestinal obstruction. The parents refused to grant permission for the operation. The child died of starvation in the hospital after fifteen days. The basic ethical question is always "What should one do?" In this case, what should the doctors have done? Or, did the parents act ethically in deciding as they did? The basic ethical question of appropriate action is always prefaced by the question of agency: Who decides? This is the first dimension of ethical discourse. In this case, should the parents be able to make the decision they did? Or should doctors decide? Or perhaps a committee? Lurking behind questions of agency are questions of criteria and certitude, two more dimensions of ethical discourse: On what basis is the case to be decided and how certain are we of the consequences of acting or not acting? In this case, the ethicist might raise the question of the criteria of personhood: Is the being in question a person? At what point or by what criteria do we attribute personhood and treat a being as if it were a person? Also, the ethicist would ask, How certain is the diagnosis? What probabilities are attached to what outcomes for various courses of action? In this case it was certain the child was mongoloid. Lack of surgical treatment for the atresia made it certain the child would die if other forms of nutrition were withheld, but just how long it would take for the child to die was uncertain. Another uncertainty was what the infant might have become if surgery had been permitted. It might have lived many years with a subnormal IQ and have been a loving child, well-integrated into the family unit despite the parents' expectations to the contrary. It might have had an IQ below 20, not ever have shown signs of self-consciousness or demonstrated typical patterns of human interaction. Assigning probabilities to outcomes like these is impossible at childbirth, and this complicates the decision.

Beyond problems of action, agency, criteria, and certitude, there are questions concerning consequences. If no surgery was done, the child would die, but who should bear the burden of his death? In this case, leaving the child in the hospital subjected most of the staff to the enormous emotional burden of treating a child in a way they found abhorrent to their own views of right and wrong and in a way that conflicted with their training as health professionals. Should they have to bear the consequences of the parents' decision, or should the child be sent home, so the parents would have to live with the slow death that was the result of their own decision not to permit the surgery? Beyond implications for the immediate situation lie questions of the consequences for other cases of adopting a particular course of action in a particular case. Does this decision set one on a "slippery slope" where the line for choosing nontreatment instead of treatment keeps slipping into other situations which, considered individually, might be decided one way, but, considered in the light of precedents, might be decided another way?

A final dimension of ethical discourse is concern over crucial distinctions in formulating descriptions of medical actions. Thus, questions about the difference between active and passive euthanasia or ordinary and extraordinary care appear in ethical discourse. In the example above is "letting die" different from "killing"? Do the circumstances of the case convert the surgery required from ordinary surgery, as it would be considered in other circumstances, into extraordinary surgery?

Ethics as a discipline revels in the many possible permutations of problems of appropriate action, agency, criteria, certitude, consequences, and crucial distinctions in descriptions of action.[44] Articles on ethics are filled with question marks following the ethical thrust in the unusual case that exposes the dilemmas and value conflicts of modern medicine. But, at its heart, ethical discourse is limited to these few dimensions.

Ethical and Medical Discourse:
Conflict and Cooperation

The modes of discourse in ethics and medicine are remarkably similar. Both tend to work inductively from the "case" to general principles and systems of knowledge rather than the other way around. The importance of learning from the difficult case in medicine, especially when one's actions are seen in retrospect to have been wrong, has been documented by Bosk and by Arluke,[45] and the importance of the case-study method of medical education is apparent in any medical journal or text. Similarly in ethics the case is paramount. The ethicist is typically concerned with those cases where one's sense of right and wrong is inadequate, or with the case which exposes inconsistencies or conflicts in one's system of values. A system of ethics is analogous to medicine's texts on physiology and anatomy; it represents the accumulated wisdom of the discipline which can be used to formulate action, although it does not necessarily dictate action itself. In all these respects medical discourse and ethical discourse are similar.

Medical and ethical discourse are brought together by medicine's new understanding of childbirth and pregnancy. It is not just the "expansionist quality of [the] technological extension of care"[46] that raises ethical problems; rather it is the expansionist quality of the medical view of pregnancy and childbirth as a process with extensions forwards and backwards through a woman's entire life, inwards to subcellular structures and outwards into the community, that provides an infinite array of nodes for the development of ethical discourse. Medicine sees the incremental steps of pregnancy and birth as an array of points of intervention in deviant processes; ethics sees the incremental steps of pregnancy and birth as an array of points of attachment to other aspects of the social order. Graphical representations of processes, like cervical dilatation over time, are "norms" for medicine; for ethics these same graphs are inappropriate isolations of a single process among many occurring in an ecological context. A medical intervention at one point in the process may correct a deviation from the natural course of the process but, ethics points out, that same intervention will have ramifications throughout layers of systems—emotional, psychological, social, economic, legal, religious, moral—which articulate with the process of pregnancy and birth at precisely the point of intervention. Seeming "goods" at the point of intervention have counterbalancing, somewhat predictable "bads" at other, more distant parts of the world which are related to the process that commands the physician's attention. Ethics does not seek a confrontation with medicine; instead, it "structures" issues and points out all the far-flung yet significant implications of medical practices. K. Danner Clouser, an ethicist who spends most of his professional life in a large medical center and whose colleagues often turn the tables on him by confronting him with the difficult case, asking "What would you do?" says this about ethics:

> We are not calling on some special sense of morality, but only on the principles or moral rules that we ordinarily acknowledge in everyday life.
> Furthermore, the reasoning about medical-ethical issues proceeds much as is already familiar to you in everyday circumstances. What do you do? Suppose you genuinely wonder if a particular action is moral. If the action occurs in a context laden with many variables, pressures and causal chains, you try to sort out all the strands of argument, and all the contingent conditions. . . . You figure out the implications of the action with the best probabilities you can—who will be hurt, how badly, which moral rules will be broken, and who will benefit. And ultimately you try to balance all this out, to determine the best action or the least immoral action you can do in the circumstances.
> "Structuring" the issues is an analytic dissection. It is a road map of the issue, showing routes, relations, functions, shortcuts, and central and peripheral locations. It shows where various arguments and actions lead, what facts would be relevant, what concepts are crucial, and what moral principles are at issue and probably in conflict.[47]

Although ethics does not actively seek a confrontation with medicine it is easy to see why they would come into conflict. Medicine would like to see the patient as an amalgam of known processes to be kept on course by selective intervention. Ethics sees the patient as a set of known processes which articulate with other structures and processes, all of which must be considered *before* an intervention is effected. Ethics insists that the physician not consider the patient in isolation. This principle puts medicine and ethics squarely in conflict with one another.

How does medicine experience this conflict? First, we must grasp the counterintuitive notion that medicine, under monitoring, feels that its range of therapeutic options has been limited. In the words of one analyst, "there may be an inverse relation between scientific, technologic medicine and freedom of therapeutic choice."[48] Scientific advances actually constrain one's range of action. By reconceptualizing pregnancy as a process, for example, monitoring provides more and more points of intervention and thus the possibility of having more and more treatment regimens, but monitoring also limits therapeutic options. If the physician has a chart of the natural course of a process—the partograph of cervical dilatation, for example—and his system of monitoring detects a deviation from that course, he must intervene in a way that will restore the process to its proper, natural trajectory designated by the graph. In this, the modern physician has no choice. He is compelled to it by monitoring. If he fails to do his duty, the record will make his failure evident. The patient's chart will testify to anyone who will read it that the patient's processes deviated from their proper course and the physician failed to do his work. By focusing attention on ever smaller increments of processes and by making treatments lighter, simpler, more precise, more efficient, more "physiologic," monitoring makes the ramifications of a given treatment regimen more peripheral to the medical project, more difficult to appreciate, and therefore more difficult to take into consideration when making medical decisions. When a cesarean-section operation meant utter disruption and perhaps destruction of the family unit, it was impossible not to consider the social ramifications of intervention. They thrust themselves in the physician's face. Today, cesarean section is well-integrated into the structure of monitoring; it is not terribly disruptive. A cesarean section can be "family-centered." Considering the broader social, economic, and perhaps even political ramifications of performing a cesarean delivery is more difficult.[49] The therapeutic option—the therapeutic freedom—of *not* keeping processes on their natural courses is not available when there are so many simple, safe ways to do so.

Medicine is torn between the physiological processes which it understands in much greater detail than ever before and which are much more easily sustained than ever before and the imperative of the ecological perspective that it pay attention to the ecological order as a whole. Ethics forces medicine down on the horns of its dilemma and medicine becomes a "double agent,"[50] an advocate for the patient on the one hand and an advocate of competing interests on the other hand. The modern physician is torn between his commitment to contribute to the knowledge base of his profession and his obligations to his patient. He may become a therapy's advocate instead of the patient's advocate. One person said that the demands of research in new fields like perinatology "set in motion a subtle, unintended, slide from patient-physician to subject-investigator styles of relation."[51] The physician also experiences the potential conflict of acting in the interest of his patient, a baby or fetus, at the same time that he must consider the child's (or fetus's) parents and family. "For whom does the doctor work?" is a question the physician must face and which often subjects him to agonizing cross-pressures. Furthermore, the physician finds himself making decisions in an economy of scarcity. Does the doctor serve his patient or the Professional Service Review Organization (PSRO) or, more recently, the Health System Agency (HSA) in the efforts of these organizations to contain costs? The constraints of the economy make rationing of medical services, a task "never before explicitly faced by medicine, except in classic triage," inevitable.[52] All of these cross-pressures result from medicine's adoption of an ecological perspective.

Even though medical reasoning and ethical reasoning often conflict, both disciplines share the goal of achieving harmony in the ecological system, and so there is a basis for cooperation. As ethicists put it, "what makes us call a judgment 'ethical' is the fact that it is used to *harmonize* people's actions," or "the object of ethics is a harmonious and just society."[53] A language of right is not a language of liberation but an "instrument of domination." Foucault says one intention of his work is to show how "right (not simply the laws but the whole complex of apparatuses, institutions and regulations responsible for their application) transmits and puts into motion relations that are not relations of sovereignty but of domination."[54] Ethics—a discourse on right—is an implement of power. It is a social device used to achieve harmony.

Ethics will harmonize the social system surrounding medicine by offering new freedom of therapeutic choice, by offering a counterpoint to the demands of monitoring. Ethics suggests that a physician may be permitted to consider peripheral ramifications of his actions and interventions and, when it seems appropriate, to accede to the

dictates of peripheral considerations and exercise therapeutic choice—
"the selection of a mode of treatment (or non-treatment) that accords
best with a realistic assessment . . . of the patient's present capabilities and future possibilities"[55]—even if such accession is inimical
to the physiological processes which traditionally had first call on
the physician's work.

Although ethical reasoning may not be any sort of special reasoning ethicists still insist that it cannot be done casually. Thus the
ethicist is insisting that he must be made part of the medical team.
Clouser, for example, is deliberate in his approach to medicine.
Noting that some people say ethics "is just a matter of his values
against mine [and] anyone's opinion is just as good as anyone else's,"
he declares that "there are better ways and worse ways to accomplish [the] harmonizing task. . . . One opinion is simply not as useful
to that end as another." He says, "Everyone is needed and each
must listen to the other."[56] Daniel Callahan agrees:

> The physician's insights and experience are as much needed
> as the philosopher's theories and constructs (and vice versa!).
> Neither can proceed well without the other, and if any wisdom
> is to be gained it will represent a shared wisdom, to which each
> has made a contribution.[57]

Medicine seems interested in the assistance ethics can provide and
has sought to resolve the conflict between itself and ethics to the
benefit of both parties.

Ethics and Medicine:
The Negotiations

During the 1970s medicine and ethics were involved in negotiations
to resolve the differences between them. While not resolved yet, the
give-and-take between medicine and ethics has refashioned some of
the basic elements of the medical encounter. In particular, the "patient" is different today because of these negotiations.

Ethics' first and unalterable position, as outlined previously, is
that medicine must pay attention to the broader implications of its
work. A 1974 conference on "critical issues in newborn intensive
care" tried to exclude major social, political, and economic dimensions of care in attempting to formulate an ethical position on neonatal intensive care, but the participants found that such issues had

to be considered because "they always lurk in the background."[58] Ethics compels medicine to acknowledge and act in cognizance of its social position. On the claim that medicine is not an isolated social entity, ethics will not compromise.

Medicine's first response to ethics' fundamental assertion was reactionary. In the early 1970s, medicine tried to isolate itself and not acknowledge the social aspects of its work. In one of the first major reviews of prenatal diagnostic capabilities, Milunsky and his colleagues urged physicians to remain impartial in genetic counseling. They said, "Our present responsibility is to establish safe technics and reliable data, which can then provide the required sound basis for legal, governmental, theologic, and other considerations."[59] The physician should seek to serve everyone without making judgments and decisions of value. Some practitioners echoed this sentiment saying, "Some new kind of physician will have to be developed if the societal imperatives are to take first place [over obligations to the individual]. As a practitioner, I hope that this kind of physician will never be necessary nor even desirable," and "I shall leave it to a separate advocate of the state to rank my patients according to their worthiness to receive care."[60]

Isolationism was intolerable, of course, for it meant giving up authority in order to maintain an autonomy that most physicians admitted was a fiction anyway. The task for medicine was to be responsive to ethics' concerns and at the same time preserve its position of relative privilege and its capacity to decide care. Dr. Franz J. Inglefinger, outspoken editor of the *New England Journal of Medicine,* devoted several editorials to the medical imperative that the doctor remain firmly in his position of decision-maker regardless of how difficult the decisions might be. Inglefinger had no time for those who suggested that anyone but the physician should make decisions concerning care. To the question, "Who decides care for the critically ill child?" his answer was unequivocal:

> The answer is "you"—you the child's doctor, for who else is in a similarly pivotal position to make sure that the proper medical consultation has been obtained in ascertaining the hopeless condition of the patient, that the parents receive sympathetic and thorough explanation, and that they are exposed to broadly based advice? Who else can lead all those involved to a decision, and who else is more responsible for consoling after a decision has been reached? Society, ethics,

institutional attitudes and committees can provide the broad guidelines, but the onus of decision making ultimately falls on the doctor in whose care the child has been put.

Inglefinger saw attempts to "de-mysticize and debase the status of the physician" as "compromising this ability to provide leadership (not exercise dictatorship!) when health and life are at stake—a function that may be the most important service that the physician renders to society."[61]

Rather than endorse an isolationist view of the profession which would require that others make the difficult decisions about care, Inglefinger endorsed the position advanced by the ethicist Paul Ramsey. Ramsey urged the profession to develop an internal solution to the challenge of moral dilemmas. He said,

> Increasingly, the medical profession—if it moves from a strictly medical to a more extensive definition of health—would have to find the sources of its medical ethics not in the culture generally but by developing within its own community a moral ethos representative of mankind's general well-being.[62]

Ramsey urged the profession to develop a new understanding of the doctor-patient relationship, one which saw doctor and patient as "joint adventurers in medical care and progress, . . . in the moral history of mankind, in the exigencies of a covenant or fiduciary relation of man with man in which they resolve to live faithfully even while not knowing the future outcome."[63]

An internal solution would increase the freedom of therapeutic choice. It would allow the physician to turn his attention from, in Inglefinger's terms, "electron-transport chains and enzymatic sequences (and often defective ones at that!)" to the "physical, intellectual, emotional, and social ingredients that make up human existence."[64] In short, an internal solution would allow medicine to be responsive to the demands of an ecological perspective, and simultaneously maintain its position of authority. From this general position medicine began to work out the specifics of an internal solution.

The first form of internal solution proposed in medicine was the creation of lists of criteria for determining appropriate care in ambiguous situations. Dr. John Lorber bemoaned the fact that in the mid-1970s there was no satisfactory treatment for infants born with spinal cord defects and the fact that some infants continue to be born with such defects despite medicine's ability to detect them in utero.[65] In response, Lorber proposed a list of criteria for deciding which infants born with myelomeningocele were to be given active treatment and which were not to be treated. His criteria were strictly medical:

> Infants who have any one or any combination [sic] of the following should not be given active treatment, but should be given normal nursing care, together with symptomatic treatment to avoid pain, discomfort, or fits. These criteria are: (1) gross paralysis of the legs. . . ; (2) thoracolumbar or thoracolumbarsacral lesions related to vertebral levels; (3) kyphosis or scoliosis; (4) grossly enlarged head. . . ; (5) intracerebral birth injury; (6) other gross congenital defects—for example, cyanotic heart disease, ectopia of bladder, and mongolism.[66]

Selection according to these criteria, he said, caused most infants to die before one month of age, although some lived for up to nine months.

Lists of treatment criteria such as Lorber's would have constituted an adequate solution to medicine's problem of social exposure, especially if a degree of consensus about the lists could have been developed in the profession. They would have allowed the physician greater freedom of therapeutic choice since he could decide not to treat in some cases and since the lists would have provided the physician the backing of a moral community if any particular decision had been challenged.

Lists of selection criteria have serious problems, though. It is often difficult to achieve consensus over any particular list. For example, Rosalyn Darling, a sociologist who studied the effects on their families of children with spinal defects, criticized Lorber's criteria because they imposed the physician's understanding of the quality of life on parents who must, after all, live with the deformed child. She suggested adding social criteria to Lorber's list but warned, "*no* pre-established criteria can adequately suggest the emergent, interactional nature of 'adjustment': parents typically learn to value and love their children as they live with them."[67] Another author, an ethicist, proposed "the potential for human relationships" as the guideline for treating or not treating but cautioned physicians not to run off and draw up scales of relational potential, for "relational capacity is not subject to mathematical analysis but to human judgment."[68]

Ethicists generally see criteria lists as, at best, unfortunate and, at worst, perverse. Robert Veatch, writing specifically about Lorber's criteria said:

We may become so infatuated with our technical abilities to accumulate data and tally scores that we run the risk of seriously misunderstanding the nature of the difficult decisions that must be made. We may succumb to what might be called the "technical criteria fallacy."

It is not the precise content of the list which is important. Rather it is the concept that *any* list of objectively measurable criteria can be translated directly into decisions about selection for treatment or nontreatment. . . .

When Lorber uses the phrase "contraindications to active therapy," he is medicalizing what are really value decisions.[69]

Ethicists will not let physicians simplify their situation by reducing it to a technical problem. They insist on making the value content and the social implications of medicine's practice available for discussion.

Disapproving such criteria lists was ethics' first response to medicine's first form of internal solution. However, by turning down this particular "ethical solution" to the internal tensions of medicine, ethics may have done medicine a favor. For while criteria lists may increase therapeutic freedom and bring greater harmony to the practice of medicine by making difficult choices easier, accepting concrete lists of treatment criteria could extend the system of surveillance which reflexively controls medical practitioners. The decisions of the doctor could be checked more easily if there were public, consensually endorsed lists of criteria for making difficult decisions. The physician might choose not to treat, but he would have to make that decision through the same restricted form of scientistic reasoning that he had had to use in deciding in favor of treatment.

The second solution proposed by medicine was legislative reform. There are two types of legislative solutions to the tensions experienced by medicine: changes in the public law governing medical practice[70] and declarations of medical ethics made by professional organizations which have, in their turn, an indirect effect on the law.

Duff and Campbell, whom most credit with "breaking the ice" on public discussion of ethical dilemmas in medicine by publishing a 1973 paper describing deaths caused by withholding treatment in an intensive care nursery, followed the first course. They argued for wide legal latitude in dealing with seriously ill or defective newborns. They concluded their article by saying, "If working out these dilemmas [of care] in ways such as those we suggest is in violation of the law, we believe the law should be changed."[71] Even if changes in laws do not necessarily make a practice ethical, legal reform at least clarifies the physician's duty and provides a degree of protection if he follows the dictates of the law. This is the advantage of a California law which clarified the legal status of a fetus born alive after an intended abortion by stipulating that a physician must make efforts to save the infant's life. Direct legal reforms like this one can relieve some of the tension in medicine.

Beyond direct action in the legal realm, medicine exerts an indirect effect on law by publishing statements of medical ethics. The American Medical Association's House of Delegates, for example, passed the following statement on euthanasia, one of the issues raised by developments in neonatal intensive care:

> The intentional termination of life of one human being by another—mercy killing—is contrary to that for which the medical profession stands and is contrary to the policy of the American Medical Association.
> The cessation of the employment of extraordinary means to prolong the life of the body when there is irrefutable evidence that biological death is imminent is the decision of the patient and/or his immediate family. The advice and judgment of the physician should be freely available to the patient and/or his immediate family.[72]

Thus there is, according to the AMA, a crucial difference between active and passive euthanasia, the former being unethical and the latter ethical. The AMA's position satisfies the requirements for a politically effective solution to medicine's problems by allowing the doctor therapeutic latitude based on a consideration of higher motives than the sustenance of bodily processes.

On the face of it, either a direct or indirect legislative solution is appealing. Legislative solutions fail, though, because they leave the ethical quandaries of most physicians unresolved even once legal responsibility is clarified. For example, the AMA's statement makes a distinction between death caused by action and death caused by inaction (by withholding therapy). But James Rachels, an ethicist, points out that withholding treatment may cause more suffering than a quick, lethal injection. He asks whether this is a distinction physicians ought to be asked to make. In condemning the AMA's attempt to distinguish between active and passive euthanasia, he says, "whereas doctors may have to discriminate between [the two] to satisfy the law, they should not do any more than that. In particular, they should not give the distinction any added authority and weight by writing it into official statements of medical ethics."[73] Dr. John Freeman, a physician at Johns Hopkins, shares Rachels's views and goes a step further, by suggesting that, after seeing infants with spinal defects selected for nontreatment linger on, "one cannot help but feel that the highest form of medical ethic would have been to end the pain and suffering, rather than wishing that the patient would go away."[74] Given these problems, legislative solutions have gone the route of criteria lists and are not the preeminent solution to emerge from the medicine-ethics dialogue.

Stanley Hauerwas, a philosopher who insists on an accurate description of a situation before invoking ethical imperatives to direct action, provides an explicit demonstration of the kind of logic needed to move away from legislative solutions and toward more effective social solutions to medicine's problems. Hauerwas argues that making distinctions between active and passive euthanasia, between acting and refraining, is just an emotional salve that helps preserve culturally shared understandings of obligations inherent in our social roles when we face decisions that force us to question the nature of those roles and those obligations. He says,

> We normally think that we do have duties to aid our children beyond our obligations to strangers. To employ the language of refraining to "solve" these neonatal dilemmas amounts to transforming our duty toward our children into the duty we acknowledge to a stranger—namely, non-interference.
> We are drawn to the idea that we are simply refraining to give care because we are concerned to describe our action in a manner congruent with our assumed roles and identities. . . .
> The distinction between acting and refraining, in the context of neonatal dilemmas, is an attempt to defeat certain ascriptions of

responsibility for two extremely significant roles: parents and doctors.[75]

Hauerwas is saying that the linguistic gymnastics of legislative so-lutions are necessary because the obligations that individuals incur, based on the social relations in which they stand to one another, are called into question by the situations faced in modern perinatology. The person who occupies the role "parent" is expected to act to save his or her "child," expending all the resources necessary to do so, because that is the socially ascribed obligation of parent to child. The "doctor" must not act to kill a "patient" because the socially ascribed obligations of doctors to patients demand just the opposite action, vigilant struggle against death. Hauerwas says that human beings tend to cast actions which run counter to their role obligations in terms of nonaction simply to preserve commonsensi-cal socially shared understandings of their roles and their attendant obligations. Legislative solutions that make distinctions between acting and refraining become balms to the consciences of people who are placed in difficult situations and who must act in ways contrary to those prescribed by their roles.

An alternative solution to criteria lists and legislative solutions is implicit in Hauerwas's argument: we must change the relations in which people stand to one another; we must change the roles of "doctor" and "patient" so the old obligations no longer apply. This is exactly what medicine has done and what ethics has endorsed. Medicine has changed the nature of the doctor-patient relationship so that the patient is no longer the individual with an illness seeking care. The patient now is the family constellation, perhaps including the individual with an illness or disability, perhaps not.

Reformulating the doctor-patient relationship is an ideal solution to the dilemmas posed by medical genetics and neonatal intensive care. It increases freedom of therapeutic choice by widening the field which commands the physicians' attention to include consid-eration of the family's interests as well as the (old) patient's interests. "Therapy" that is clearly detrimental to the individual with an illness or to the "potential individual" with potential problems becomes ethically permissible under the reformulation because it can be seen as being in the best interests of the (new) patient, the wider family network. Physicians need not fear accusations of overstepping their bounds of expertise when they consider family dynamics in a medical decision because family dynamics—bonding, divorce, child abuse, and so one—are simply processes that occur inside the space of the "body" of the new patient, the family, in the same way physiological processes occurred inside the physical body of the old patient. Physicians have not only the conceptual apparatus for understanding such social processes, but they claim to have scientifically based expertise in that realm as well, as the chapter on bonding showed.

The new form of patient was proposed relatively early in the medical-ethical dialogue, but it took some time for it to be endorsed and widely accepted. Dr. Raymond Duff, a physician who has ventured outside his discipline on a number of occasions by writing on medical sociology and medical ethics, was the main proponent of the "family as patient" concept. Arguing against prevailing wisdom, Duff and A. G. M. Campbell said that parents *can* understand the long-term implications of serious medical disorders if they "are heard sympathetically and at length and are given information and answers to their questions in words they understand."[76] Not only can they understand the situation, they are the ones who *must* make the difficult decisions:

> We believe the burdens of decision making must be borne by families and their professional advisers because they are most familiar with the respective situations. Since families primarily must live with and are most affected by the decisions, it therefore appears that society and the health professions should provide only general guidelines for decision making.[77]

In two other articles,[78] Duff spelled out the implications of what he calls a "person-oriented" philosophy of deciding care, a philosophy which involves families in the incremental process of "muddling through" to a therapeutic choice. The rent in the doctor-patient relationship caused by the divergent interests and commitments of physicians and parents can be repaired if the physician gives up some degree of control and, for example, "grant[s] patients and families the autonomy to protect the family commons,"[79] the pool of limited resources available to a family which could be easily drained away if a defective fetus were allowed to be born or a critically ill child kept alive. In short, a new order must emerge in which the basis of medical work—a doctor-patient relationship based on trust and cooperation to the exclusion of all antagonistic elements including the law or society at large—is constructed anew.

Some physicians have resisted involving families in difficult decisions,[80] but general sentiment seems to have swung away from defense of the status quo toward the view that parents must be involved. One physician goes even further in this view, arguing that, in cases of severely deformed infants:

> The only persons involved in such situations . . . are the physicians, nurses, parents and siblings of the patient. The child itself (and to make the point more forcefully, I should not even call it a "child") is not a person, and the fundamental error of our ways consists in thinking that it is one.[81]

The physician in this recast role can treat his patient humanely by "easing death" for "human forms" because the human form, previously the patient, has a diminished place in calculations for care.

The individual case takes on renewed importance under this scheme. Thus, Anthony Shaw writes that the philosophy of care appropriate in this era is "one that tries to find a solution, humane and loving, based on the circumstances of each case rather than by means of a dogmatic formula approach."[82] Each case must be located precisely. Committees and review boards, which might undermine the authority of the physician, are excluded from the doctor-patient relationship by this new vision. The physician, and only the physician, knows his patient well enough to judge what a good regimen of care is, and the physician cannot be accused anymore of narrowly biological/physiological interests since the patient is no longer a strictly biological/physiological entity.

Under the new regime, "informed consent" takes on a new meaning. The new "patient" must actively participate in decisions about "its" care. The new type of informed consent is one "that goes far beyond the traditional presentation of complications of surgery, length of hospitalization, cost of the operation, time lost from work, and so on."[83] As a strong, concerned critic of obstetrics put it: "It cannot be hurried, and it cannot be printed up in a form because informed consent is an *exchange* between care-giver and care-receiver."[84] A new form of autonomy can be achieved[85] which will provide a new space within which the physician can still exercise a degree of professional prerogative and control, but which also will provide the physician a degree of protection from unwanted inquiry about the ramifications of his actions at peripheral locations throughout the layers of systems articulated with the physiological processes that used to be his sole concern.

Ethicists have endorsed medicine's reformulation of the patient. In 1979, the genetics research group of the Hastings Center defined the "patient" in genetic screening programs as "the mother of the fetus and, in most cases, the father as well";[86] in the same year, the NIH consensus-development task torce implicitly adopted this view. The new view of the patient also seems to have wide acceptance within perinatology and even outside it.[87]

The new doctor-patient relationship helped reestablish a boundary around the profession of obstetrics. The new boundary encompassed the patient—the family—and made the patient a joint adventurer in the obstetrical project. The boundary protected the profession from the inquiry and scrutiny of committees, ethical review boards, and "society" in general. The space in which obstetricians work was expanded, but with the help of ethics the profession was able to encase the expanded space rather than leaving it open to view. The profession has a new boundary *and* a new partner in the defense of the boundary in ethics. Medicine and ethics have not completely resolved their conflicts nor have they cemented their partnership firmly. A degree of antagonism still remains between the disciplines, but the cooperative, negotiated solution of the inherent conflict solved medicine's most pressing problem by reducing the possibility of criticism from outside the profession.

With the profession more securely bounded, obstetrics could once again turn its attention inward to the organization of the professional space and begin to deal with new internal problems caused by the technical and conceptual developments of the preceding thirty years. Two problems were prominent. First, medicine could offer women or families a position as joint adventurer in the obstetrical project, but nothing guaranteed their acceptance of the offer. How to get women to cooperate, to take a share in the control of childbirth and become a joint adventurer in the preservation of the obstetrical project, became an important issue. The other internal problem for obstetrics stemmed from the development of new specialties and new technologies that monitoring brought with it. New specialties and new technologies threaten to make some physicians *just* team members with limited parts to play rather than to leave all physicians in their traditional post of team leader. How obstetrics solved this problem while simultaneously making women active participants in obstetrical work is the subject of the final chapter.

7 Modern Women and Modern Obstetricians
The Development of a Univocal Discourse

The natural childbirth movement from the 1940s onwards was an organized manifestation of a conflict between women and obstetricians, a conflict that obstetrics had been able to suppress since the formation of the profession in the early part of the century. Obstetricians had captured childbirth and had kept it in their domain for some thirty to fifty years. In focusing exclusively on childbirth, though, obstetrics had forgotten one thing: the woman. While obstetricians directed their attention to the passages, the passenger, and the powers of birth, women were left to themselves, alone and faceless, at the other end of the delivery table. Natural childbirth involved more than just a demand that *birth* be treated differently; it presented a demand that *women* be treated differently. Through natural childbirth women brought a negative meaning to obstetrically managed childbirth and asserted that their experiences of childbirth, their psychology, they themselves, were valuable and valued aspects of birth. The discovery of the fetus in the 1940s might be considered a response to women's assertions, but obstetricians were not just demonstrating their political understanding and their ability to undermine a salient challenge to obstetrical work; they were simply making their orientation and their allegiances known. Obstetricians were there to take care of birth, not the woman. Once women made it clear that

Parts of this chapter appeared in a paper coauthored with Jane Neill, ''The Location of Pain in Childbirth: Natural Childbirth and the Transformation of Obstetrics,'' *Sociology of Health and Illness* 4, no. 1 (March 1982): 1–24.

there were sides to be taken in the obstetrical encounter—the woman or the fetus, the psychosocial or the physiological—obstetricians chose as they had to choose and sided with the fetus.

The relationship between women and obstetricians did not end on this irreconcilable point, though. Obstetrics offered to make women "joint adventurers" in the obstetrical project. In fact, obstetrics embraced natural childbirth almost as quickly as it had embraced its own technical developments in the past. Rather than leading to an all-out war between women and their obstetricians, the confrontation between them led to a surprising conjunction of interests and to some mutually acceptable reforms of obstetrical work.

The continuing language of conflict between modern women and modern obstetricians is, in fact, a univocal discourse. Beneath a thin veneer of belligerence lies one common goal: the development of a flexible system of obstetrical alternatives in which women's enjoyment of the psychosocial and even sexual experience of childbirth is balanced against obstetrical safety.

This chapter is about natural childbirth, and what obstetrics did with women once they became new members of the obstetric team, but the chapter is also about recent developments in the organization of obstetrical care and what obstetrics has done with physicians displaced from their traditional position as leaders of obstetrical team by the deployment of the monitoring concept. One does not usually think that topics like natural childbirth and the regionalization of perinatal services go together, but the regionalization of services and the development of new modes of delivering obstetrical care are practical responses to the demand that a flexible system of obstetrical alternatives be available to women. Neonatal intensive-care nurseries, alternative birthing centers, the revitalization of the midwife, and the discovery and enjoyment of psychosexual aspects of birth are all parts of a single, albeit rather intricate, whole.

Two-Dimensional Childbirth

Natural childbirth was *not,* as the Wertzes claimed, women's attempt to "regain possession of their bodies and of the life they had lost."[1] For in truth women had not lost their lives to obstetricians and, furthermore, they had lost only a small part of their bodies—the region around the uterus, cervix, and vaginal outlet—and that for only a severely delimited period of time in their lives. Women retained their lives, their psychology, and most of their bodies by default. Obstetricians only took control of childbirth. They tamed the savage which they had confronted as they formed their profession and which remained a sublimated threat inside all women, and they did this not by chaining the savage down, but by carefully isolating the obstetrical component of women for a very short, obstetrically appropriate, period and by submerging all other parts of women that threatened interference with obstetrical work beneath a heavy veil of anesthesia or under delivery-table drapes and restraints. By their use of birth position and other technologies of control, obstetricians made the women on the delivery tables faceless so that women's heads—their psychology and their subjective experiences—literally and metaphorically never entered into obstetrical decision-making.

Early obstetricians tacitly recognized that birth was a two-dimensional phenomenon, that women had a psychological side as well as a physical side to their existence. Professional obstetrics, however, did not permit the psychological side of women to interfere with its work since the psychological component of birth had negative obstetrical value. Uncontrolled emotionalism might interfere with obstetrical work that had to be done on the physiological component of birth. Against this position natural childbirth advocates simply asserted that the psychological component of birth had positive value. They insisted, very simply, that a woman had a face, a psychology, and important subjective experiences that deserved to be taken into consideration. Paralleling this simple principle were simple proposals for reform. Grantly Dick-Read, for example, wanted women to give birth in a position which "allows a woman to see and hear her attendant," which "enables her to collaborate with her attendant." He wanted her face to be seen because "her wishes must be considered."[2] The challenge of natural childbirth was simple: that a woman's wishes, her desires, her psychological side, be accorded positive value in the obstetrical encounter—that the obstetrician look the woman in the face.

Grantly Dick-Read, whose book *Childbirth without Fear* first appeared in 1933,[3] argued that the dual dimensions of birth had a reflection in the dual dimensions of pain. He felt that the "mind" side of the mind-body dichotomy had to be resurrected from the depths to which obstetricians had tried to banish it if obstetricians were to understand the experience of pain in childbirth and treat it properly. Pain may have a physiological component but, according to Dick-Read,

> Superstition, civilization, and culture have brought influences to bear upon the minds of women which have introduced justifiable fears and anxieties concerning labor. The more cultured the races of the earth have become, so much more the positive have they been in pronouncing childbirth to be a painful and dangerous ordeal.[4]

Society and culture label childbirth painful and condition women to anticipate pain, and then "fear and anticipation [give] rise to natural protective tensions in the body. . . . Fear inhibits; that is to say, gives rise to resistance at the outlet of the womb." Resistance causes pain because "fear, tension, and pain go hand in hand."[5] The mind, conditioned by culture, thus plays a part in the production of pain.

During the 1950s many people in and out of obstetrics studied the two-dimensional character of pain and refined Dick-Read's notion of pain. If, as he seemed to say, psychology was causally prior to physiology, then reducing fear would break the fear-tension-pain chain and a woman could experience not just "childbirth without fear" but "childbirth without pain." Obstetricians could not believe birth could be painless, so they started asking women what they felt. Work in the 1950s concluded that women "were certainly experiencing pain . . . but they were nevertheless enthusiastic about the regime [of natural childbirth]."[6] This was curious indeed. Physicians wondered how women could give birth using techniques which caused them to experience pain—the old ubiquitous threat to obstetrical work and presumed threat to women's well-being—and still enthusiastically endorse the techniques they used. Physicians concluded, "There is a difference between *feeling* and *minding* pain."[7] Women might experience pain but physicians had to ask a new question: "Can she bear the pain?, Can she cope with it?"[8] A 1957 review of more than a hundred years of research on pain concluded that the experience of pain has two components, the "original sensation" and the "psychic reaction component."[9] Stimuli alone did not *cause* pain, the new view argued. Instead the stimuli had to be processed through the mind and given meaning, either positive or negative. If, but only if, the mind attached a strictly negative meaning to a stimulus would it be experienced as "painful." Otherwise, a stimulus might be experienced as part of an ecstatic experience or as pleasurable, or perhaps not even experienced at all.

The dual dimensionality of pain was so well accepted by the mid-1950s that even critics of natural childbirth had to mount their arguments in terms of the new conceptualization. Drs. Duncan Reid and Mandel Cohen, in a review critical of the research on the obstetrical effects of childbirth education, admitted that two disciplines, "scientific psychology" and "scientific obstetrics," had interests in and contributions to make toward understanding birth. As critics of natural childbirth, though, they claimed "it is not clear whether the 'psychologically based' practices represent good obstetrics," and they tried to assert the greater importance of the obstetrical component of birth over the psychological component.[10] Still, they were compelled to acknowledge that birth had two dimensions. Models of women's birth experiences that appeared in the 1970s crystallized the dual dimensionality of pain. As one study put it, "Pain and enjoyment emerge as two distinct, though related, dimensions of the birth experience. Social-psychological and medical factors are relatively independent of each other."[11]

Two-dimensional childbirth immediately appeared in the antenatal educational literature of the post–World War II period. Hilary Graham[12] has shown how a new romanticism emerged in the antenatal literature of postwar Britain. She found that the physiological, active aspects of birth, like going to one's doctor to be examined, obeying the doctor's orders, following prescribed diets, and doing recommended exercises, were complemented in the 1950s by the appearance of a psychological, passive side of birth. Antenatal literature even used a new medium—photographs—to portray the new, romantic, feminine essence of the state of simply *being* pregnant. Line drawings and cartoons illustrated the active aspects of pregnancy in which the woman does something as an object of medical attention and inquiry. Photographs showed women doing nothing except being pregnant and being ultimately feminine against out-of-focus, brightly lit fields of wheat, pine forests, or other scenes evocative of images of life.

> In photographs, pregnancy appears narcissistic and contemplative . . . and healthy. In drawings, pregnancy is seen as physiological and practical, and the possibility of ill health, although not explicitly spelt out, can be inferred from non-

performance of the antenatal routines that the cartoon figures demonstrate.[13]

The physiological and psychological components were separate, distinct aspects of birth that mirrored the pain and enjoyment of delivery that had their bases in the psychological and physiological dimensions of pain.

One-dimensional pain, pain that is the logical and necessary result of physiological responses to physical stimuli, has significance and meaning only within the spaces of the body. Two-dimensional pain achieves meaning because of its location in the patient's socio-psycho-biochemical ecology. A randomized study of the effectiveness of one approach to prepared childbirth concluded, "the woman's past experiences and present situation influenced her experience of childbirth pain [even more than childbirth education training]. The woman's attitude toward pregnancy and motherhood seemed to be of special importance in this connection."[14] To understand a woman's pain one must know her location in the world, her relationships to everything else. A woman's past experiences and present situation must be assessed in order to know her present location properly. After all, the mind, which now has a role in the experience of pain, articulates with the entire "exoteric cosmos and its ecological processes."[15] The woman's location in her "cosmos"—her relationship to social support, her relationship to her body which is determined in part by her knowledge of bodily functions and physiological processes, her relationship to obstetrical attendants, even her relationships with her mother and father as manifest in her attitudes toward childbirth—determines the significance and meaning of pain and her experience of it. Pain that is situationally determined can be altered by changing the situation, by changing a woman's relationships to everything else. Childbirth education changes a woman's relationship to her body by making the alien sensations of the contracting uterus familiar; the presence of her husband or labor coach at delivery changes her relationship to social supports; delivery at home, where medicine is a guest in the house of woman, rather than in the hospital, where woman is a guest in the house of medicine, changes her relationship to obstetrical attendants. Managing pain by changing a woman's location may even be more economical than the rather brutal regimens of care which treat pain as if it were located strictly within the body, as if it were one-dimensional. The dual dimensionality of childbirth, which had its basis in the dual dimensionality of pain, opened up the possibility that childbirth could be treated differently than obstetricians had treated it since they assumed sovereignty over birth. Opening this possibility was the challenge of natural childbirth in its several forms.

Despite their differences, "natural childbirth" methods followed two basic schools of thought. One school, to which Dick-Read belonged, emphasized the importance of the external world in the generation of fear and ultimately pain. If fear and anxiety resulted from learning, this line of thought suggested, then fear and anxiety could be reduced or eliminated through counteractive education and training, and pain could be eliminated or controlled. This school told women what was going on inside them, what they could expect during labor and delivery, what could go wrong, and what they could reasonably expect to happen if anything did go wrong. Above all, though, natural childbirth emphasized the beauty of birth. Dick-Read waxed biblical in his effort to reinvest childbirth with a positive image. He wrote his philosophy of childbirth, he tells us, "in terms of a belief in God," and said, "We must bring a fuller life to women who are called upon to reproduce our species. The joy of new life must be the vision of motherhood, instead of the fear of death that has clouded it since civilization developed."[16] He explained the problem of contemporary woman in almost mystical terms:

> What manner of thing is this love that leads its most natural and perfect children to the green pastures of all that is beautiful in life, and urges them on by a series of ever increasing delights until their ultimate goal is in sight, then suddenly and without mercy chastises and terrifies them before hurling them unconscious, injured and resentful into the new world of motherhood. I strongly suggest that there is only one answer— this is not the course of the Power of Love. This is not the purposeful design of creation. Somewhere, for some reason, an interloper has crept in, and must be eradicated. Something stands in the way which, through blindness and ignorance in the development of our civilization, has been allowed to grow and impede the natural course of events.[17]

The interloper, of course, was unnatural fear and tension that could be eradicated by replacing them with "physical *and* mental relaxation." Educating women to anticipate the sensations of pregnancy and delivery, training them in techniques of relaxation, and developing a new romanticism about pregnancy, birth, and motherhood all would contribute to relaxation, enabling women to "have their babies and themselves [be] born again."[18]

The second school of thought invoked a much less romantic vision of pregnancy but respected its psychological dimension just the same. The psychoprophylactic school of childbirth education traces its origins to the work of the physiologist Pavlov, who showed that both pain and the inhibition of pain could be made conditional responses in subjects. "Psychoprophylactic" methods of pain relief condition women to inhibit the experience of pain. Exercises teach women to control specific muscle groups as necessary and as called for by her labor coach or obstetrician. Breathing techniques both provide oxygen to tissues and take a woman's mind off the pain of birth. The psychiatrist Platonov was Dick-Read's opposite number in Russia, where obstetrical hypnosis and psychological conditioning were developed first. Platonov fought the resistance of the medical establishment to give his procedures a fair hearing in Russia, just as Dick-Read had to do in England. Through the work of the obstetrician Nicolaiev psychoprophylaxis gained such credibility that hypnotariums were established in Russia for women who wanted to use this new approach to childbirth. Other early advocates of the psychoprophylactic method included the obstetrician Velvovsky in Russia and Fernand Lamaze, Lamaze's student Pierre Vellay, and Leon Chertok in France.[19]

Psychoprophylaxis came to the United States in force with the publication of Majorie Karmel's book *Thank You, Dr. Lamaze: A Mother's Experiences in Painless Childbirth*.[20] Her book described Mrs. Karmel's trips to France and her deliveries under Dr. Lamaze and created an immediate demand for the new techniques in this country. A number of groups formed during the late 1950s and early 1960s to prepare women for natural childbirth and to provide them with *monitrices,* childbirth educators who would act as women's labor coaches. The American Society for Psychoprophylaxis in Obstetrics was among the first groups on the scene, but its efforts were encumbered by its inability to provide enough *monitrices* to meet the demands of women who had taken preparation classes. In the words of Elisabeth Bing, one of the most noted childbirth educators in the United States, "A new idea, therefore, presented itself to us: We had to make the husband a wife's coach."[21] Women went to classes with their husbands where both learned the exercises—one so she could use them, the other so he could monitor them—and both became active participants in the childbirth experience.

A number of other approaches to natural childbirth have appeared since the early 1960s but all of them derive from either Dick-Read's romanticism or the Pavlov/Lamaze conditioning, or a combination of the two. For example, Sheila Kitzinger, whose work will be discussed in more detail below, is a proponent of the "psychosexual" approach to childbirth and emphasizes the psychosexual beauty, wonder, and thrill of childbirth. Her procedures follow in the tradition of Dick-Read.[22] The psychoprophylactic approach has evolved a systematic desensitization technique which treats pregnancy and delivery like a phobia and through which women overcome their fears by being systematically desensitized to all the elements of a psychologist-constructed anxiety hierarchy of pregnancy.[23] Little attention is given to education; one simply has to overcome fear and anxiety without necessarily understanding their origins. Another approach to pyschoprophylaxis uses biofeedback to gain control over one's physiological responses to pregnancy.[24] Despite the claims that are usually made about each new technique opening up a "new era" in childbirth, all approaches to childbirth training are based on the forty-year-old notion of two-dimensional childbirth and all share a respect for the second dimension, the psychological, of pregnancy and birth.

Now I must make a statement that will surprise some people. Obstetrics, the profession, accepted natural childbirth with surprising quickness.[25] Early studies done by the profession showed that women trained in psychoprophylactic techniques had shorter labors and a lower incidence of operative intervention in labor than untrained women, that trained women required less anesthesia and less analgesia, that they experienced less blood loss, and that they had a lower incidence of gestational hypertension. They tended to experience more perineal tears, but they had no more serious complications of pregnancy than their untrained counterparts. Trained women's reactions to their deliveries, both in terms of satisfaction and happiness and in terms of convalescence, were better than untrained women's reactions. Babies produced by women using natural childbirth techniques were happier and healthier, too.[26] The early research insisted that women prepared under one of the natural childbirth regimens not only had a better time in childbirth but also were better patients, obstetrically speaking.

There were critics, of course, and many of their criticisms of their colleagues' research were not without support. Reid and Cohen's article, for example, reviewed the obstetrical literature and concluded that there was no reliable and valid evidence that uterine contractions were painless, that there was no evidence to indicate that pain in labor is psychologically desirable, and that on the basis of the available evidence "one cannot draw any conclusion regarding the soundness of the obstetrics of 'natural' childbirth."[27] They were right. As a 1978 review of the obstetrical literature on natural childbirth showed, most studies—even those done in the 1970s—suffered from major methodological flaws.[28] The only mistake Reid and Cohen made in their critical assessment of trends in obstetrics evident in the early 1950s was to claim that there was scientific support for the surgico-prophylactic methods of DeLee and his colleagues. They could have said there was equal support for surgico-prophylaxis and psychoprophylaxis or they could have said there was no reliable, scientific support for either set of techniques; then they would have been correct.

Obstetrics has always accepted innovation on the most meager of evidence, provided that it has the appearance of being scientific. Just as with episiotomies, prophylactic forceps operations, and other innovations, the profession embraced the innovation offered by psychoprophylaxis and natural childbirth, the critics had their say, and then the profession reformed itself to incorporate the new development.

Even Reid and Cohen agreed that "scientific psychology and scientific obstetrics are not incompatible." They felt that eventually "certain techniques may be developed which appear to abolish fear and readily establish confidence." Once "further scientific work" discovered such techniques, obstetricians would be forced to recognize the psychological side of birth in new management schemes.[29] Clyde Randall, in a 1959 paper called "Childbirth Without Fear of Interference," even began to divide up the obstetrical territory. He wanted to work out a truce with women:

> Let us hope that the proponents of natural childbirth will eventually be willing to see their philosophic approach revolutionize our former conduct of the first stage of labor, and accept the evidence that actual delivery, even of the normal

case, can be most safely accomplished by the prophylactic measures recommended by DeLee two generations ago.[30]

Women could have part of childbirth and obstetricians could retain another part, Randall said, in laying his proposal on the table. The antagonist's terms in the struggle—natural childbirth's two-dimensional birth—had been accepted by obstetrics and the only possible avenue left open to the profession was to accommodate natural childbirth's challenge by working out a plan that met the demands of women while still preserving the obstetrical project for obstetricians.

Women's Interests and Obstetricians' Interests

Women had specific interests around childbirth that conflicted with obstetricians' historically conditioned interests. Obstetrics, however, did not meet women's demands with obstinancy and counterforce. Instead, the profession reformulated its practices to accommodate women's interests.

What did women want? They wanted to be active participants in birth; they wanted a sense of mastery over birth; they wanted to feel as if they were in control. In short, they wanted a piece of the action. This is the message implicit in natural childbirth's reconceptualization of pain. Alleviating one-dimensional pain was the principal entrée to the active control of labor and delivery. When obstetricians relieved women of their pain, they relieved them of childbirth as well. Two-dimensional pain is pain that women experience as their own pain, the pain that accompanies active participation in attempts to master a challenge. Just like Virginia Woolf's character Lily Briscoe, a woman artist who lifts her brush only to have it "for a moment [stay] trembling in a painful but exciting ecstacy in the air,"[31] a woman can now experience that *painful* but exciting *ecstacy* that signals her active participation in the delivery of her child.

"Women are no longer willing to be dependent in the doctor-patient relationship," contemporary commentators tell us. "This generation of women wants physicians who will treat them as equals and expects the medical profession to meet their changing needs."[32] Just as Lily Briscoe wishes to master a challenging painting, women wish to master birth. "Everything that is done with or for a pregnant woman should be done to increase rather than decrease her sense of mastery,''[33] for a woman who achieves this sense may have a wonderful and even orgasmic birth:

> Several authors, as well as many women in our study, report that they enjoy their second stage (the pushing part) of labor, often describing it as feeling "great" or "wonderful," even to the point (for a few) of referring to it as the "birth orgasm." The very positive attitudes of these fully conscious women can be attributed to the rewards of their active achievement: they describe working very hard to push out their own babies and feel afterward, that they have truly *given* birth. . . . The rewards of active achievement compared with passive observation are clear.[34]

Obstetricians' initial hostility toward natural childbirth techniques and their frustrations with the women who wanted to use them arose from a sense of alienation from what had been their work. Women were taking over parts of their jobs:

> Obstetricians felt threatened in their authority. They were suddenly asked to relinquish a most rewarding role, namely, that of being not only the expert, but also of being the wise father figure, the all knowing, benevolent friend, or even the lucky chap who was allowed to kiss and certainly be kissed by grateful young women, to whom he had just delivered a healthy baby. He was now asked to become a member of the team, to share his knowledge, and above all to become involved in a very emotional and significant event in a young couple's life, where *he* was not kissed at the birth of the child, but the husband was. And he did not like it. The great scientist became emotional and said louder and louder that he would not sacrifice his great skill to some emotional nonsense, such as keeping the family unit together.[35]

In 1952, members of the profession criticized their colleagues' reluctance to accept natural childbirth techniques and noted that obstetricians were angry because they were losing control:

> We believe that the few people who are criticizing the method have not given it a fair trial, or else may have had a deflation of the ego when they saw how successfully a patient could accomplish, with proper preliminary training, what a physician

has been trained for years to do with all sorts of specialized drugs and instruments.[36]

But women, along with the opinion leaders and innovators in the profession, had momentum and the early scientistic studies of natural childbirth on their side, so turning back the tide was to be for obstetrics, as it is for anyone, an impossible task. Obstetrics had to search out a compromise position.

Certainly there was a basis for compromise. Women's interests were remarkably consistent with obstetrics' interests. Women wanted controlled births without intolerable pain. While women's methods of control differed from obstetricians' methods and women's demands were clouded by a veil of emotionalism and talk of subjective experiences which had never had a place in scientific obstetrics, natural childbirth appeared to embody a set of interests consistent with those held by obstetrics since its earliest days. If women could help control birth, as "control" was understood by obstetricians, and if they could do it without drugs and instrumental interference, that is, if they could do it more economically, why not let them share the responsibility for birth? Birth would be so much the better for it.

Modern obstetrics and modern women have implicitly agreed upon a rule which underlies the contemporary joint adventure of preserving the obstetrical project. The rule, simply stated, is that *birth should occur within a flexible system of obstetrical alternatives in which a woman's experiences can take prominence against a background of obstetrical expertise and safety.* Around this rule modern women and modern obstetricians have begun a univocal discourse over childbirth. They are ostensibly engaged in a dialogue, but in the exchanges only a single voice is heard.

That women wrote the rule in the first place is clear. An article called "The Sense of Mastery in the Childbirth Experience," published in 1978, began this way:

> There are three basic goals in attempts to assist the process of labor: (1) enhancing safety for mother and child; (2) allowing freedom from undue pain without the loss of positive and indeed ecstatic aspects of the experience; and (3) setting or maintaining the best foundation for a solid, exuberant relationship between mother and child (and the rest of the family).[37]

The task women are setting for themselves is to construct a system in which a proper balance is struck among these goals. To achieve this, women believe that obstetrics has to be reformed at three levels. Reform has to occur at the psychological level by emphasizing and respecting a woman's desires for a sense of mastery and participation; at the interactional-ethical level by organizing the doctor-patient relationship around the old ethical dictum *primum non nocere* (first, do no harm); and at the organizational level by delineating "first, second, and third-line services (i.e., primary care for normal situations with several levels of expert backup as necessary)."[38] The women's health-care and natural childbirth movements do not fail to recognize the possibility of difficulties and disasters in pregnancy and birth nor do they fail to recognize the importance of obstetrical expertise in crises. Contemporary critics of obstetrics simply want obstetrical expertise to be applied intelligently, conservatively, and with respect for women's experiences and understanding of birth.

But this is not inconsistent with what modern obstetrics wants. In fact, obstetrics has come forward with a plan to reform the profession that is almost identical to that proposed by women and the natural childbirth movement. In 1976 five professional organizations established an Interprofessional Task Force on Health Care of Women and Children. The task force, composed of representatives from the American Academy of Pediatrics, the American College of Nurse-Midwives, the American College of Obstetricians and Gynecologists, the Nurses Association of the American College of Obstetricians and Gynecologists, and the American Nurses' Association, evaluated traditional childbirth practices in hospitals. Two years later, in June, 1978, the task force issued a *Joint Position Statement on the Development of Family-Centered Maternity/Newborn Care in Hospitals*. The statement defined family-centered care as "the delivery of safe, quality health care while recognizing, focusing on, and adapting to both the physical and psychological needs of the client-patient, the family, and the newly born." "The emphasis," said the task force, "is on the provision of maternity/newborn health care which fosters family unity while maintaining physical safety."[39] The language is familiar since this is the same set of goals proffered by "critics." The recommendations by the task force for implementing family-centered care paralleled almost exactly Anne Seiden's recommendations for fostering a sense of mastery in childbirth which were published at about the same time as the task-force statement. The task force recognized that "health includes not only physical dimensions, but social, economic, and psychological dimensions as well," and went on to recommend a reorganization of obstetrical care that would be responsive to all these levels of health. At the psychological level, the task force said health care must permit women to "achieve their own goals within the concept of a high level of wellness, and within the context and cultural atmosphere of their choosing." At the interactional-ethical level, the task force urged practitioners to recognize that "the provision of maternity/newborn care requires a team effort of the woman and her family, health care providers, and the community." At the organizational level, the task force suggested the provision of a flexible system of obstetrical alternatives which "includes the cooperative interrelationships of hospitals, health care providers, and the community so as to provide for the total spectrum of maternity/newborn care within a particular geographic region."[40] The Joint Position Statement specifically endorsed the recommendations for regionalization of perinatal services formulated by the Committee on Perinatal Health of The National Foundation–March of Dimes and the Committee on the Fetus and Newborn of the American Academy of Pediatrics, both of which endorsed the idea of having primary, secondary, and tertiary care available and well coordinated within a given geographic region, just as the critics wished.[41] The present orientation of obstetrics is completely congruent with the interests of some of its most vocal critics. Both obstetrics and its critics want a flexible system of obstetrical alternatives in which women's experiences of their births can be treated as valuable.

The conjunction of obstetricians' and women's interests was crystallized in the mid to late 1970s, but as early as the 1950s obstetricians were beginning to announce and applaud the shift from obstetrician-centered, or at least pelvis/uterus/fetus-centered, birth to family-centered, or at least woman-centered, birth. A 1956 article described (and endorsed) the shift by saying:

> Considering the fact that, for the vast majority of married women, having a baby is the most important thing that they do . . . our domination of their pregnancy and delivery thus robs them of a considerable amount of the psychological satisfaction they might derive from the process. More and more we, and less and less they, are having the baby.
> Natural childbirth seems to reverse this situation, so that the

women, despite the fact that we still play an important part, feel that they are having the baby, and that we are simply auxiliaries to the fact.[42]

And Herbert Thoms said in 1951, "it is important that the prospective mother recognize more fully that bringing a child into the world is a cooperative endeavor in which she plays the most important role."[43] Family-centered maternity care acquired real meaning early, too, as the husband became part of the obstetrical team. Including husbands on the team may have been the result of an afterthought when childbirth education groups could not provide enough *monitrices* to meet the demand, but by 1965 the concept of the husband-coach was so well accepted that popular books were written about it.[44] By the early 1970s husband-wife teams were teaching childbirth education classes jointly and the husband was so accepted that one commentator could outline the role of the father in detail:

> [The father's] role does not interfere with good obstetrical care. Rather, the presence of a prepared father enhances and complements the quality of obstetrics.
> The father's role in the delivery room is very specific. He is there as a coach, supporter, and reporter to his wife. . . . He is there to share the joy, the excitement, and the sense of accomplishment when their baby is born.[45]

With the husband accorded his proper place, the joint adventure of childbirth could proceed smoothly with each joint adventurer certain of his or her position on the team.

Developing family-centered maternity and newborn care held three distinct advantages for the profession. First, responsibility for birth became diffused. The Interprofessional Task Force put it simply:

> While physicians are responsible for providing direction for medical management, other team members share appropriately in managing the health care of the family, and each team member must be individually accountable for the performance of his/her facet of care.[46]

This does not, of course, absolve the physician from his legal responsibility for birth, but it makes women partially acountable for the quality of the birth experience. Obstetricians could no longer be blamed for all bad things that happened. One group even said, "ultimately, the care of even very sick newborns is the responsibility of the parents and . . . the medical and nursing staff exist to assist them in doing what needs to be done while not usurping the parents' role."[47]

Second, regionalization of perinatal care, required by family-centered care, rationalized the distribution and use of resources, gave the physician displaced from the directorship of the obstetrical team a new, still-valued position, and cut costs.

The provision of a high level of perinatal care over large geographic regions requires a cooperation and organization never before practiced in medicine. Hospitals are designated Level 1, 2, or 3, depending on their capacity to provide specific kinds of care. Level 1 hospitals provide services for uncomplicated deliveries and for early detection of problem pregnancies. Problem cases are referred to Level 2 or 3 hospitals for assessment and sometimes care. This flexible system of obstetrical alternatives forces some hospitals to handle only routine cases and refer elsewhere all the "interesting" cases, those that present a challenge, that occur only rarely in community hospital settings, and that break up the routine of day-to-day obstetrical work. Health professionals are often reluctant to loose interesting cases and sometimes fail to follow DeLee's dictum that every man act according to his limitations. The challenge of establishing a regionalized perinatal care system is to "improve the delivery of patient care while simultaneously providing an intellectually satisfying milieu for the professional."[48] Elaborate systems of communication and referral/transport link hospitals in a regionalized care area in order to insure that mothers and babies get good care while all physicians in an area are made to feel that they are an important part of the team. The principles which inform regionalization are shown in figure 7.1. There is reciprocity in terms of care and referral, but there is also reciprocity in terms of criticism and compliments even though the medical-center staff sits at the apex of a pyramidal regional system of care.

Regionalization optimizes the use of scarce resources, both economic and intellectual. Regional assessments of needs, deployment of resources, and continuous evaluation of services all insure that women get all the care they need, but just the care they need. Regionalization provides for the early identification and proper routing of all patients through the system so that precise, individualized management schemes can be designed.

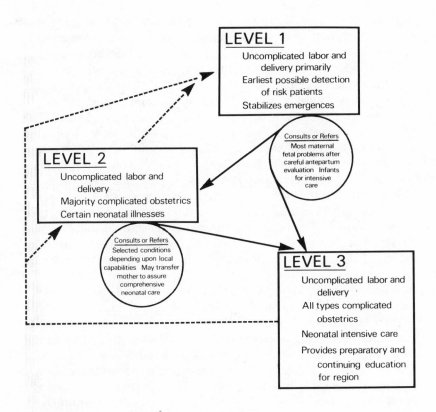

Schematic representation of regionalized perinatal care.
Note equal responsibility and reciprocal interaction between levels.

Figure 7.1 The regionalization of perinatal care. (From George A. Little and Joseph L. Butterfield, "Regionalization of Perinatal Care," in Robert A. Hoekalman et al., *Principles of Pediatrics: Health Care of the Young* [New York: McGraw-Hill, 1978], pp. 415–20. Used by permission.)

Furthermore, regionalization "frees" obstetricians from the burdens of routine care. Other team members, the mother and the obstetrically supervised midwife, can take care of the routine cases outside a technologically intensive labor and delivery milieu. In 1971, John Van S. Maeck, an obstetrician at the medical center in Burlington, Vermont, urged the profession to forge a partnership with the midwife so that the obstetrician can "function primarily as a skilled professional" devoting most of his efforts to the patient at risk. "The obstetrician-midwife team," Maeck wrote, "will provide maximum utilization of each partner's skills. Its obvious benefits to patients and team members should help us to bring into obstetrics men and women of the highest caliber."[49] By the last part of the decade many physicians and physician-midwife teams had established alternative birthing centers both in and out of hospitals. "[The midwife's] motivation and background bring to this professional care an important aspect of psychological and educational support which is often neglected by the busy obstetrician."[50] Midwives assumed responsibility for screening and routine care and the physician moved into the background. In fact, controlled trials of care by midwives, in which clinic patients were randomly assigned to care by a nurse-midwife or care by hospital staff, showed that the only detectable differences in outcomes favored the midwives. Midwife-delivered patients had a lower incidence of forceps delivery and came to the clinic more often than the usual antenatal routines of the clinic required.[51] Midwives have been particularly useful in areas and practices unable to attract qualified obstetricians, such as those in rural and inner-city areas.[52] In this context, it was claimed "the consumer . . . seems delighted to have total management by a midwife, with the knowledge that instant assistance is available. . . . This type of midwifery service not only provides the consumer . . . what she wants but also protects her from what she does not know can happen."[53]

Obstetrics is not just paying lip service to the rule of a "flexible system of obstetrical alternatives in which a woman's experiences can achieve prominence against a backdrop of obstetrical expertise." It is implementing it with good success, since rationalizing care seems to have improved the outcomes of pregnancy. The few systematic evaluations of regionalized care that have been done indicate that, in fact, regionalization does decrease infant mortality and that regionalization's effects are independent of technological advances.[54]

The third advantage accruing to obstetrics from the implementation of family-centered care, besides diffusing responsibility for birth and rationalizing care, is that family-centered care cuts costs. An alternative birthing center in New York City, one not located in a hospital but closely tied into the regionalized system of care, charges one-third to one-half the average hospital rate for a normal delivery.

Because women who deliver in birthing rooms do not use anesthesia and only occasionally use medication, these costs are eliminated. . . . There are no separate fees for well-equipped labor, delivery, and recovery rooms as there are in regular maternity departments. Nursery costs are also lowered because families keep their babies with them for the entire hospital stay. With the early discharge pattern in the birthing rooms, families can leave the hospital one to two days earlier than those who deliver in the traditional setting. This practice produces savings in daily room charges.[55]

Cost containment is valuable in itself, but in today's economy achieving that goal will give the profession credibility and needed support from both consumers and government agencies.

The conjunction of women's and obstetricians' interests is strong but it is not yet perfect. Women and obstetricians agree on the "flexible system of obstetrical alternatives" rule, but some details of its implementation are still in dispute. For example, whether or not obstetricians should or will move into the background of the obstetrical encounter so that women's experiences can gain prominence is disputed. John Tomkinson, a member of the Central Midwives' Board in England, responded to American efforts to "glamorize" the midwife out of her proper role by saying that the midwife's place is "as a member of a team headed as always by the obstetrician who remains in the background to deal with complications."[56] The ambivalence of his statement captures the discomfort the profession is experiencing as it tries to balance obstetrical safety with the experiential aspects of pregnancy. Does the obstetrician head the team or does he give up his position, recede into the background, and let the team run itself? Some obstetricians want to maintain their status as team leader because they feel that if they relinquish that position much more will be lost as well:

If we cannot have everything, we must make a decision as to whether we are going to give away "normal" obstetrics. If we are, then I think the time will come that we must also decrease residency programs by a third or by 50 percent.

We cannot flood an already saturated system. A [survey in Ohio which asked] people what they really wish reveals, at least in Ohio, that patients really want doctors.[57]

A second tension in the compromise worked out between obstetricians and women centers on the proper setting for birth. Medicine will agree to a flexible system of obstetrical alternatives, but flexibility can only occur within strict limits. The Interprofessional Task Force was unequivocal on one point: "the hospital setting provides the maximum opportunity for physical safety and for psychological well-being."[58] Obstetricians have drawn the line at the hospital door, or at the door of the alternative birthing center not more than thirty seconds away from a well-equipped delivery suite, as one physician put it. Obstetrics refuses to recognize the value of a home birth, even if a woman makes an informed choice to have her baby at home:

> Since the return of home delivery unmonitored and outside the existing system raises the specter of increased maternal and perinatal mortality, obstetricians and pediatricians are trying to make hospital delivery as acceptable and pleasant as possible. Flexibility and responsiveness to patient needs will be keys to mutually satisfactory solutions. Toward this end, family-centered care in hospitals is being encouraged.
>
> It is hoped the implementation of a family-centered philosophy and care within innovative and safe hospital settings will actively provide the public with the services they need, request, and demand, and make it unnecessary for them to seek unconventional facilities for childbirth.[59]

The fetal advocate comes out when women express a preference for home birth. Jerold Lucey, editor of *Pediatrics,* said:

> I think every baby in this state is entitled to have the safest kind of delivery possible. And when somebody denies him that by crawling up into a cave or a log cabin without a telephone or electricity or running water—as we've seen happen—they are just not considering that infant's right to an intact birth.[60]

Yet some women want to have their babies at home and are doing so, even though some of them are unable to secure adequate medical back-up services.

A third tension exists over the rationales given for using natural childbirth and for developing family-centered care. The profession has seized on the obstetrical benefits of the new developments as the basis for its rationale and appreciates the economic savings that institutional reforms can effect. Women justify the techniques and the reforms in experiential terms. They have laid a claim for the value of the psychological, subjective side of pregnancy and appear willing to assume risks on the obstetrical-physiological side that their claim sometimes forces them to incur. So even though obstetricians agree on a common rule to inform obstetrical practice we cannot say that women's interests and obstetricians' interests coincide exactly. The arguments that remain are significant and constitute important fractures in the otherwise strong coalition between women and obstetricians that formed under the umbrella of the monitoring concept.

Arguments will probably continue over the question "Who *should* control birth?" and over the advantages and disadvantages of different team configurations, different divisions of responsibility, and different settings for birth. There is a prior question, however, that we must ask: "Who (or what) *does* control birth?" By trying to answer this analytical question we may be able to shed some light on contemporary debates over the normative question.

Who (or What) Controls Birth?

Diana Scully titled her recent book *Men Who Control Women's Health* and leaves no doubt about who controls birth. She allows that obstetrics has some internal regulating mechanisms, but according to her they are weak, ineffective, and, most important, in the wrong hands. In her view, men control women's health and are subject to little control themselves.[61] Hilary Graham, after demonstrating that antenatal literature purveys an "ambivalence" about the two-sided nature of pregnancy, says, "the doctor appears to have surrendered a considerable portion of power to the woman and her husband who are granted a license to manage and enjoy the emotional and relational aspects of pregnancy." But appearances, to Graham, are deceptive, for "a narcissistic and self-directed approach to pregnancy is conditional upon and secondary to the woman's acceptance of a higher medical prerogative."[62] In both views the obstetrician is in control. The reality of childbirth, according to critics, is a harshly "medicalized" antenatal, intrapartum, and postpartum course in which the little control allowed to women is a public relations device.

Without question, obstetricians controlled birth after they had eliminated their major competitor, the midwife, at the beginning of this century. They maintained control of birth at least through the end of World War II. Their approach to childbirth, their modality of social control, then changed as they deployed social technologies of monitoring and surveillance rather than technologies of domination and control. The monitoring concept exposes women to a constant field of visibility and implements its control through natural childbirth training as well as through traditional obstetrical means, but the same concept casts the health-care team into a field of visibility as well. Control acts reflexively. Obstetrical history has moved past the point where we can identify an agent of control, but never before has it been so manifestly evident that birth *is* controlled. Monitoring is in control and women and obstetricians are joint adventurers in the obstetrical project, both subject to monitoring's controlling oversight.

By using natural childbirth techniques a woman submits to a panoptic regime of control. Natural childbirth requires women to place themselves on view, exposing their innermost fears, anxieties, joys, and pleasures to external, normalizing gazes. By submitting to the confessional mode of interaction structured by natural childbirth training, a woman allows herself to be positioned (or may position herself) in terms of her deviations on normalizing distributions of experience and subjects herself to new technologies of normalization.

We need not dwell on the claim that to use natural childbirth is to submit to a regimen of control. Control was the motivating interest behind natural childbirth as well as being one reason obstetrics could accept the techniques quickly. The practical parts of Dick-Read's writing stress the need to control birth: "Loss of control allows stimuli to run riot"; "when control is maintained, it is quickly realized that the sense of impending pain experienced at the acme of uterine contraction does not materialize." Controlled but "natural" childbirth was designed with a single goal: "progress, both moral and physical," was to be achieved through the "perfection of motherhood."[63] Dick-Read wanted to shift the balance of power and responsibility for control from obstetricians to women, but that birth should be controlled was never a question for him.

The issue we must spend some time on is the nature of the control to which women submit by using natural childbirth. I said that natural childbirth establishes a "panoptic regime of control." What, exactly, does that mean?

Foucault spells out the ultimate power of the Panopticon when he says,

A real subjection is born mechanically from a fictitious relation. So it is not necessary to use force to constrain the convict to good behavior, the madman to calm, the worker to work, the schoolboy to application, the patient to observation of the regulations. . . . The efficiency of its power, its constraining force have, in a sense, passed over to the other side—to the side of its surface of application. He who is *subjected to a field of visibility, and who knows it,* assumes responsibility for the constraints of power; he makes them play spontaneously upon himself; he inscribes in himself the power relation in which he simultaneously plays both roles; he becomes the principle of his own subjection.[64]

In the panopticon, a guard need not be the immediately and constantly present expression of power, the evident "other" in the power relationship to which the prisoner is subject. The tower in the middle of the machine casts prisoners into a field of visibility in which they know their behavior can be seen even though their behavior might not be under surveillance at any given moment. The prisoner obeys the rules, not under threat of punishment, but under threat of observation. The prisoner creates for himself a "fictitious relation" in which he plays both parts in the control of his own behavior, the role of the governed and the role of the governor. Likewise, the guards know the effects of their work are potentially visible to anyone who cares to look and they create a similar relation with and for themselves.

Who is in control? Certainly not the prisoner; but not the guards either. To speak of an agent of control in the panopticon is absurd since the machine is in control. As when a man walks a dog that carries its own leash in its mouth, neither party can claim to be in control. Rather the *situation is controlled* by the fictitious relationships created through history, in our case through the deployment of monitoring with its reformation of the doctor-patient relationship.

In a more recent work, *The History of Sexuality,* Foucault discussed what happens to one subjected to a field of visibility. A field of visibility creates an ever present "incitement to discourse"; it contains technologies for extracting information. "Not only will you confess to acts contravening the law, but you will seek to transform your desire, your every desire, into discourse." One is caused to confess all so that, first, a "grid of observations" about behavior, desires, fantasies, and so on, to the most minute details of life, can be constructed, and so that later, each individual can be precisely located on that grid. The smallest details of the most intimate parts of life must be known so that the "controllers" of social life may make use of the behavior "but also [so] that each individual [may] be capable of controlling the use he [makes] of it."[65] The ideal, then, becomes behavior that is controlled by the actors but in ways consistent with social interests, the interests embedded in the structure of the machine and the presumably shared interests of controllers and controlled. The interests and even desires of controllers and controlled mirror one another and all are subject to technologies of monitoring so that the least deviation can be noted immediately and can be quickly subjected to technologies of normalization. Behavior becomes "a thing to be . . . managed, inserted into systems of utility, regulated for the greater good of all, made to function according to an optimum." "Sex," according to Foucault's history of it in the Victorian era, "was not something one simply judged; it was something one managed."[66] Childbirth today is not something to be judged and categorized according to archaic schemes like normal/abnormal, at risk or not; childbirth now is something to be managed. In fact, it is many things—psychological, physiological, and ecological—to be managed.

In natural childbirth "subjecting women to a constant field of visibility" becomes "providing women with social support during labor and delivery." Obstetrics recognized early the value of having women constantly visible and it realized natural childbirth provided this service. Herbert Thoms said in 1951 that " 'support' during active labor is the most important single factor in our program."[67] "Support" meant then as it does now letting a woman have as much privacy during labor as she wants, but making sure that that privacy is constantly monitored. "As nearly as possible, we try to have someone with the patient during her entire labor, whether it be friend, nurse, husband, or intern."[68] The woman remains in a field of visibility but it is a calm field in which "activity and busyness on the part of those attending [the woman] are kept to a minimum."[69] The guard need not be present constantly for, "In a normal labor, the prepared couple are in control and can manage for long periods with intermittant professional supervision. They do what is normal and will call for help if they suspect anything is amiss."[70] If the field of visibility, the provision of adequate support, breaks down, control dissipates and delivery becomes painful: "A feeling of inadequate support from the midwives correlated with the experience of delivery as painful."[71] Control can be reinstituted efficiently and without resort to old regimes of control by simply fortifying the field of visibility:

> We have on many occasions been called to a patient who has lost control toward the end of labor. She was crying out with her contractions, thrashing around on the table in the intervals, thoroughly out of control. But after talking with her for a few minutes, sitting with her through a couple of contractions, reassuring her about the progress of labor, we have been amazed to see this woman regain control, become relaxed and free of tension during the intervals, and bear down with her contractions with little evidence of the pain that had previously seemed so severe.[72]

Subjecting women to constant visibility brings about the control of birth and reestablishes control if it is ever lost.

Making women aware of the field of visibility and placing them on normalizing grids of observation are the tasks of childbirth education classes. To accomplish these tasks the classes are constructed in the form of a confessional. "Classes encourage women and their partners to *air their concerns* ahead of time, and teach pregnant women and their partners many techniques that will help during childbirth."[73] Ideally, group members lead other group members in their respective searches for placement on distributions of experiences known to childbirth educators and in their searches for techniques to optimize experiences. This is better than having to be led by childbirth educators: "we always hope to find among our listeners a real group-leader capable of stimulating discussion."[74] And groups need to be tailored to the characteristics of participants just as the priest must tailor the penance to the person and not just to the sin: "it would sometimes be desirable to educate separately certain women."[75] Women who are less developed intellectually, who might be on the verge of a neurosis, or simply women who have had one baby previously all need special instruction and special attention.[76] Ideally, education and preparation programs would be designed for the individual, and all of her individual concerns could be aired, accommodated, normalized, and managed.

Natural childbirth controls women, but by the same mechanisms it acts reflexively to reform hospitals and change staffs as well. A lot of sociology has come from criticizing institutions that lay the blame for their failures at the feet of their clients, institutions that try to "blame the victim." In the case of natural childbirth, however, members of the profession have attributed failure to the "impatient doctor"[77] or to "poor communication of the obstetric team" and "lack of adequate and honest feedback between consumers and teachers."[78] The profession has attributed failure to the structure of the system:

> We have found the hospital the most difficult part of our natural childbirth technique. To make sure that nothing happens to the woman in the hospital to increase her fears or anxieties, to have someone with her or at her call throughout the entire labor, to arrange the hospital physically so that she does not have to be in close proximity to the delivery rooms until she needs to go there, to protect her from the behavior of the less disciplined woman who is making outcry, to instill into the hospital personnel the philosophy necessary, all these things are not easy of achievement and take a great deal of time and attention.[79]

The hospital had to be restructured to accommodate natural childbirth, even if it meant rebuilding the entire physical space to include birthing rooms or to relocate labor suites.

Natural childbirth, as a component of the monitoring concept, can do more than move hospital walls; it can also command reformulations of relationships of health professionals. "Natural childbirth, with its emphasis on the normal and natural, on teaching, and on the development of good relationships brings together the specialists in the various departments of the hospital and helps to focus their skills and knowledge on the mother, her baby, and her family."[80] To achieve Dick-Read's cardinal requisites for the obstetrician and midwife—patience, peacefulness, personal interest, confidence, concentrated observation, and cheerfulness[81]—physicians and staff must also enter confessional as penitents: "Teaching physicians to *become conscious* of their sexual biases and to *talk* about sexuality in a relaxed manner should ideally begin at the medical school level";[82] "The future doctor must have some understanding of the dynamic determinants of his own personality and especially of his *unconscious*."[83] Medical schools must be made into instruments which incite doctors-to-be to air *their* feelings and desires and to subject themselves to normalizing distributions and technologies. If medical schools fail, regional programs' evaluations of cases referred to Level 3 hospitals or analyses of perinatal deaths in the region reveal problems after the fact. Perinatal programs thus constitute a technology for extracting confessions if other aspects of the system fail to work. Hospital staffs must be trained, educated, and subjected to systems of surveillance, just as women must be trained, educated, and subjected to systems of surveillance, in order to assume their proper places in the new system of obstetrical alternatives.

Monitoring subjects women and staffs to its control, extracting information as necessary, subjecting all to analysis, location, and normalization for one purpose: that childbirth be manageable. Management is thought to benefit all:

> Psychoprophylaxis as currently taught in the United States focuses mainly upon providing a more satisfying birth experience. For the woman herself, through education it reduces anxiety due to lack of knowledge about the birth process. . . . For the married couple, it gives the husband ways of helping his wife and allows both to share in the birth experience. Furthermore, medical benefits including shorter labors, lower levels of medication and anesthesia in labor and delivery, and fewer operative deliveries have been claimed for the psychoprophylactic method.[84]

> Childbirth education appears to be an appropriate procedure for maximizing a positive beginning to family life.[85]

Even conceptualizing birth as a psychosexual experience is done with the goal of management in mind:

> In the management of reproductive behavior, the underlying similarities of all three [behaviors, i.e., coitus, birth, and lactation] should be kept in mind. It is of biological and clinical significance that coitus, birth, and lactation appear to have a common neurohormonal base and share the tendency to be inhibited by environmental disturbance. All three appear, under some circumstances, to trigger caretaking behavior, which is an essential part of mammalian reproduction.[86]

The psychosexual aspects of birth are fitted into schemes of utility at the psychosexual level, the economic aspects of birth are optimized at the same time, and all attention is focused through natural childbirth and family-centered care on the optimization of the obstetrical project at many levels.

This approach undoubtedly frees women from the brutality of old-time obstetrics, but it replaces that brutality with a secure set of chains, in the fashioning of which women have participated. When pain was one-dimensional and birth likewise, surrendering pain to obstetrical relief from it meant surrendering childbirth to obstetrics. With two-dimensional pain and two dimensional childbirth, submitting to a regimen that will control pain and control childbirth means surrendering not just childbirth but the woman's mind, her experiences, her subjective self, to the regimen of control as well. Under the new order women do, in fact, surrender the possibility of making themselves their own point of reference for the assessment of their own experiences in relation to an external order. Women have participated in obstetrics' act of replacing one system of control over childbirth with another, more totalizing system. This is admittedly an interpretation, but the character of two responses to the rise of natural childbirth—the response of the profession of obstetrics and the variety of responses originating in the women's health movement—supports it.

The remarkable aspect of obstetrics' response to natural childbirth was not its quick acceptance of the techniques, but the rapidity with which the profession mobilized its own inquiry into the techniques. The profession did not engage in a "rush to judgment" of natural childbirth so much as it engaged in a "rush to knowledge." The techniques of natural childbirth simply *had* to be investigated. Everything had to be made known. Why is this so remarkable, though? It is remarkable in the same sense that the enormous mobilization of inquiry into the life of M. Jouy, a nineteenth-century French farmhand, the "village half-wit," was remarkable. Foucault describes the judicial action, medical intervention, detailed clinical examination, the entire "theoretical elaboration," and the final creation of M. Jouy as a perpetual object of medical knowledge through his lifetime incarceration in a hospital (despite his acquittal on all charges) that followed M. Jouy's arrest for soliciting sexual favors from young village girls. The authorities of the village of Lapcourt deployed a "rush to knowledge" around a petty, inconsequential "everyday occurrence in the life of village sexuality."[87]

In like manner obstetrics deployed its "rush to knowledge" in response to a very simple, most certainly "petty" (in the eyes of obstetrics), request that women's experiences be accorded value in the obstetrical encounter. Women wanted obstetricians to look them in the face. What could be simpler? But the response was anything but simple. The profession has devoted years of inquiry to ferreting out the most minute details of the conscious woman's experience of childbirth. Sociologists have joined in and constructed models of the determinants of the quality of the childbirth experience,[88] making it absolutely clear that quality of experience can be made to have an external referent. Women, under the extractive mechanisms of positivistic social and obstetrical science, provide the data which are subjected to analysis only to come back and haunt women in the guise of scientifically known distributions of possible experiences. Women are offered the "free choice" of moving themselves to the apex of scientifically known distributions of experience to optimize their experience of childbirth. But this is not a choice. The woman's task becomes not the human task of assessing of her own experience but the scientific task of locating herself in terms of deviations on normalizing distributions and participating in exercises, techniques, and rituals to correct and optimize her situation. She molds her desires, interests, and behavior to standards laid before her in order to produce an optimal experience in an economical way. Obstetrics' response, then, to the challenge of natural childbirth was the creation of a new science of birth around the new form of birth proposed by the profession's antagonists.

Responses from within the women's health movement have typically taken the form of alternatives to traditional medical care. In fact, though, present alternatives are not alternatives at all, for they all obey the "flexible system of obstetrical alternatives" rule and all require the woman to submit to external regimes of control. A brief examination of three contemporary childbirth alternatives— birth in an out-of-hospital alternative birthing center, spiritual midwifery on the Farm in Tennessee, and Sheila Kitzinger's "psychosexual approach" to childbirth education—will support this claim.

The Maternity Center Association (MCA) established the Childbearing Center in New York City in 1975. The MCA has consistently been a leader in the development of progressive programs in obstetrics. The MCA established the first antenatal clinics in the United States in 1918, was involved with nurse-midwife training in 1931, and began childbirth education programs in 1948. MCA's Childbearing Center carefully selects patients for normal obstetrical care.

In the Center nurse-midwives, physicians, and para-medical and support staff provide care that, so far as possible, conforms to women's desires. The Center, however, follows the "flexible systems" rule absolutely:

> The center is a maxi-home and not a mini-hospital. . . . The birth is managed at the center, with a return home in up to 12 hours. No rigid procedures are used: A woman can give birth in the position of her choice as long as her safety and that of her baby are ensured. Pitocin is never used to stimulate labor in the setting, nor are forceps ever used.[89]

Safety, satisfaction, and economy, in that order, are the priorities of the Center. To the first end the Center is involved in the regional system for providing sophisticated perinatal care as necessary. "A childbearing center . . . can serve as an effective support of regionalization concepts, screening and referring families to appropriate levels of care."[90]

The Childbearing Center offers parents a significant and relatively inexpensive alternative to in-hospital care, but it offers no alternative to the degree of submission demanded of women under other circumstances. "Safety first," as safety is understood by obstetrics, is the part of the motto that clarifies the Center's orientation. The Center, in fact, is a practical manifestation of Hilary Graham's assessment of all of modern obstetrics which understands the possibility of value being accorded to women's experiences as conditional upon and secondary to the acceptance of the preeminence of obstetrical control. Control, and submission to it, are the themes which inform this alternative just as they are the themes that inform all postwar obstetrics.

The "spiritual midwifery" practiced on the Farm, a charismatic, spiritual community in Summertown, Tennessee, arose in response to the usurpation of the rights of women, families, and newborns by a "predominantly male and profit oriented medical establishment."[91] The Farm offers its members a childbirth that emphasizes the spiritual, mystical aspects of birth but which backs up that spirituality with a physician, two paramedics, six nurses, forty emergency medical technicians, a lab, an intensive-care nursery, an outpatient clinic, and two ambulances.[92] The Farm does not violate the rule which insists that birth occur in a setting where the experiential aspects of birth are balanced against obstetrical safety. Birth on the Farm follows no rigid rules; there is, instead, an emphasis on togetherness, the importance of loving energy, support of friends, family, and obstetrically knowledgeable people, and on patience. Radical though this may sound, the degree of submission required is perhaps greater in this setting than in more traditional ones. One's whole life must be reoriented according to the dicta of the community:

> Those who come to the Farm to have their babies can be lacto-vegetarians up to the last six weeks of pregnancy; when they come to the Farm they are then total vegetarians. Our diet is based on the soybean and we supplement it with vitamin B12. We believe that a high-protein diet, no exogenous cholesterol, no tobacco smoking, and no alcohol are factors that at least partially contribute to our low incidence of toxemia and other complications of pregnancy.[93]

The flexibility of the Farm occurs within very strict limits. A woman's experience is clearly not allowed to speak for itself there.

Consider, finally, the "psychosexual approach" to childbirth education proffered by Sheila Kitzinger.[94] Kitzinger's approach celebrates the individuality of experiences of childbirth with an eye to its psychosexual dimensions. She says, "There are many ways of having a baby, and they vary from woman to woman," and "Women express their own personalities with infinite variety in childbirth."[95] She thinks a flexible system of obstetrical alternatives should be available so that a woman's desires can be accommodated without difficulty. So where in Kitzinger's scheme is the submission? One takes classes to learn the psychosexual method, but one surrenders experience not to the educator but to something quite different:

> Part of the task of the new art of childbirth education can be to help women become more aware of these psychosexual aspects of birth, of the continuity of their psychosexual lives, and of how, even with the first baby, the experience is not a complete novelty for them; how they can trust their bodies then as they also must be able to in lovemaking if they are to achieve *complete surrender*.[96]

A woman does not surrender to her partner in lovemaking, she surrenders to her body, to the biological law embedded within her. This is rhetoric not unlike the sociobiological writing on bonding. The task of the human being is to strip away all that keeps us from being in tune with the rhythms of our inner cosmos so that we may respect and obey the rules which our biology lays down for us. And to optimize experience requires, we are told, *complete* surrender to those rules.

Alternatives in birth have arisen not in opposition to the rule that birth should occur within a flexible system of obstetrical alternatives in which a woman's experience can gain prominence against a background of obstetrical expertise and safety; alternatives have arisen *within* this rule. The rule informs and facilitates alternatives, and the rule, in turn, is strengthened by their existence as they push the apparent limitations imposed by the rule farther and farther outward. The rule comes to resemble a liberating rather than a constraining force. The constraint passes over to the other side, so that the person who is constrained assumes responsibility for her own discipline. The rule creates alternatives which present the possibility of more humane care which increases the tacit acceptance of the rule which makes it ever harder to break out of the confines of the rule. The world of imaginable possibilities comes to be defined in terms of the options available under the rule. The "flexible systems" rule constrains imagination and becomes the force that holds together the panoptic machine that controls birth.

The Future

After authors have reshaped the present by writing their history, a desire to frame the future seems to compel them to finish with a section on *the* future or on alternative futures. They either project existing trends forward to a usually dismal, often cataclysmic end, or they paint pictures of the future inspired by hopes and romantic visions. "The future" sections of interpretive histories usually examine the embryonic forms of existing alternatives and either applaud their existence and the courage they show or bemoan the waste of human and other resources they represent and decry the irresponsibility they embody.

I will not present either a projection or a vision of the future. The future remains an empirical question, conditioned by history, for which we will collectively provide an answer. Besides, if I were to give my own vision of the future, would I not be engaging in exactly the same kind of behavior of which I have been so critical throughout this work? To write down an idea of the future is to constrain the world of possibility, to limit imaginable possibilities, for others who will have to live the future.

As a social analyst I have outlined the situation as I see it. Women today have many more options in childbirth than ever before. These options exist, however, in and because of an extraordinarily tightly controlled situation. Power is present throughout and around the experience of childbirth. It extends up and down, outward and inward. It crisscrosses itself to form entangling webs of constraining force in which we are all caught up but within which we enjoy many alternatives and more "humane"[97] treatment, an enjoyment that was not available to our forebears throughout history. Some would say we enjoy more freedom. But we enjoy a freedom within which all must be known. The one freedom we do not have is the freedom of remaining unseen. The obstetrical horror today is not the botched or the tragic case. Distributions of survival probabilities inform us to expect deaths even in those categories where death is the rarest of events. It happens, the charts tell us. The horror for modern obstetrics is, instead, the *unseen birth,* the birth that occurs "unmonitored and outside the existing system"; such a birth raises a "specter" over obstetrical work, as Dr. Young put it.[98] We enjoy a special kind of freedom today, the freedom to have a fully monitored, well-managed, optimized birth with a guarantee that no specter shall appear to haunt the experience. That is the situation today.

There are two possible futures. That is to say, there are only two futures that can be conceived according to the dictates of logic. In the first, everyone—women, men, obstetricians—will agree to conduct their discourse on a common ground, will work out the tensions in the structure of the existing coalition around birth; birth will become even more "humane," even more alternatives will appear, women will enjoy themselves more, and obstetricians will have work that is more satisfying to them. All of this will occur within the tight and demanding constraints of the "flexible systems" rule. The other alternative is to go absolutely in the opposite direction and not imagine another system in which birth can occur, for "if you wish to replace an official institution by another institution that fulfills the same function—better and differently—then you are already being reabsorbed by the dominant structure." The opposite direction is toward the rejection of all "theory and forms of general discourse."[99] Such a rejection would commit women and men to an unknown and unknowable situation which contains risks (and possibly joys) that

are literally unimaginable under existing conditions. Like Lily Briscoe, Virginia Woolf's artist, as she faced a blank canvas, every
woman in or contemplating childbirth would have to face the terrifying question, "Where to begin?" And if one should choose to
begin, one would thereby make a commitment, as Lily realized:
"One line placed on the canvas committed her to innumerable risks,
to frequent and irrevocable decisions. All that in idea seemed simple
became immediately complex." To begin would require that a
woman, in William Smellie's words, "consult her own ease," and
do so in opposition to an absolute assurance of an optimal birth
experience. Lily Briscoe decided "the risk must be run; the mark
made."[100] If faced with that simple yet enormous decision, I am not
sure how I would decide.

Notes

Chapter One

1. I also realize that future historians of histories will not get the quotation marks off my "true," just as I am unable to get the quotation marks off the "true" I might use in my interpretations of others' work.

2. Theodore Cianfrani, *A Short History of Obstetrics and Gynecology,* Springfield, Ill.: Charles C. Thomas, 1960.

3. Ibid., p. v.

4. Barbara Ehrenreich and Deirdre English, *For Her Own Good: 150 Years of the Experts' Advice to Women,* Garden City, N.Y.: Anchor Press, 1978, pp. 84–88. See also the notes in Chapter 2 below.

5. Ibid., p. 62.

6. Ann Oakley, *Women Confined: Towards a Sociology of Childbirth,* Oxford: Martin Robinson, 1980, p. 97.

7. Mary Daly, *Gyn/Ecology: The Metaethics of Radical Feminism,* Boston: Beacon Press, 1978, p. 226.

8. Ibid., p. 228.

9. Figure 1.1 periodizes history. This is always unfair to the record even though periodizing remains a practice which has a magnetic attraction for historians.

The preprofessional period of medicine ended roughly with the end of the nineteenth century as regular medicine undermined all of its competitors, including the midwife, and gained control over the medical marketplace. The ascendancy of modern, scientific-rational medicine began with the rise of European rationalism centuries before, and it did not culminate in America until the two decades around the turn of this century. The key events which mark the end of the preprofessional era are the rise to dominance over access to medical practice of the medical societies, which was facilitated by the enactment of state licensing laws (1890–98), and the rise to dominance of the American Medical Association over medical education, which was facilitated by its own Committee on Medical Education (1907) and the Flexner Report (1910).

The second period in medical history, the intertransitional period, extended at least through World War II and perhaps into the early 1950s. Pressures began mounting in medicine's environment in the period from 1910 to 1940, though. Britain implemented a national health insurance scheme in 1911 and recommended regionalization of medical services in 1920. During the 1930s and 1940s third-party payers, group-practice schemes, and other threats to the autonomy of medicine appeared. The government took a more active role in medical education during the war itself. The second transformation of medicine may have been a response to the accumulation of pressures and threats, but to argue that there was any direct causal link would be difficult. What is clear is that by the early 1950s medicine had changed in the ways described in the text. Periodization may be unfair, but as a first approximation and a heuristic device it is helpful.

10. Michel Foucault, *The Birth of the Clinic: An Archeology of Medical Perception*, New York: Vintage Books, 1973.

11. Barry Barnes, *Interests and the Growth of Knowledge*, London: Routledge & Kegan Paul, 1977, p. 2.

12. Ibid., pp. 16, 38. See also Barry Barnes, *Scientific Knowledge and Sociological Theory*, London: Routledge & Kegan Paul, 1974.

13. Barnes, 1977, p. 6.

14. Michel Foucault, "History of Systems of Thought: Summary of a Course Given at Collège de France—1970–1971," pp. 199–204 in Donald F. Bouchard, ed., *Michel Foucault: Language, Counter-Memory, Practice: Selected Essays and Interviews*, Ithaca, N.Y.: Cornell University Press, 1977, pp. 202–3.

15. Michel Foucault and Gilles Deleuze, "Intellectuals and Power: A Conversation," pp. 205–17 in Donald F. Bouchard, ed., *Michel Foucault: Language, Counter-Memory, Practice: Selected Essays and Interviews*, Ithaca, NY: Cornell University Press, 1977, pp. 206–7; Deleuze is the speaker.

16. Foucault and Deleuze, 1977, p. 208; Foucault is the speaker.

17. Ibid., p. 208; Deleuze is the speaker.

18. Thomas J. Cottle, "The Politics of Pronouncement: Notes on Publishing in the Social Sciences," pp. 50–62 in *Science, Heritability, and IQ*, Cambridge, Mass.: Harvard Educational Review, 1969, pp. 51–52.

19. Foucault and Deleuze, 1977, p. 209; Deleuze is the speaker.

20. Ibid., pp. 207–8; Foucault is the speaker.

21. Michel Foucault, "Truth and Power: An Interview," pp. 109–33 in Colin Gordon, ed., *Power/Knowledge: Selected Interviews and Other Writings, 1972–1977,* New York: Pantheon, 1980, p. 133.

22. Arthur L. Stinchcombe, *Theoretical Methods in Social History,* New York: Academic Press, 1978, p. 21.

23. Ibid., p. 17.

24. Ibid., p. 22.

25. Barnes, 1974, p. 57.

26. Foucault, 1977, pp. 199–201.

27. Alessandro Fontano and Pasquale Pasquino, "Interview with Foucault: Truth and Power," pp. 29–48 in Meaghan Morris and Paul Patton, eds., *Michel Foucault: Power, Truth, and Strategy,* Sydney, Australia: Feral Publications, 1979, p. 31.

28. Donald F. Bouchard, "Introduction," pp. 15–25 in Donald F. Bouchard, ed., *Michel Foucault: Language, Counter-Memory, Practice: Selected Essays and Interviews,* Ithaca, N.Y.: Cornell University Press, 1977, p. 16.

29. Oakley, 1980.

30. Charles L. Bosk, *Forgive and Remember: Managing Medical Failure,* Chicago: University of Chicago Press, 1979.

31. Diana Scully, *Men Who Control Women's Health: Education of Obstetricians and Gynecologists,* Boston: Houghton Mifflin, 1980. See also Nancy Stoller Shaw, *Forced Labor: Maternity Care in the United States,* New York: Pergamon, 1974. For studies of women's experiences see Oakley, 1980, or Ann Oakley, *Becoming a Mother,* Oxford: Martin Robinson, 1979. For a survey approach to the same issue see Ann Cartwright, *The Dignity of Labour?: A Study of Childbearing and Induction,* London: Tavistock, 1979.

Part One

1. Alessandro Fontano and Pasquale Pasquino, "Truth and Power: Interview with Foucault," pp. 29–48 in Meaghan Morris and Paul Patton, eds., *Michel Foucault: Power, Truth, Strategy,* Sydney, Australia: Feral Publications, 1979, p. 33.

Chapter Two

1. Jane B. Donegan, *Women and Men Midwives: Medicine, Morality, and Misogyny in Early America,* Westport, Conn.: Greenview Press, 1978; Judy Barrett Litoff, *American Midwives: 1860 to the Present,* Westport, Conn.: Greenview Press, 1978; Jean Donnison, *Midwives and Medical Men: History of Inter-Professional Rivalries and Women's Rights,* London: Heinemann, 1977; Richard W. Wertz and Dorothy C. Wertz, *Lying-In: A History of Child-*

birth in America, New York: The Free Press, 1977; Catherine Scholten, "On the Importance of the Obstetrick Art: Changing Customs of Childbirth in America, 1760–1825," *William and Mary Quarterly* 34 (1977): 426–45; Francis E. Kobrin, "The American Midwife Controversy: A Crisis of Professionalization," *Bulletin of the History of Medicine* 40 (1966): 350–63. These are the major works in the field. I draw freely from them and other works noted.

2. See the pamphlet by Barbara Ehrenreich and Deirde English, *Witches, Midwives, and Nurses: A History of Women Healers,* Old Westbury, N.Y.: The Feminist Press, 1973, and the book by the same authors, *For Her Own Good: 150 Years of the Experts' Advice to Women,* New York: Doubleday, 1978. Also see Thomas R. Forbes, *The Midwife and the Witch,* New Haven: Yale University Press, 1966.

3. Jeffrey Lionel Berlant, *Profession and Monopoly: A Study of Medicine in the United States and Great Britain,* Berkeley, Calif.: University of California Press, 1975, p. 134.

4. Donnison, p. 6; Donegan, p. 12.

5. For a review of the kinds of operations performed and pictures of the instruments used by the barber-surgeons, see Harold Speert, *Historie Illustrée de Gynecologie et de Obstétrique,* Paris: Roger Dacosta, 1973, chap. 9. Also cf. Kedarnath Das, *Obstetric Forceps: Its History and Evolution,* Calcutta: The Art Press, 1929.

6. For a brief review of the developments at the Hotel-Dieu, see Walter Radcliffe, *Milestones in Midwifery,* Bristol: John Wright and Sons, 1967, chap. 3, or for the early history of the Hotel-Dieu, Henriette Currier, *Origines de La Maternité de Paris: Les Maîtresses Sages-Femmes et L'Office Des Accouchées de L'Ancien Hôtel-Dieu (1378–1796),* Paris: Georges Steinheil, 1888.

7. Speert, chap. 7, shows the plan of the pelvis as conceived by Levret, the instruments used by Baudelocque, and many of the deformities described by the latter.

8. Terms like "science" and "rationality" are used to indicate forms of knowledge and approaches to the world which are symmetric with other forms of knowledge. To strip them of the privilege which they carry in our culture and to remind the reader that they are treated in this way, they are often enclosed in quotation marks throughout the narrative.

9. Barry Barnes, in *Scientific Knowledge and Sociological Theory,* London: Routledge and Kegan Paul, 1974, develops the connection between theory and metaphor, claiming that all theory is metaphor. This is the basis for the quick jump from "metaphor" to "theory" in the text. See chapter 1 above.

10. Wertz and Wertz, pp. 31–34.

11. This is not to say that they were not used at all. In fact, the Library of the National Academy of Science speculates that very few copies of

Culpepper's *Directory for Midwives* are extant because they may have been "thumbed" out of existence through use. Such a book could have had this kind of use over its long life and still have been relatively unread during the period in question.

12. Donegan, 1978, pp. 22–25; Irving S. Cutter and Henry R. Viets, *A Short History of Midwifery,* Philadelphia: W. B. Saunders, 1964, pp. 77–82.

13. James Hobson Aveling, *The Chamberlens and the Midwifery Forceps: Memorials of the Family and an Essay on the Invention of the Instrument,* London: J. H. Churchill, 1882; Walter Radcliffe, *The Secret Instrument: The Birth of the Midwifery Forceps,* London: Heinemann, 1947; Cutter and Viets, 1964, pp. 44–69. For a recent and readable version of the story, see Adrienne Rich, *Of Woman Born: Motherhood as Experience and Institution,* New York: Norton, 1976, pp. 133ff.

14. Edmund Chapman, *A Treatise on the Improvement of Midwifery, Chiefly with Regard to the Operation,* London, 1733.

15. Donegan, 1978, p. 47.

16. Philip Thicknesse, *Man-Midwifery Analysed,* London, 1765, p. 39.

17. Cutter and Viets, 1964, pp. 44–69.

18. Rich, 1976, pp. 138–42.

19. Elizabeth Nihell, *A Treatise on the Art of Midwifery,* London, 1760, pp. 461–62.

20. Donegan, 1978, p. 33.

21. Charles White, *A Treatise on the Management of Pregnant and Lying-in Women,* 2d ed., London: Edward and Charles Dilly, 1773, pp. xi–xii, viii, 329–42.

22. Hugh Chamberlen, "Translator to the Reader," in his translation of François Mauriceau, *The Diseases of Women with Child, and in Child-bed,* London: John Darby, 1683.

23. William Smellie, *A Treatise on the Theory and Practice of Midwifery,* 3d ed., London: Wilson and Durham, 1756, p. 248.

24. Berlant, 1975, pp. 64–127.

25. Donegan, 1978, pp. 80–83.

26. Donnison, 1977, p. 57.

27. James Hobson Aveling, *English Midwives: Their History and Prospects,* reprint of the 1872 edition with additions, London: Hugh K. Elliot, 1967.

28. Robert Barnes, Obstetric Physician to St. George's Hospital, London, "On the Relations of Pregnancy to General Pathology," an address to an unspecified American medical society, 1876, held by the Wellcome Institute for the Study of the History of Medicine, London.

29. Donnison, 1977, p. 130.

30. Berlant, 1975, pp. 190ff.

31. See Donegan, 1978, pp. 91–94, for a discussion of the origins of the oaths used in the colonies.

32. Ibid., pp. 117–18.

33. Wertz and Wertz, 1977, pp. 55–56.

34. Ehrenreich and English, 1978.

35. Thomas Ewell, M.D., proposed such a school in 1817.

36. See E. Richard Brown, *Rockefeller Medicine Men: Medicine and Capitalism in America,* Berkeley, Calif.: University of California Press, 1979, or Steven Jonas, *Medical Mystery: The Training of Doctors in the United States,* New York: W. W. Norton, 1978.

37. Harriot K. Hunt, *Glances and Glimpses; or Fifty Years Social, Including Twenty Years Professional Life,* Boston: John P. Jewitt and Co., 1856, pp. 265–67.

38. Donegan, 1978, p. 148.

39. Barbara Ehrenreich and Deirdre English, *Complaints and Disorders: The Sexual Politics of Sickness,* Old Westbury, N.Y.: The Feminist Press, 1973; Rich, 1976, chap. 7.

40. Frederick T. Parsons, stenographer, *Report of the Trial: The People versus Dr. Horatio N. Loomis for Libel,* Buffalo: Jewitt, Thomas, and Co., 1850, pp. 26, 23, reprinted in *The Male-Midwife and the Female Doctor,* New York: Arno Press, 1974.

41. Hugh L. Hodge, *Introductory Lecture to the Course on Obstetrics and the Diseases of Women and Children, Delivered in the University of Pennsylvania, November 7, 1838,* Philadelphia: J. G. Auner, 1838, p. 11, emphasis added.

42. William Potts Dewees, *A Compendious System of Midwifery,* Philadelphia: Carey and Lea, 1824, pp. 1–2.

43. Oliver Wendell Holmes, "The Contagiousness of Puerperal Fever," *New England Quarterly Journal of Medicine and Surgery* 1 (1843): 503–30, reprinted as *Puerperal Fever as a Private Pestilence,* Boston, 1855.

44. Litoff, 1978, pp. 18ff.

45. Berlant, 1975, chap. 5.

46. William G. Rothstein, *American Physicians in the Nineteenth Century: From Sects to Science,* Baltimore: The Johns Hopkins University Press, 1972, pp. 211–12.

47. Thomas Darlington, "The Present Status of the Midwife," *American Journal of Obstetrics and Diseases of Women and Children* 63 (1911): 870–76.

48. Brown, 1979.

49. J. Whitridge Williams, "Medical Education and the Midwife Problem in the United States," *Journal of the American Medical Association* 58 (1912): 1–7.

50. Joseph B. De Lee, "Progress toward Ideal Obstetrics," *Transactions of the American Association for the Study of the Prevention of Infant Mortality* 6 (1915): 117. For later assertions of this sort, see, for example, George C. Marlett, "Discussion," in response to E. R. Hardin, "The Mid-

wife Problem," *Southern Medical Journal* 18 (1925): 350, and John F. Moran, "The Endowment of Motherhood," *Journal of the American Medical Association* 64 (1915): 122–26.

51. Litoff, 1978, p. 113.

52. This is the argument of both Litoff and Kobrin.

53. See, for example, John Van S. Maeck, "Obstetrician-Midwife Partnership in Obstetric Care," *Obstetrics and Gynecology* 37 (1971): 314–19.

Chapter Three

1. For a personal view of DeLee, see the article by M. Edward Davis, "Joseph Bolivar DeLee, 1869–1942: As I Remember Him," *Lying-In: The Journal of Reproductive Medicine* 1 (1968): 33–44.

2. Joseph B. DeLee, "The Prophylactic Forceps Operation," *American Journal of Obstetrics and Gynecology* 1 (1920): 39–40.

3. Joseph B. DeLee, *The Principles and Practice of Obstetrics,* 1st ed., Philadelphia: W. B. Saunders, 1913, p. xiii.

4. Ibid., p. 291.

5. Joseph B. DeLee, *The Principles and Practices of Obstetrics,* 4th ed., Philadelphia: W. B. Saunders, 1924, p. iii; emphasis added.

6. American Gynecological Association, "Society Transactions," meeting of May 24–26, 1920, published in *American Journal of Obstetrics and Gynecology* 1 (1920): 76.

7. J. Whitridge Williams, *Obstetrics: A Text-Book for the Use of Students and Practitioners,* 1st ed., New York: D. Appleton, 1903, p. 175.

8. Rudolph W. Holmes, "The Fads and Fancies of Obstetrics: A Comment on the Pseudoscientific Trend of Modern Obstetrics," *American Journal of Obstetrics and Gynecology* 2 (1921): 233.

9. Ibid., p. 228.

10. Irving W. Potter, "Discussion" of the series of papers critical of aggressive operative obstetrics, *American Journal of Obstetrics and Gynecology* 2 (1921): 297–98.

11. American Gynecological Association, 1920, p. 79.

12. W. J. Blevins, "Episiotomy with Modified Operative Technic," *American Journal of Obstetrics and Gynecology* 17 (1929): 197; Charles A. Gordon, "The Conduct of Labor and the Management of Obstetric Emergencies," *American Journal of Obstetrics and Gynecology* 13 (1927): 505.

13. DeLee, 1920, p. 43.

14. Joseph B. DeLee, "Discussion," of the series of papers critical of aggressive operative obstetrics, *American Journal of Obstetrics and Gynecology* 2 (1921): 298; DeLee, 1920, p. 43. This interpretation is in accord with the personal view of DeLee by Davis in the article cited in note 1 above.

15. Gordon, 1927, p. 505.

16. B. P. Watson, "The Responsibility of the Obstetric Teacher in Relation to Maternal Mortality and Morbidity," *American Journal of Obstetrics and Gynecology* 14 (1927): 285–86.

17. J. Wesley Bovee, "Discussion," of the series of papers critical of aggressive operative obstetrics, *American Journal of Obstetrics and Gynecology* 2 (1921): 304.

18. Arthur H. Bill, "The Choice of Methods for Making Labor Easy," *American Journal of Obstetrics and Gynecology* 3 (1922): 71.

19. J. M. Munro Kerr, James Haig Ferguson, James Yorun, James Hendry, *A Combined Text-Book of Obstetrics and Gynecology,* Edinburgh: E. & S. Livingstone, 1923, p. 153.

20. Thomas Watts Eden, *A Manual of Midwifery,* 2d ed., London: J. A. Churchill, 1908, p. 163.

21. Ibid., p. 230.

22. Ibid, pp. vi–vii.

23. DeLee, 1913, p. 270.

24. Virtually all recent books on obstetrics (those written from a sociological or historical point of view, that is) discuss the use of "birthing stools" and positions assumed by women under the care of midwives. These women and their childbirth positions can, I suppose, be included among the practices and the knowledge embedded in the practices that obstetrics confronted at this point. Kathleen Vaughan (*Safe Childbirth: The Three Essentials,* Baltimore: William Wood and Co., 1937, p. 108) for example sees the conflict of doctors and midwives as turning on the "secret" of the midwives, namely, "the position natural to women during childbirth" and the willingness of midwives to accommodate various positions. I hesitate to make too much of this because the knowledge—the secret—was not codified and probably did not constitute a serious point of conflict in practice. The important challenges to professional discretion came, I think, from the treatises written primarily by men directly challenging popular obstetrical practice and calling for changes.

25. George J. Englemann, *Labor among Primitive Peoples,* St. Louis: J. H. Chambers, 1883, pp. 54, 149.

26. Ibid., p. 149.

27. Edward A. Schumann, *A Textbook of Obstetrics,* Philadelphia: W. B. Saunders, 1936, pp. 206, 216.

28. J. Whitridge Williams, *Obstetrics: A Text-Book for the Use of Students and Practitioners,* 6th ed., New York: D. Appleton Century, 1930, p. 377.

29. William Thompson Lusk, *The Science and Art of Midwifery,* New York: D. Appleton, 1882, p. 109.

30. Karl Schroeder, *A Manuel of Midwifery Including the Pathology of Pregnancy and the Puerperal State,* from the 3d German ed., London: Churchill, 1873, pp. 90–91.

31. William Potts Dewees, *A Compendious System of Midwifery,* London: John Miller, 1825, p. 189.

32. Williams, 1903, p. 285; for a more recent version see Louis M. Hellman and Jack A. Pritchard, *Williams Obstetrics,* 14th ed., London: Butterworth's, 1971, p. 407.

33. Joseph B. DeLee, *The Principles and Practice of Obstetrics,* 7th ed., Philadelphia. W. B. Saunders, 1940, p. 338.

34. Joseph B. DeLee and J. P. Greenhill, *The Principles and Practice of Obstetrics,* 8th ed., Philadelphia: W. B. Saunders, 1944.

35. Emmanuel A. Friedman, *Biological Principles and Modern Practice of Obstetrics,* 13th ed., Philadelphia: W. B. Saunders, 1974, p. 258.

36. William George Lee, *Childbirth: An Outline of Its Essential Features and the Art of Its Management,* Chicago: University of Chicago Press, 1928, p. 275.

37. George Gallhorn, "Item: A new delivery bed," *American Journal of Obstetrics and Gynecology* 12 (1926): 301; emphasis added.

38. A. C. Williamson, "A new obstetric bed," *American Journal of Obstetrics and Gynecology* 17 (1929): 876.

39. Claude J. Meyer, "Letter: The Continental Delivery Bed," *Obstetrics and Gynecology* 30 (1967): 757.

40. Forest H. Howard, "Delivery in the Physiologic Position," *Obstetrics and Gynecology* 11 (1958): 318.

41. For an example where generally accepted rules for the creation of knowledge were broken, and for an interpretation of why, see Chapter 5, below.

42. Roberto Caldeyro-Barcia, Luis Noriega, Luis A. Cibils, et al., "Effect of Position Changes on the Intensity and Frequency of Uterine Contractions during Labor," *American Journal of Obstetrics and Gynecology* 80 (1960): 203–17, is perhaps the best-known early study of the subject in the American literature, but this paper cites studies published in Britain in 1952, in Switzerland and Germany in 1954, and in Mexico in 1958 which make similar claims. The research continued throughout the 1960s and even included direct radiographic observation of the deleterious effects of the recumbent position on maternal circulation (J. Bieniarz, J. J. Crottogini, E. Curuchet, et al., "Aortacaval Compression by the Uterus in Late Human Pregnancy," *American Journal of Obstetrics and Gynecology* 100 [1968]: 203–17). But even such direct evidence of cause and effect led the authors to the highly scientistic, almost apologetic conclusion that "These circulatory disturbances . . . may have their functional and hormonal implications for the homeostasis and pathology of the pregnant woman" (p. 217). Theirs was certainly not a call for action or change.

For a more social psychological assessment of birth positions, which also was ignored, see Michael Newton and Niles Newton, "The Propped

Position for the Second Stage of Labor," *Obstetrics and Gynecology* 15 (1960): 28–34.

43. Nubar G. O. Tchilinguir, "Fetal Monitoring in High-risk Pregnancy," *Clinics in Obstetrics and Gynecology* 16, 1 (1973): 339.

44. Sir Andrew Claye and Aleck Bourne, eds., *British Obstetric and Gynecological Practice*, 3d ed., London: Heinemann, 1963, p. 198. Texts which recommend the left lateral position for delivery usually also recommend turning the woman onto her back for delivery of the placenta and for the repair of any perineal or cervical tears.

45. Jean Towler and Roy Butler-Manuel, *Modern Obstetrics for Student Midwives*, London: Lloyd-Luke, 1973, pp. 359–60.

46. R. W. Johnstone and R. J. Keller, *A Text-Book of Midwifery*, London: Adam and Charles Black, 1968, p. 574.

47. W. N. Leak, "Letter: Position for Delivery," *British Medical Journal* 2 (1955): 735–36.

48. Grantly Dick-Read, "Letter: Position for Delivery," *British Medical Journal* 2 (1955): 850–51.

The debate continued through several numbers and included this statement from Kathleen Vaughan: "I would like to say that we seem to be the only people in the world who do not use the squatting position for childbirth. . . . And I ask once more, if Newton's tree had been laid on the ground how could the apple have fallen?" (*British Medical Journal* 2 [1955]: 967–68). The debate was closed nine weeks later, before a query about the positions adopted by the anthropoid apes could be answered.

49. For a brief historical review, see Robert H. Barter, John Parks, and Charles Tyndal, "Median Episiotomies and Complete Perineal Lacerations," *American Journal of Obstetrics and Gynecology* 80 (1960): 654–62. Stahl's paper appeared in the *Annals of Gynecology and Pediatrics* 8 (1895): 674.

50. Brooke M. Anspach, "The Value of a More Frequent Employment of Episiotomy in the Second Stage of Labor," *American Journal of Obstetrics and the Diseases of Women* 72 (1915): 711–14.

51. Ralph H. Pomeroy, "Shall We Cut and Reconstruct the Perineum for Every Primipara?" *American Journal of Obstetrics and the Diseases of Women* 78 (1918): 213.

52. DeLee, 1920, pp. 39, 43, 79.

53. Nicholson J. Eastman, "Editorial Comment," *Obstetrical and Gynecological Survey* 3 (1948): 160; emphasis added.

54. Wallace B. Schute, "Episiotomy: A Physiologic Appraisal and a New Painless Technic," *Obstetrics and Gynecology* 14 (1959): 468.

55. DeLee, 1920, pp. 42–43.

56. Ibid., p. 298.

57. Williams, 1930, p. 383.

58. Fred B. Nugent, "The Primiparous Perineum after Forceps Delivery: A Follow-up Comparison of Results with and without Episiotomy," *American Journal of Obstetrics and Gynecology* 30 (1935): 249–56.

59. Polak, 1927.

60. Kenneth R. Niswander and Myron Gordon, "Safety of the Low-Forceps Operation," *American Journal of Obstetrics and Gynecology* 117 (1973): 619–27.

61. Ibid., p. 625.

62. Ibid., p. 626.

63. Robert E. Harris, "An Evaluation of the Median Episiotomy," *American Journal of Obstetrics and Gynecology* 106 (1970): 660–65.

64. J. Bright Banister, Aleck W. Bourne, Trevor B. Davies, et al., *The Queen Charlotte's Practice of Obstetrics,* London: J. A. Churchill, 1927, p. 255.

65. Towler and Butler-Manuel, 1973, p. 487.

66. Claye and Bourne, 1963, p. 203.

67. See Sidney R. Sogolow, "An Historical Review of Oxytocin Prior to Delivery," *Obstetrics and Gynecological Survey* 21 (1966): 155–72; Ralph A. Reis, "A Comparative Study Based on Five Hundred Consecutive Cases of Induction of Labor," *American Journal of Obstetrics and Gynecology* 17 (1929): 392–400; and Schroeder, 1873, pp. 166–194.

68. W. Blair Bell, "The Pituitary Body and the Therapeutic Value of the Infundibular Extract in Shock, Uterine Atony, and Intestinal Paresis," *British Medical Journal* 2 (1909): 1609–13. See also H. H. Dale, "On Some Physiological Actions of Ergot," *Journal of Physiology* 34 (1906): 163–206.

69. B. P. Watson, "Pituitary Extract in Obstetrical Practice," *Canadian Medical Association Journal* 3 (1913): 739; George W. Kosmak, "The Use and Abuse of Pituitary Extract," *Journal of the American Medical Association* 71 (1918): 1117–20; Edward P. Davis, "The Induction, Complicated by Hemorrhage, of Labor," *American Journal of Obstetrics and Gynecology* 2 (1921): 1–5, and discussion, pp. 313–16.

70. Williams, 1903, pp. 283, 294.

71. DeLee, 1913, pp. 351, 364, 428, 443.

72. J. Hofbauer and J. K. Hoerner, "The Nasal Application of Pituitary Extract for the Induction of Labor," *American Journal of Obstetrics and Gynecology* 14 (1927): 148; emphasis added.

73. Williams, 1930, pp. 458, 461.

74. DeLee, 1933; Henricus J. Stander, ("Obstetric Education" and "The Present Trend of Obstetrics," *American Journal of Surgery* 35 [1937]: 221–22) reported a widespread conservative attitude toward induction during this period.

75. Ernest W. Page, "Response of Human Pregnant Uterus to Pitocin Tannate in Oil," *Proceedings of the Society for Experimental Biology and Medicine* 52 (1943): 195–97.

76. DeLee and Greenhill, 1943, pp. 1060, 1064.

77. Nicholson J. Eastman, *Williams Obstetrics,* 10th ed., New York: Appleton-Century-Crofts, 1950, p. 1046.

78. Reed, 1920, p. 33.

79. Harry Fields, John W. Green, and Robert R. Franklin, "Intravenous Pitocin in Induction and Stimulation of Labor: A Study of 3,754 Cases," *Obstetrics and Gynecology* 13 (1959): 353–59.

80. Nicholson J. Eastman, *Williams Obstetrics,* 12th ed., New York: Appleton-Century-Crofts, 1961, p. 1120.

81. J. P. Greenhill, *The Principles and Practice of Obstetrics,* 13th ed., Philadelphia: W. B. Saunders, 1965, p. 436.

82. All of these procedures will be discussed in subsequent chapters.

83. Hellman and Pritchard, 1971, p. 1094; emphasis added.

84. Greenhill and Friedman, 1974, p. 304.

85. See, for example, Claye and Bourne, 1963, pp. 1068–69.

86. M. P. M. Richards, "Innovation in Medical Practice: Obstetricians and the Induction of Labor in Britain," *Social Science and Medicine* 9 (1975): 595–602.

87. For a concise review, see Ann Cartwright, *The Dignity of Labour?: A Study of Childbearing and Induction,* London: Tavistock, 1979. For other perspectives, see Sally MacIntyre, "The Management of Childbirth: A Review of Sociological Research Issues," *Social Science and Medicine* 11 (1977): 477–84, and Royal College of Obstetricians and Gynecologists, *The Management of Labour: Proceedings of the Third Study Group,* London: Royal College of Obstetricians and Gynecologists, 1975.

88. Iain Chalmers, J. G. Lawson, and A. C. Turnbull, "Evaluation of Different Approaches to Obstetric Care: Part I," *British Journal of Obstetrics and Gynecology* 83 (1976): 921–29; idem, "Evaluation of Different Approaches to Obstetric Care: Part II," Ibid., 83 (1976): 930–33.

89. Vincent Tricomi, "Induction of Labor: A Contemporary View," *Clinics in Obstetrics and Gynecology* 16, 4 (1973): 233.

90. William Young, "The Birth Process: Labor and Delivery," pp. 429–43 in R. A. Hockelman, S. Blatman, P. A. Brunell, et al., eds., *Principles of Pediatrics: Health Care of the Young,* New York: McGraw-Hill, 1978, p. 433.

91. Helmuth Vorheer, "Induction and Stimulation of Labor," *Obstetrics and Gynecology Annual* 3 (1974): 283–344.

92. Royal College of Obstetricians and Gynecologists, 1975, p. 8.

Part Two

1. David Armstrong, "Madness and Coping," *Sociology of Health and Illness* 2 (1980): 293–316.

2. Michel Foucault, *Discipline and Punish: The Birth of the Prison,* London: Allen Lane, 1977, p. 209.

3. N. Destounis, "On Teaching Psychosomatic Medicine to Medical Students," pp. 68–70 in *Psychosomatic Medicine in Obstetrics and Gynaecology, Third International Congress, London, 1971,* Basel: Karger, 1972, pp. 68–69.

4. Ibid., p. 69.

5. The translator of Foucault's *Discipline and Punish* made it clear that "discipline," the word that describes the set of techniques and activities outlined in the text, is the wrong word. Foucault's title was *Surveiller et Punir.* There is just no word in English to convey the sense of the French *"surveiller."* Neither "surveillance," "supervise," "inspect," or "observe" captures the full sense of the word. I feel that using "monitoring" and "surveillance" together is a reasonable representation. I will use the word "monitoring" alone to describe the entire structure of control and the two words together to represent the activities, mechanisms, and techniques of the structure.

The important point about panopticism, the mechanism underlying monitoring, is that the panopticon is a structure of control, a machine that carries out monitoring, surveillance, and normalization independent of agents of control.

6. Henry M. Seidel and Robert A. Hoekelman, "Ecology of Patient Care," pp. 3–17 in Robert A. Hoekelman, Saul Blatman, Philip A. Brunell, Stanford B. Friedman, and Henry M. Seidel, eds., *Principles of Pediatrics: Health Care of the Young,* New York: McGraw-Hill, 1978.

7. Ibid., p. 3.

8. Ibid., p. 8.

9. Ibid., p. 8.

10. Ibid., p. 16

11. Ibid., p. 7.

12. Hans O. Mauksch, "A Social Science Basis for Conceptualizing Child Health," *Social Science and Medicine* 8 (1974): 521–28, quoted in Seidel and Hoekelman, 1978, p. 8.

13. Seidel and Hoekelman, 1978, p. 9.

14. Ibid., p. 3.

15. Ibid., p. 6.

16. E. O. Wilson, *Sociobiology: The New Synethesis,* Cambridge, Mass.: Harvard University Press, The Belknap Press, 1975.

17. Jürgen Habermas, *Knowledge and Human Interests,* Boston: Beacon Press, 1971, p. 310. See also John P. Sisk, "The Tyranny of Harmony," *American Scholar* 46 (1977): 193–205.

18. Seidel and Hoekelman, 1978, pp. 4–6.

19. Alice Rossi, "A Biosocial Perspective on Parenting," *Daedulus,* (Spring 1977): 25.

20. Selma Fraiberg, *Every Child's Birthright: In Defense of Mothering,* New York: Basic Books, 1977, p. 5.

21. Ernst Becker, *Escape from Evil,* New York: The Free Press, 1975.

22. Seidel and Hoekelman, 1978, p. 13.

23. Ibid., p. 17.

24. Michel Foucault, "History of Systems of Thought: Summary of a Course Given at Collège de France—1970–1971," pp. 199–204 in Donald F. Bouchard, ed., *Michel Foucault: Language, Counter-Memory, Practice: Selected Essays and Interviews,* Ithaca, N.Y.: Cornell University Press, 1977, p. 200.

25. J. Whitridge Williams, *Obstetrics: A Textbook for the Use of Students and Practitioners,* 6th ed., New York: Appleton-Century, 1930, p. 376; emphasis added.

26. John S. Tomkinson, "Discussion" of Thomas F. Dillon, Barbara A. Brennan, John F. Dwyer, Abraham Risk, Alan Sear, Lynne Dawson, Raymond Vande Wiele, "Midwifery, 1977," *American Journal of Obstetrics and Gynecology* 130 (1978): 924.

Chapter Four

1. R. T. H. Lannec, *D l'Auscultation Mediate,* Paris: J. A. Brossen, 1819. Also see J. A. Lejeaneau: *Memoire sur l'Auscultation, Appliqué d l'Etude de la Grossesse,* Paris, 1822.

2. Edward H. Hon and O. W. Hess, "Instrumentation of Fetal Electrocardiography," *Science* 125 (1957): 553–54.

3. Michael R. Neuman, Jacques F. Roux, Malcolm G. Munro, Stephen M. Owen, and Harold E. Fox, "Evaluation of Fetal Monitoring by Telemetry," *Obstetrics and Gynecology* 54 (1979): 249–54.

4. J. Whitridge Williams, *Obstetrics: A Textbook for the Use of Students and Practitioners,* 1st ed., New York: D. Appleton, 1903.

5. Edward H. Hon, "The Fetal Heart Rate Patterns Preceding Death in Utero," *American Journal of Obstetrics and Gynecology* 78 (1959): 47–56.

6. For a discussion of these patterns, see the brief review in National Institutes of Health, *Antenatal Diagnosis: Task Force on the Predictors of Fetal Distress,* Washington, D.C.: U.S. Department of Health, Education, and Welfare, April, 1979.

7. The Boston Women's Health Book Collective, *Our Bodies, Ourselves: A Book by and for Women,* rev. ed., New York: Simon and Schuster, 1976, p. 286.

8. Ibid., p. 286.

9. Philip J. Steer, "Monitoring in Labor," *British Journal of Hospital Practice* 17 (1977): 219–25.

10. Edward J. Quilligan and Richard H. Paul, "Fetal Monitoring: Is it Worth It?," *Obstetrics and Gynecology* 45 (1975): 96–100.

11. H. David Banta and Stephen B. Thacker, *Costs and Benefits of Electronic Fetal Monitoring: A Review of the Literature,* NCHSR Research Report Series, Washington, D.C.: U.S. Department of Health, Education, and Welfare, April, 1979. Virtually all of the assumptions used to arrive at the cost estimate in this report have been challenged in an editorial in *Obstetrics and Gynecology.* John C. Hobbins, Roger Freeman, and John T. Queenan ("The Fetal Monitoring Debate," *Obstetrics and Gynecology* 54 [1979]: 103–9) say, "Probably the only valid analysis [in Banta and Thacker's report] involves the actual cost of EFM—that is, $35–$50 per patient" (p. 107). They add, "In summary, the cost of EFM shrinks from $411 million to $80 million per year, roughly equivalent to the cost of a B1 bomber" (p. 108).

12. National Institutes of Health, 1979, pp. III:133–III:144.

13. The courts are clearly involved in the control of obstetrical work, and government documents like these play a role in court cases. H. David Banta and Stephen B. Thacker, in "Policies toward Medical Technology: The Case of Electronic Fetal Monitoring," *American Journal of Public Health* 69 (1979): 931–35, comment on some of the legal cases involving fetal monitoring on which they have already been asked to consult. They say, "More than ten malpractice suits have been brought against institutions and physicians in cases where a newborn had died or been born mentally retarded and EFM had not been used. At least one suit has been brought against a physician for the use of EFM which alledgedly caused a fatal infection of the mother" (p. 934). Dr. Keith P. Russell, commenting on a 1977 analysis of fetal heart patterns (discussion of Robert C. Goodlin and Hanns C. Haesslin, "When Is It fetal distress?," *American Journal of Obstetrics and Gynecology* 128 [1977]: 440–47) said, "My own concern with this phenomenon has become accentuated by the medical-legal implications. . . . What we are seeing is the increased introduction of an abnormal fetal heart tracing as prima facie evidence of any resultant abnormality" (p. 445).

Women are encouraged to use these documents to effect change in obstetrical practice through editorials like that of Madeleine H. Shearer, "Auscultation Is 'Acceptable' in Low-Risk Women," *Birth and the Family Journal* 6 (1979): 3–5, which encouraged childbirth educators to use the government's Task Force Report in their classes and to send its recommendations to doctors and legislators.

14. (a) *Experimental Studies: Randomized Designs:* Albert D. Haverkamp, Horace E. Thompson, John G. McFee, and Curtis Cetrulo, "The Evaluation of Continuous Fetal Heart Rate Monitoring in High-Risk Pregnancy," *American Journal of Obstetrics and Gynecology* 125 (1976): 310–20; Albert D. Haverkamp, Miriam Orleans, Sharon Langendoerfer, John McFee, James Murphy, and Horace E. Thompson, "A Controlled Trial of the Differential Effects of Intrapartum Fetal Monitoring," *American Journal of Obstetrics and Gynecology* 134 (1979): 399–412; Peter Renou, Allan

Chang, Ian Anderson, and Carl Wood, "Controlled Trial of Fetal Intensive Care," *American Journal of Obstetrics and Gynecology* 126 (1976): 470–76; Ian M. Kelso, R. John Parsons, Gordon F. Lawrence, Shyam S. Arora, D. Keith Edmonds, and Ian D. Cooke, "An Assessment of Continuous Fetal Heart Rate Monitoring in Labor: A Randomized Trial," *American Journal of Obstetrics and Gynecology* 131 (1978): 526–32.

   (b) *Experimental Studies: Non-randomized Designs:* Wan H. Chan, Richard H. Paul, and Judy Toews, "Intrapartum Fetal Monitoring: Maternal and Fetal Morbidity and Perinatal Mortality," *Obstetrics and Gynecology* 41 (1973): 818–24; Richard H. Paul, James R. Huey, and Carl F. Yaeger, "Clinical Fetal Monitoring: Its Effect on Cesarean Section Rate and Perinatal Mortality: Five-Year Trends," *Postgraduate Medicine* 61 (1977): 160–66; Gino Tutera and Robert L. Newman, "Fetal Monitoring: Its Effect on the Perinatal Mortality and Cesarean Section Rates and Its Complications," *American Journal of Obstetrics and Gynecology* 122 (1975): 750–54; Jack C. Amato, "Fetal Monitoring in a Community Hospital: A Statistical Analysis," *Obstetrics and Gynecology* 50 (1977): 269–74.

   (c) *Quasi-experimental Studies:* P. T. Edington, J. Sibanda, and R. W. Beard, "Influence on Clinical Practice of Routine Intrapartum Fetal Monitoring," *British Medical Journal* 3 (1975): 341–43; K. S. Koh, D. Greves, S. Yung, and L. J. Peddle, "Experience with Fetal Monitoring in a University Teaching Hospital," *Canadian Medical Association Journal* 112 (1975): 455–60; Lewis Shenker, Robert C. Post, and Jerome S. Seiler, "Routine Electronic Monitoring of Fetal Heart Rate and Uterine Activity during Labor," *Obstetrics and Gynecology* 46 (1975): 185–89; Wing K. Lee and Michael S. Baggish, "The Effect on Unselected Intrapartum Fetal Monitoring," *Obstetrics and Gynecology* 47 (1976): 516–20; Raymond R. Neutra, Stephen E. Feinberg, Sander Greenland, and Emmanuel A. Friedman, "Effect of Fetal Monitoring on Neonatal Death Rates," *New England Journal of Medicine* 299 (1978): 324–26.

   15. Lee and Baggish, 1976, p. 516.

   16. See, for example, Dr. Robert A. Munsick's discussion of the Haverkamp et al. 1979 study, *American Journal of Obstetrics and Gynecology* 134 (1979): 409–11.

   17. Lee and Baggish, 1976, p. 519.

   18. Edward J. Quilligan, "The Obstetric Intensive Care Unit," *Hospital Practice* 7, 6 (1972): 61–69.

   19. Paul, Huey, and Yaeger, 1977, p. 166.

   20. National Institutes of Health, 1979, pp. III:197–III:198.

   21. Neutra et al., 1978, p. 325.

   22. Banta and Thacker, 1979, p. 18.

   23. R. Alan Baker, "Technologic Intervention in Obstetrics: Has the Pendulum Swung too Far?," *Obstetrics and Gynecology* 5 (1978): 241–44.

24. Leader, "Intrapartum Fetal Monitoring for All?" *British Medical Journal* 2 (1976): 1466.

25. Hobbins, Freeman, and Queenan, 1979, p. 108.

26. National Institutes of Health, 1979, p. III:166.

27. *British Medical Journal* Leader, 1976, p. 1466.

28. National Institutes of Health, 1979, p. III:165; Baker, 1978, p. 243.

29. David Armstrong, "Clinical Sense and Clinical Science," *Social Science and Medicine* 11 (1977): 601.

30. M. P. M. Richards, "Innovation in Medical Practice: Obstetricians and the Induction of Labor in Britain," *Social Science and Medicine* 9 (1975): 595–602, is just one example of this kind of argument.

31. Richard W. Wertz and Dorothy C. Wertz, *Lying-In: A History of Childbirth in America,* New York: The Free Press, 1977, pp. 132–77.

32. Ibid., p. 173. As I suggest in chapter 7, this is an overstatement. Women had not lost their *bodies.* They had lost only part of their bodies—the obstetrically important part—and for only a short period of time, the obstetrically appropriate period.

33. That the transformation of the hospital was a matter of national policy in Britain makes its history easier to document, but the course of British and American obstetrics with regard to the development of mechanisms of surveillance and monitoring were so similar from the 1950s onwards that the conclusion that a similar transformation was occurring in the United States is at least reasonable. A later section on monitoring's control over physicians and staff in American obstetrics shows how developments in the two countries paralleled one another.

34. Royal College of Obstetricians and Gynecologists, *Report on a National Maternity Service,* London, May, 1944; Ministry of Health, *Report of the Maternity Services Committee,* London: HMSO, 1959. (This is the *Cranbrook Report,* so called because the committee was chaired by the Earl of Cranbrook.) Standing Maternity and Midwifery Advisory Committee, *Domiciliary Midwifery and Maternity Bed Needs: Report of the Subcommittee,* London: HMSO, 1970. (This is the *Peel Report,* so called because the subcommittee was chaired by Sir John Peel.)

35. Royal College of Obstetricians and Gynecologists, 1944, p. 6; emphasis added.

36. Ibid.

37. Ibid., pp. 8–9.

38. Ibid., pp. 22, 38.

39. Ibid., pp. 8–9.

40. Ibid., p. 41.

41. Ministry of Health, 1959, p. 19.

42. Ibid.

43. Ibid., pp. 83–84.

44. Standing Maternity and Midwifery Advisory Subcommittee, 1970, p. 54.

45. Ibid., p. 60.

46. Ibid., pp. 10, 60.

47. Michel Foucault, *Discipline and Punish: The Birth of the Prison,* London: Butterworth, pp. 197, 198, 198, 202, 203.

48. Joint Committee of the Royal College of Obstetricians and Gynecologists and the Population Investigation Committee, *Maternity in Great Britain,* London: Oxford University Press, 1948, pp. 1–2, vi.

49. Ibid., pp. 22–47, vi, 215–16.

50. See, for example, the studies in George McLachlan and Richard Shegog, *In the Beginning: Studies of Maternity Services,* London: Nuffield Provincial Hospitals Trust, 1970; N. R. Butter and D. G. Bonham, *Perinatal Mortality: First Report of the 1958 British Perinatal Mortality Survey,* Edinburgh: Livingstone, 1963; and N. R. Butter and E. D. Alberman, *Perinatal Problems: The Second Report of the 1958 British Perinatal Mortality Survey,* Edinburgh: Livingstone, 1969.

51. Ursula M. Anderson, Rachel Jenss, William E. Mosher, Clyde L. Randall, and Edward Marra, "High-Risk Groups: Definition and Identification," *New England Journal of Medicine* 273 (1965): 308.

52. Ibid., p. 312.

53. Jacques F. Roux, Michael R. Newman, and Robert C. Goodin, "Monitoring of Intrapartum Phenomena," *CRC Critical Reviews in Bioengineering* 2 (1975): 120.

54. Standing Maternity and Midwifery Advisory Subcommittee, 1970, p. 27.

55. Williams, 1903, p. 750; Henricus J. Stander, *Williams Obstetrics,* 8th ed., New York: D. Appleton-Century, 1941, p. 1103.

56. Jack A. Pritchard and Paul C. MacDonald, *Williams Obstetrics,* 15th ed., New York: Appleton-Century-Crofts, 1976, p. 265.

57. Curtis L. Cetrulo and Roger K. Freeman, "Problems and Risks of Fetal Monitoring," pp. 82–103, in Silvio Aladjem, ed., *Risks in the Practice of Modern Obstetrics,* vol. 2, St. Louis: Mosby, 1975.

58. Quilligan, 1972, p. 69.

59. Harvey A. Galbert and Morton A. Stenchever, "Continuous Electronic Monitoring of Fetal Heart Rate during Labor," *American Journal of Obstetrics and Gynecology* 115 (1973): 919–23. See also Paul, Huey, and Yaeger, 1977, pp. 165–66.

60. Kieran O'Driscoll, Malachi Coughlan, Vincent Fenton, and Maire Skelly, "Active Management of Labor: Care of the Fetus," *British Medical Journal* 2 (1977): 1452.

61. Clyde L. Randall, "Childbirth without Fear of Interference," *Clinics in Obstetrics and Gynecology* 2 (1959): 366.

62. Quilligan and Paul, 1975, pp. 96–97.

63. William Young, "The Birth Process: The Setting," pp. 425–27 in R. A. Hoekelman, S. Blatman, P. A. Brunell, S. B. Friedman, and H. M. Seidel, *Principles of Pediatrics: Health Care of the Young,* New York: McGraw-Hill, 1978. Young says, "The physician responsible for newborn care must remember that he or she is the baby's advocate" (p. 427).

64. Pritchard and MacDonald, 1976, p. vii.

65. Kelly and Kulkarni, 1973, pp. 822–23.

66. Tutera and Newman, 1975, p. 752.

67. Pritchard and MacDonald, 1976, p. 323; Quilligan, 1972, p. 69.

68. Ralph C. Benson, Frank Shubek, Jerome Deutschberger, William Weiss, and Heinz Berendes, "Fetal Heart Rate as a Predictor of Fetal Distress: A Report from the Collaborative Project," *Obstetrics and Gynecology* 32 (1968): 259–66. Hon, 1957, also felt the fetal monitor would help chart the limits of normalcy.

69. Stander, 1941, pp. 1103–4.

70. Jack A. Pritchard, *Williams Obstetrics,* 14th ed., New York: Appleton-Century-Crofts, 1971. The thirteenth edition, by Nicholson Eastman and Louis Hellman, published in 1966, is almost identical in this passage.

71. Pritchard and MacDonald, 1976, p. 787.

72. R. I. Lowensohn, S. Y. Yeh, A. Forsythe, and E. H. Hon, "Computer-Assessed Fetal Heart Rate Patterns and Fetal Scalp pH," *Obstetrics and Gynecology* 46 (1975): 190–93.

73. Sidney F. Bottoms, Mortimer G. Rosen, and Robert J. Sokol, "The Increase in the Cesarean Section Birth Rate," *New England Journal of Medicine* 302 (1980): 559–63.

74. David J. Nochimson, Jane S. Turbeville, Joan E. Terry, Ray H. Petrie, and Laurence E. Lundy, "The Non-Stress Test," *Obstetrics and Gynecology* 51 (1978): 419. Also see Donna Pratt, Frayda Diamond, Harry Yen, Joseph Bieniarz, and Lawrence Burd, "Fetal Stress and Nonstress Tests: An Analysis and Comparison of Their Ability to Identify Fetal Outcome," *Obstetrics and Gynecology* 54 (1979): 419–23.

75. Goodlin and Haesslin, 1977.

76. James W. Goodwin, James T. Dunne and Bruce W. Thomas, "Antepartum Identification of the Fetus at Risk," *Canadian Medical Association Journal* 101 (1969): 458–64; emphasis added.

77. Robert E. L. Nesbitt and Richard H. Aubry, "High-Risk Obstetrics II. Value of a Semiobjective Grading System in Identifying the Vulnerable Group," *American Journal of Obstetrics and Gynecology* 103 (1969): 972.

78. Ian Morrison and Joan Olsen, "Perinatal Mortality and Antepartum Risk Scoring," *Obstetrics and Gynecology* 53 (1979): 362–66. These authors say, "Risk scoring is better suited to the role of screening and identification for investigation than as a basis for directly affecting treatment and management of pregnancy. . . . The collection of this information on a regional basis in the pregnant population can identify the distribution of risk preg-

nancies. . . . The function of a numerical scoring system will be to refine [the process of referring high-risk women to regional centers for care] by more clearly and urgently identifying the high risk group" (p. 365).

79. Emmanuel A. Friedman, "Primigravid Labor: A Graphicostatistical Analysis," *Obstetrics and Gynecology* 6 (1955): 567–89.

80. R. H. Philpott and W. M. Castle, "Cervicographs in the Management of Labor in Primigravidae," in two parts, *Journal of Obstetrics and Gynecology of the British Empire* 79 (1972): 529–98 (Part I) and 599–602 (Part II).

81. John Studd, "The Partographic Control of Labor," *Clinics in Obstetrics and Gynecology* 2 (1975): 127–51.

82. Williams, 1903, pp. 402–3.

83. Bottoms, Rosen, and Sokol, 1980, p. 561. See also Lester T. Hibbard, "Changing Trends in Cesarean Section," *American Journal of Obstetrics and Gynecology* 125 (1976): 798–804.

84. Hani Haddad and Laurence E. Lundy, "Changing Indications for Cesarean Section: A 38-Year Experience at a Community Hospital," *Obstetrics and Gynecology* 51 (1978): 136.

85. Murray W. Enkin, "Having a Section is Having a Baby," *Birth and the Family Journal* 4 (1977): 99–105; emphasis added.

86. Dyane D. Affonso and Jaynelle F. Stichler, "Exploratory Study of Women's Reactions to Having a Cesarean Birth," *Birth and the Family Journal* 5 (1978): 88—94.

87. Pritchard and MacDonald, 1976, p. 903.

88. James Walker, Ian MacGillivray, and Malcolm Macnaughton, *Combined Textbook of Obstetrics and Gynecology,* 9th ed., Edinburgh: Churchill Livingstone, 1976, p. 313.

89. Steer, 1977, p. 224. Most of the list of monitoring devices is taken from this article.

90. Haverkamp et al., 1976, p. 316.

91. Munsick, 1979, p. 410–11: "I would like you to entertain a hypothesis which will explain on the basis of dehumanization with EM [electronic monitoring] the increased rates of both fetal distress and cesarean section. We begin by restraining a woman early in her labor. We allow her to see the EM's chattering stylus and winks; often we even torture her unnecessarily with hours of its staccato sounds at 150 beeps per minute and we watch the monitor and not her. She dare not interrupt our silent vigil. Anxiety gives way to fright and anger. Something—possibly cathecholamines—causes her to have abnormal contractions and those in turn cause arrest of labor and sometimes uteroplacental blood flow. And then we apply the modern-day obstetric panacea—cesarean section."

92. Neuman et al., 1979, pp. 252–53.

93. Barbara Ehrenreich, "Birth Is Their Business," *Seven Days,* May 5, 1978: 26–27, p. 27.

94. Newman et al., 1979, p. 254; Anna Flynn and John Kelly, "Continuous Fetal Monitoring in the Ambulent Patient in Labor," *British Medical Journal* 2 (1976): 843.

95. Jane E. Brody, "Routine Fetal Monitoring is Termed Costly and Unsafe," *New York Times*, January 2, 1979.

96. Steer, 1977, p. 219.

97. Haverkamp et al., 1976, p. 316.

98. Foucault, 1977, pp. 197, 204, 207.

99. Roux, Newman, and Goodlin, 1975, p. 129; emphasis added.

100. Haverkamp et al., 1979, p. 406; emphasis added.

101. Lee and Baggish, 1976, p. 520.

102. Koh et al., 1975, pp. 457–60.

103. Quilligan, 1972, p. 62.

104. Ibid., p. 64.

105. Ibid.

106. Leon I. Mann and Janice Galbert, "Modern Indications for Cesarean Section," *American Journal of Obstetrics and Gynecology* 135 (1979): 437.

Chapter Five

1. Vermont Educational Television, "Home Births in Vermont: New Odds for an Old Gamble?" 1978. Quote is from an independent midwife practicing in Vermont.

2. Marshall H. Klaus and John H. Kennell, Maternal-Infant Bonding: The Impact of Early Separation or Loss on Family Development, St. Louis: Mosby, 1976; Edward O. Wilson, *Sociobiology: The New Synthesis,* Cambridge: Harvard University Press, 1975.

3. Klaus and Kennell, 1976, p. 22.

4. Ibid., p. 28.

5. Alice Rossi, "A Biosocial Perspective on Parenting," *Daedalus,* 106, 2 (1977): 9–11.

6. Klaus and Kennell, 1976, p. 37.

7. John Bowlby, "Nature of a Child's Tie to His Mother," *International Journal of Psychoanalysis* 39 (1958): 350–73; John Bowlby, *Attachment and Loss,* vol. 1, New York: Basic Books, 1969; Arthur J. Brodbeck and Orvis C. Irwin, "The Speech Behavior of Infants without Families," *Child Development* 17 (1946): 145–56; Anna Freud and Dorothy Burlingham, *Infants Without Families,* New York: International Universities Press, 1944; René A. Spitz, "Hospitalism," *Psychoanalytic Study of the Child* 2 (1946): 113–17.

8. Leon J. Yarrow, "Maternal Deprivation: Toward an Empirical and Conceptual Re-evaluation," *Psychological Bulletin* 58 (1961): 459–90.

9. Alison Clarke-Stewart, *Child Care Policy in the Family: A Review of Research and Some Propositions for Policy,* New York: Academic Press, 1977, p. 12.

10. M. H. Klaus, R. Jerauld, N. C. Kreger, W. McAlpine, M. Steffa, and J. H. Kennell, "Maternal Attachment: Importance of the First Post-partum Days," *New England Journal of Medicine* 286 (1972): 460–63.

11. Ibid., p. 461.

12. Norma M. Ringler, John H. Kennell, Robert Jarvella, Billie J. Navojosky, and Marshall H. Klaus, "Mother-to-Child Speech at 2 Years: Effects of Early Postnatal Contact," *Journal of Pediatrics* 86 (1975): 141–44; Norma Ringler, Mary Ann Trause, and Marshall H. Klaus, "Mother's Speech to Her Two-Year-Old, Its Effect on Speech and Language Comprehension at 5 Years," *Pediatric Research* 10 (1976): 307.

13. Klaus and Kennell, 1976, p. 59.

14. Ibid., pp. 65–66.

15. Clarke-Stewart, 1977, p. 6.

16. Klaus and Kennell, 1976, p. 2.

17. Leslie Jordon Cohen, "The Operational Definition of Human Attachment," *Psychological Bulletin* 81 (1974): 207–17; Jacob L. Gewirtz, "Attachment, Dependence, and Distinction in Terms of Stimulus Control," pp. 139–215 in Jacob L. Gewirtz, ed., *Attachment and Dependency,* Washington: Winston, 1972; Michael E. Lamb, "A Defense of the Concept of Attachment," *Human Development* 17 (1974): 376–85; John C. Masters and Henry M. Wellman, "The Study of Human Attachment: A Procedural Change," *Psychological Bulletin* 81 (1974): 218–37; Miriam K. Rosenthal, "Attachment and Mother-Infant Interaction: Some Research Impasses and a Suggested Change in Orientation," *Journal of Child Psychology and Psychiatry* 14 (1973): 201–7; Marsha Weinraub, Jeanne Brooks, and Michael Lewis, "The Social Network: A Reconsideration of the Concept of Attachment," *Human Development* 20 (1977): 31–47; Tannis MacBeth Williams, "Infant Development and Supplemental Care: A Comparative Study of Basic and Applied Research," *Human Development* 20 (1977): 1–30.

18. Rosenthal, 1973, pp. 201–2.

19. Weinraub, Brooks, and Lewis, 1977.

20. Andrew Whitten, "Assessing the Effects of Perinatal Events on the Success of Mother-Infant Relationships," pp. 403–25 in H. R. Schaffer, ed., *Studies in Mother-Infant Interaction,* London: Academic Press, 1977.

21. Masters and Wellman, 1974, p. 218.

22. Ibid., p. 228.

23. A. D. Leifer, P. H. Leiderman, C. R. Barnett, and J. A. Williams, "Effects of Mother-Infant Separation on Maternal Attachment Behavior," *Child Development* 43 (1972): 1203–18.

24. Ibid., pp. 1213–14; emphasis added.

25. Ibid., p. 1214.

26. Klaus, Jerauld et al., 1972.

27. See Judith Bernal Dunn and M. P. M. Richards, "Observations on the Relationship between Mother and Baby in the Neonatal Period," pp. 427–55 in H. R. Schaffer, ed., *Studies in Maternal-Infant Interaction,* London: Academic Press, 1977, for this criticism and an exception.

28. Selma Fraiberg, *Every Child's Birthright: In Defense of Mothering,* New York: Basic Books, 1977, p. 56; emphasis added.

29. Ibid., p. 34.

30. Ibid., p. 49.

31. Ibid., p. 47.

32. Robert W. ten Bensel and Charles L. Paxson, "Clinical Notes: Child Abuse Following Early Postpartum Separation," *Journal of Pediatrics* 90 (1977): 490; Margaret A. Lynch, "Ill-Health and Child Abuse," *Lancet* 2 (1975): 317–19; Avroy A. Fanaroff, John H. Kennell, and Marshall H. Klaus, "Follow-up on Low Birth Weight Infants: The Predictive Value of Maternal Visiting Patterns," *Pediatrics* 49 (1972): 287–90.

33. Klaus and Kennell, 1976, p. 53.

34. Richard M. Wertz and Dorothy C. Wertz, *Lying-In: A History of Childbirth in America,* New York: The Free Press, 1977.

35. Ibid., p. 179.

36. Klaus and Kennell, 1976, pp. 6ff.

37. Jeffrey Lionel Berlant, *Profession and Monopoly: A Study of Medicine in the United States and Great Britain,* Berkeley: University of California Press, 1975.

38. Joann S. Lublin, "The Birthing Room: More Hospitals Offer Maternity Facilities That Feel Like Home," *Wall Street Journal* 193 (February 15, 1979): 1, 22.

39. Klaus and Kennell, 1976, p. 41.

40. ten Bensel and Paxson, 1977.

41. Leader, "Helping Mothers to Love Their Babies," *British Medical Journal* 2 (1977): 595.

42. Fraiberg, 1977, p. 62.

43. Ibid., p. 76.

44. Jeffrey M. Blum, *Pseudoscience and Mental Ability: The Origins and Fallacies of the IQ Controversy,* New York: Monthly Review Press, 1978.

45. Ibid., p. 146.

46. Ibid., p. 156.

47. Leta S. Hollingsworth, "Social Devices for Impelling Women to Bear and Rear Children," *American Journal of Sociology* 22 (1916): 21; emphasis in the original.

48. Ibid., pp. 20–21.

49. Ibid., p. 29.

50. Jacques Donzelot, *The Policing of Families,* New York: Pantheon, 1979, p. xxvi.

51. Christopher Lasch, *Haven in a Heartless World: The Family Besieged,* New York: Basic Books, 1977.

52. Bias is different from error. Research can be well done and still be biased. Methodological errors were discussed earlier. Errors are important in this context because they force one to ask why rules of inquiry were violated. Bias points one in the direction of answers to this crucial question.

53. Klaus, Jerauld et al., 1972.

54. Wini Breines, Margaret Cerullo, and Judith Stacey, "Social Biology, Family Studies, and Anti-Feminist Backlash," *Feminist Studies* 4 (1978): 43–67.

55. Clarke-Stewart, 1977, p. 21.

56. Rossi, 1977, p. 25.

57. Breines et al., 1978, p. 43.

58. Jürgen Habermas, *Knowledge and Human Interests,* Boston: Beacon Press, 1971, p. 310. My discussion of the social uses of theory draws on the excellent appendix to this book.

Chapter Six

1. Daniel Callahan, "To Confront Ethical Issues in Medicine," *New England Journal of Medicine* 292 (1975): 315–16.

2. Bentley Glass, "Maupertius and the Beginnings of Genetics," *Quarterly Review of Biology* 22 (1947): 196–210.

3. R. A. Fisher, "Has Mendel's Work Been Rediscovered," *Annals of Science* 1 (1936): 115–37.

4. A. H. Sturtevant, *A History of Genetics,* New York: Harper and Row, 1965.

5. National Institutes of Health, *Antenatal Diagnosis: Task Force on the Predictors of Hereditary Disease or Congenital Defects,* Washington, D.C.: U.S. Department of Health, Education, and Welfare, April, 1979.

6. The NICHD National Registry for Amniocentesis Study Group, "Midtrimester Amniocentesis for Prenatal Diagnosis: Safety and Accuracy," *Journal of the American Medical Association* 236 (1976): 1476.

7. Nancy E. Simpson, L. Dallaire, J. R. Miller, L. Siminovitch, and J. L. Hamerton, "Prenatal Diagnosis of Genetic Disease in Canada: Report of a Collaborative Study," *Canadian Medical Association Journal* 115 (1976): 739–48.

8. A. C. Turnbull, D. V. I. Fairweather, B. M. Hibbard, et al., "An Assessment of the Hazards of Amniocentesis: Report to the Medical Research Council by Their Working Party on Amniocentesis," *British Journal of Obstetrics and Gynecology* 85 (1978): supplement no. 2, pp. 1–2.

9. National Institutes of Health, 1979, pp. I:63–I:66.

10. Tabitha M. Powledge, "Genetic Screening as a Political and Social Development," pp. 25–55 in Daniel Bergsma, ed., *Ethical, Social, and Legal*

Dimensions of Screening for Human Genetic Disease, New York: Stratton, 1974, pp. 46, 34.

11. John W. Littlefield, "The Pregnancy at Risk for a Genetic Disorder," *New England Journal of Medicine* 282 (1970): 627–28, in describing the results of the first series of amniocenteses says, "Of course, amniocentesis should not be undertaken unless the family is committed to subsequent intervention [if the test indicates intervention is] appropriate."

12. Tabitha M. Powledge, "Amniocentesis Is Shown Safe and Effective: From Experimental Procedure to Accepted Practice," *Hastings Center Report* 6 (1976): 7.

13. Rosalyn Benjamin Darling, "Parents, Physicians, and Spina Bifida," *Hastings Center Report* 7 (1977): 10–14.

14. World Health Organization, *Genetic Disorders: Prevention, Treatment, and Rehabilitation,* Technical Report No. 497, Geneva: World Health Organization, 1972.

15. National Institutes of Health, 1979, pp. I:72–I:73.

16. Ibid., p. I:76.

17. Ronald Conley and Aubrey Milunsky, "The Economics of Prenatal Genetic Diagnosis," pp. 442–55 in Aubrey Milunsky, ed., *The Prevention of Genetic Disease and Mental Retardation,* Philadelphia: W. B. Saunders, 1975.

18. William B. Nelson, J. Michael Swint, and C. Thomas Caskey, "An Economic Evaluation of a Genetic Screening Program for Tay-Sachs Disease," *American Journal of Human Genetics* 30 (1978): 160–66; Richard P. Inman, "On the Benefits and Costs of Genetic Screening," *American Journal of Human Genetics* 30 (1978): 219–23; J. Michael Swint, Judith M. Shapiro, Virginia L. Corson, Linda W. Reynolds, George W. Thomas, and Haig H. Kazazian, "The Economic Returns to Community and Hospital Screening Programs for Genetic Disease," *Preventive Medicine* 8 (1979): 463–70.

19. Samuel P. Bessman and Judith P. Swaezy, "PKU: A Study of Biomedical Legislation," pp. 49–76 in Everett Mendelsohn, Judith P. Swaezy, and Irene Taviss, eds., *Human Aspects of Biomedical Innovation,* Cambridge: Harvard University Press, 1971.

20. Neil R. M. Buist and Banoo M. Jhaveri, "A Guide to Screening Newborn Infants for Inborn Errors of Metabolism," *Journal of Pediatrics* 82 (1973): 511–22.

21. Ernest B. Hook, "Behavioral Implications of the Human XYY Genotype," *Science* 179 (1973): 139–50.

22. George Stamatoyannopolous, "Problems of Screening and Counseling in the Hemoglobinopathies," pp. 268–76 in Arno G. Motulsky and W. Lenz, eds., *Birth Defects: Proceedings of the 4th International Conference,* Vienna, 1973, Geneva: Exerpta Medica, 1974.

23. Claire O. Leonard, Gary A. Chase, and Barton Childs, "Genetic Counseling: A Consumer's View," *New England Journal of Medicine* 287 (1972): 436; M. Neil Macintyre, "Problems and Limitations of Prenatal Genetic Evaluation," pp. 104–24 in Silvio Aladjem, ed., *Risks in the Practice of Modern Obstetrics,* volume 2, St. Louis: Mosby, 1975.

24. Michael B. Mosher, "Sickle Cell Trait," *New England Journal of Medicine* 282 (1970): 1157–58. The National Academy of Science (*The S-Hemoglobinopathies: An Evaluation of Their Status in the Armed Forces,* Washington, D.C.: National Academy of Science—National Research Council, 1973) recommended that everyone be screened for sickle cell trait, i.e., for heterozygosity for sickle cell disease, before induction into the armed services.

25. Barbara J. Culliton, "Sickle Cell Anemia: National Program Raises Problems as Well as Hopes," *Science* 178 (1972): 283–86.

26. A number of people have noted this benefit of screening. See, for example, R. Guthrie, "Mass Screening for Genetic Disease," *Hospital Practice* 7 (1972): 93–100, or H. M. Nitowsky, "Prescriptive Screening for Inborn Errors of Metabolism," *American Journal of Mental Deficiency* 77 (1973): 538–50.

27. Harvey L. Levy, "Newborn Screening for Metabolic Disorders," *New England Journal of Medicine* 288 (1973): 1299–1300; Robert Hecker, "The Investigation of the Patient: Modern Developments Including Automated Multiphasic Health Screening and the Use of the Computer in Medicine," *Medical Journal of Australia* 2 (1972): 492–96.

28. Robert F. Murray, "The Practitioner's View of the Values Involved in Genetic Screening and Counseling: Individual vs. Societal Imperatives," pp. 185–99 in Daniel Bergsma, ed., *Ethical, Social, and Legal Dimensions of Screening for Human Genetic Disease,* New York: Stratton, 1974, p. 189. Also see Macintyre, 1975.

29. Powledge, 1974, p. 27.

30. National Institutes of Health, 1979, pp. I:24, I:81–I:82.

31. Murray, 1974, pp. 189–90.

32. Howard Brody, "Teaching Medical Ethics: Future Challenges," *Journal of the American Medical Association* 229 (1974): 177–79.

33. James R. Sorenson, "Some Social and Psychological Issues in Genetic Screening: Public and Professional Adaptation to Biomedical Innovation," pp. 165–84 in Daniel Bergsma, ed., *Ethical, Social, and Legal Dimensions of Screening for Human Genetic Disease,* New York: Stratton, 1974, pp. 165–66.

34. Talcott Parsons, "Research with Human Subjects and the 'Profession Complex,' " *Daedalus* 98 (1969): 325–60, has argued that the patient/lay person *must* be made a quasi-colleague in the research enterprise in order for the research function, "the most important single spearhead of the trend of progressive advance in modern societies," to proceed smoothly (p. 356).

35. National Institutes of Health, 1979, p. I:88.

36. Leonard, Chase, and Childs, 1972.

37. C. E. Dent, "Preface," to D. C. Cusworth, ed., *Biochemical Screening in Relation to Mental Retardation,* New York: Pergamon, 1971.

38. Marc Lappe and Richard O. Robbin, "Newborn Genetic Screening as a Concept in Health Care Delivery: A Critique," pp. 1–23 in Daniel Bergsma, ed., *Ethical, Social, and Legal Dimensions of Screening for Human Genetic Disease,* New York: Stratton, 1974.

39. Alexander J. Schaffer and Mary Ellen Avery, *Diseases of the Newborn,* 4th ed., Philadelphia: W. B. Saunders, 1977, p. 849.

40. Stanley J. Dudrick, Douglas W. Wilmore, Harry M. Vars, and Jonathan E. Rhoads, "Long-term Total Parenteral Nutrition with Growth, Development, and Positive Nitrogen Balance," *Surgery* 64 (1968): 134–42.

41. B. S. Lindblad, G. Settergren, H. Feychting, and B. Persson, "Total Parenteral Nutrition in Infants," *Acta Pediatrica Scandanavia* 66 (1977): 409–19.

42. Schaffer and Avery, 1977, pp. 530, 533; emphasis mine.

43. James M. Gustafson, "Mongolism, Parental Desires, and the Right to Life," *Perspectives in Biology and Medicine* 16 (1973): 529–57.

44. See Warren T. Reich and David E. Ost, "Infants: Ethical Perspectives on the Care of Infants," pp. 724–35 in Warren T. Reich, ed., *Encyclopedia of Bioethics,* vol. 2, New York: The Free Press, 1978, for a discussion of various approaches to medical ethics.

45. Charles L. Bosk, *Forgive and Remember: Managing Medical Failure,* Chicago: University of Chicago Press, 1979; Arnold Arluke, "Social Control Rituals in Medicine," pp. 108–25 in Robert Dingwall, Christian Heath, Margaret Reid, and Margaret Stacey, *Health Care and Health Knowledge,* London: Croom Helm, 1977.

46. Stanley Hauerwas, "The Demands and Limits of Care: Ethical Reflections on the Moral Dilemma of Neonatal Intensive Care," *American Journal of the Medical Sciences* 269 (1975): 224.

47. K. Danner Clouser, "Medical Ethics: Some Uses, Abuses, and Limitations," *New England Journal of Medicine* 293 (1975): 385.

48. Albert R. Jonsen, "Scientific Medicine and Therapeutic Choice," *New England Journal of Medicine* 292 (1975): 1126.

49. One hesitates to include personal anecdotes in academic works, but on occasion they can be informative. When my wife had her first prenatal examination, the obstetrician said, "Well, your pelvis is a little small and we may have to do a cesarean section. I don't want to worry you. Everything will probably proceed just fine and we'll have no problems. I just think it is better to let people know early that the possibility exists." My wife and I, of course, appreciated his willingness to let us know about possibilities and his clear concern for keeping us informed. But this incident illustrates how the therapeutic choices, not just of the patient *but of the physician,*

are limited by modern developments in medicine. Some might say that this was an instance of a physician foreclosing a patient's therapeutic options prematurely. This would not be a completely inaccurate interpretation. But one must realize that the foreclosing of the patient's options derives directly from the doctor's sense that his options are foreclosed, in this case by the small pelvis for which the appropriate management, according to "scientific" medicine, is a cesarean section.

The full force of monitoring as a structure which "controls the controllers" can be appreciated by considering the physician's options in this particular case. First, he could have withheld the information about the small outlet and about the possibility of a cesarean section. If everything went smoothly, he would have had no difficulties. If, however, a cesarean delivery had been required, he would have had to contend with a surprised, perhaps angry, woman who might have an effect on his practice through her network of friends in the natural childbirth movement, in the medical community, and elsewhere. If he had arrived at the point of delivery and chosen not to do a cesarean section and something had gone awry, my wife might have sued, probably would have found a notation of "small pelvis" in her record, and probably would have won her case by reference to the "common practices" dictated by the medical literature. This little incident shows that while concerns over the "medicalization" of life might be appropriate, "medicalization" is only one aspect of a structure of control which exerts its influence on the medical profession as well as on the life of the patient.

50. John F. Burnum, "The Physician as Double Agent," *New England Journal of Medicine* 297 (1977): 278–79.

51. Jonsen, 1975, p. 1127.

52. Ibid.

53. Stephen E. Toulmin, *An Examination of the Place of Reason in Ethics,* Cambridge: Cambridge University Press, 1950, p. 202; Clouser, 1975, p. 387; emphasis added.

54. Michel Foucault, "Two Lectures," pp. 78–108 in Colin Gordon, ed., *Power/Knowledge: Selected Interviews and Other Writings, 1972–1977,* New York: Pantheon, 1980, pp. 95–96.

55. Jonsen, 1975, p. 1126.

56. Clouser, 1975, pp. 387, 386.

57. Callahan, 1975, p. 316.

58. A. R. Jonsen, R. H. Phibbs, W. H. Tooley, and M. J. Garland, "Critical Issues in Newborn Intensive Care: A Conference Report and Policy Proposal," *Pediatrics* 55 (1975): 759.

59. Aubrey Milunsky, John W. Littlefield, Julian N. Kanfer, Edwin H. Kolodny, Vivian E. Shih, and Leonard Atkins, "Prenatal Genetic Screening" (in three parts), *New England Journal of Medicine* 283 (1970): 1502, 1503.

60. Murray, 1974, p. 198; Burnum, 1977, p. 279.

61. F. J. Inglefinger, "Bedside Ethics for the Hopeless Case," *New England Journal of Medicine* 289 (1973): 914, 915.

62. Paul Ramsey, "The Ethics of a Cottage Industry in an Age of Community and Research Medicine," *New England Journal of Medicine* 284 (1971): 701.

63. Ibid., pp. 705.

64. F. J. Inglefinger, "Medical Obligations Imposed by Abortion," *New England Journal of Medicine* 284 (1971): 727.

65. John Lorber, "Selective Treatment of Myeolomeningocele: To Treat or Not to Treat," *Pediatrics* 53 (1974): 307.

66. Ibid., p. 308.

67. Darling, 1977, p. 13.

68. Richard A. McCormick, "To Save or Let Die: The Dilemma of Modern Medicine," *Journal of the American Medical Association* 229 (1974): 175.

69. Robert M. Veatch, "The Technical Criteria Fallacy," *Hastings Center Report* 7 (1977): 15.

70. Some might complain that legislation is not an ethical solution. This is true, but legislative reform is one solution, though never a very satisfactory or necessarily stable one, to the ethical problems of medicine. It is one strategy which the profession can use.

71. Raymond S. Duff and A. G. M. Campbell, "Moral and Ethical Dilemmas in the Special Care Nursery," *New England Journal of Medicine* 289 (1973): 890–94.

72. American Medical Association, "Guideline for the Physician Confronted with Ethical Problems Related to Euthanasia and Death with Dignity," *Journal of the American Medical Association* 227 (1974): 728.

73. James Rachels, "Active and Passive Euthanasia," *New England Journal of Medicine* 292 (1975): 80.

74. John M. Freeman, "Is There a Right to Die—Quickly?" *Journal of Pediatrics* 80 (1972): 905.

75. Hauerwas, 1975, p. 229.

76. Duff and Campbell, 1973, p. 753.

77. Ibid., p. 894. See also their letter in the *New England Journal of Medicine* 290 (1974): 520.

78. Raymond S. Duff and A. G. M. Campbell, "On Deciding the Care of Severely Handicapped or Dying Persons: With Particular Reference to Infants," *Pediatrics* 57 (1976): 487–93; Raymond S. Duff, "On Deciding the Use of the Family Commons," *Birth Defects: Original Articles* 12 (1976): 73–84.

79. Duff, 1976, p. 82.

80. Michael Hemphill and John M. Freeman, "Ethical Aspects of the Newborn with Serious Neurological Disease," *Clinics in Perinatology* 4 (1977): 207.

81. John Lachs, "Humane Treatment and the Treatment of Humans," *New England Journal of Medicine* 294 (1976): 839.

82. Anthony Shaw, "Dilemmas of 'Informed Consent' in Children," *New England Journal of Medicine* 289 (1973): 889.

83. Ibid., p. 890.

84. Madeleine H. Shearer, "Some Deterrents to Objective Evaluation of Fetal Monitors," *Birth and the Family Journal* 2 (1975): 61.

85. Eric J. Cassell, "Autonomy and Ethics in Action," *New England Journal of Medicine* 297 (1977): 333–34.

86. Tabitha Powledge and John Fletcher, "Guidelines for the Ethical, Social and Legal Issues in Prenatal Diagnosis: A Report from the Genetics Research Group of the Hastings Center, Institute of Society, Ethics, and Life Sciences," *New England Journal of Medicine* 300 (1979): 169.

87. See the views of medical practitioners in Jonsen et al., 1975, and Bosk, 1979, pp. 132–34, where he reports on the ethical dilemmas of a surgeon who ultimately decided on a course of care by reconceptualizing the patient as the patient (that person who originally sought care) and his family.

Chapter Seven

1. Richard W. Wertz and Dorothy C. Wertz, *Lying-In: A History of Childbirth in America,* New York: The Free Press, 1977, p. 173.

2. Grantly Dick-Read, Letter, "Position for Delivery," *British Medical Journal* 2 (1955): 850, 851.

3. Grantly Dick-Read, *Childbirth without Fear,* 1st ed., London: Heinemann, 1933. It is interesting that Dick-Read dedicated his book to Joseph B. DeLee.

4. Grantly Dick-Read, *Childbirth without Fear: The Principles and Practice of Natural Childbirth,* 3d ed., London: Heinemann, 1956, p. 10.

5. Ibid., p. 10.

6. Carl Tupper, "Conditioning for Childbirth," *American Journal of Obstetrics and Gynecology* 71 (1956): 734.

7. Ibid., p. 735.

8. "Coping" with pain is a relatively new term. The literature of the 1950s spoke of women being able to *bear* pain. The physicians asked, "Can women *tolerate* pain?" "Bearing" pain connotes that pain has a life of its own, that it is still somewhat independent of the woman and her psychology. "Coping" with pain seems more sensitive to the fact that stimuli are processed psychologically before something becomes painful. Women who "cope" with pain may either "bear" it, "suppress" it, "transform" it, "transcend" it, or do any number of things to it. Coping recognizes the psychically internal character of pain. During the 1970s papers apeared that had titles like Susan G. Doering and Doris G. Entwisle's "Preparation during Pregnancy and

Ability to Cope with Labor and Delivery," *American Journal of Orthopsychiatry* 45 (1975): 825–37.

9. Henry K. Beecher, "The Measurement of Pain: Prototype for the Quantitative Study of Subjective Responses," *Pharmacological Reviews* 9 (1957): 59–209.

10. Duncan E. Reid and Mandel E. Cohen, "Evaluation of Present Trends in Obstetrics," *Journal of the American Medical Association* 142 (1950): 622.

11. Kathleen L. Norr, Carolyn R. Block, Allan Charles, Suzanne Meyering, and Ellen Meyers, "Explaining Pain and Enjoyment in Childbirth," *Journal of Health and Social Behavior* 18 (1977): 270.

12. Hilary Graham, "Images of Pregnancy in Antenatal Literature," pp. 15–37 in Robert Dingwall, Christian Heath, Margaret Reid, and Margaret Stacey, eds., *Health Care and Health Knowledge*, London: Croom Helm, 1977.

13. Ibid., p. 32.

14. Per Nettelbladt, Carl-Fredrik Fagerstrom, and Nils Uddenberg, "The Significance of Reported Childbirth Pain," *Journal of Psychosomatic Research* 20 (1976): 220.

15. N. Destounis, "On Teaching Psychosomatic Medicine to Medical Students," pp. 68–70 in *Psychosomatic Medicine in Obstetrics and Gynaecology, Third International Congress, London, 1971*, Basel: Karger, 1972, p. 68.

16. Dick-Read, 1956, p. 4.

17. Linton Snaith and Alan Coxon, eds., *Dick-Read's Childbirth without Fear: The Principles and Practice of Natural Childbirth*, 5th ed., London: Heinemann, 1968, p. 5.

18. Dick-Read, 1956, pp. 10, 50.

19. Ivan Petrovich Pavlov, *Conditioned Reflexes: An Investigation of the Physiological Activity of the Cerebral Cortex*, London: Oxford University Press, 1927; A. P. Nicolaiev, *Obezbolievanie Rodov* [Obstetrical analgesia], Leningrad: Meditzina, 1959; K. Platonov, *The Word as a Physiological and Psychological Factor*, Moscow: Foreign Language Publishing House, 1959; I. Z. Velvovsky, *Painless Childbirth through Psychoprophylaxis*, Moscow: Foreign Language Publishing House, 1960; Leon Chertok, *Motherhood and Personality: Psychosomatic Aspects of Childbirth*, Philadelphia: J. B. Lippincott, 1969; L. Chertok, "Psychosomatic Methods of Preparation for Childbirth: Spread of the Methods, Theory, and Research," *American Journal of Obstetrics and Gynecology* 98 (1967): 698–706; Fernand Lamaze, *Painless Childbirth: Psychoprophylactic Method*, London: Burke Publishing Company, 1958; Pierre Vellay, *Childbirth without Pain*, New York: E. P. Dutton, 1960.

20. Marjorie Karmel, *Thank You, Dr. Lamaze: A Mother's Experiences in Painless Childbirth*, Philadelphia: J. B. Lippincott, 1950.

21. Elisabeth D. Bing, "Psychoprophylaxis and Family-centered Maternity," pp. 71–73 in *Psychosomatic Medicine in Obstetrics and Gynaecology, Third International Congress, London, 1971*, Basel: Karger, 1972, p. 72.

22. Sheila Kitzinger, *The Experience of Childbirth*, London: Victor Gollancz, 1962; idem, *Education and Counselling for Childbirth*, London; Balliere Tindall, 1977; idem, *Giving Birth: The Parents' Emotions in Childbirth*, New York: Schocken, 1977.

23. Ondrej Kondas and Bozena Scetnika, "Systematic Desensitization as a Method of Preparation for Childbirth," *Journal of Behavioral Therapy and Experimental Psychiatry* 3 (1972): 51–54.

24. Lawrence M. Frazier, "Using Biofeedback to Aid Relaxation during Childbirth," *Birth and the Family Journal* 1 (1974): 15–17.

25. I do not mean to imply that all obstetricians endorsed natural childbirth and encouraged their patients to use the method, or even that all obstetricians allowed patients the opportunity to use the method of their choice. As illustrated by the case of a friend seeking obstetrical care in Macon, Georgia, which occurred as this book was being written in 1980, there is still open hostility to patient's desires to practice the Lamaze technique or other procedures recommended by childbirth educators. My friend was so humiliated and infuriated by her obstetrician's reaction to her questions that she changed physicians. She secured obstetrical care from a person who would accommodate her needs and desires, but she could do so only by driving one and a half hours from her home.

Everyone has her or his horror story about mistreatment at the hands of modern obstetricians. But the statement still means what it says: "*Obstetrics*—the profession—accepted natural childbirth, quickly." Opinion leaders endorsed the techniques in journals, scientific investigations approved the techniques, and the small band of critics, some of whose opinions are discussed in the text, were shouted down and forced to retire to their private and clinic practices to deliver care in ways inconsistent with the direction the profession was taking.

26. See Michael J. Hughey, Thomas W. McElin, and Todd Young, "Maternal and Fetal Outcomes of Lamaze-prepared Patients," *Obstetrics and Gynecology* 51 (1978): 643–47, or Niels C. Beck, "Natural Childbirth: A Review and Analysis," *Obstetrics and Gynecology* 52 (1978): 371–79, for reviews of this literature.

27. Reid and Cohen, 1950, pp. 618, 619, 622.

28. Beck, 1978.

29. Reid and Cohen, 1950, pp. 622, 623.

30. Clyde L. Randall, "Childbirth without Fear of Interference," *Clinical Obstetrics and Gynecology* 2 (1959): 366.

31. Virginia Woolf, *To the Lighthouse*, New York: Harcourt, Brace and World, 1927, p. 235. My thanks to Jane Neill for bringing this reference to my attention.

32. Lillie Weiss and Rosalyn Meadow, "Women's Attitudes toward Gynecological Practice," *Obstetrics and Gynecology* 54 (1979): 110–11.

33. Anne M. Seiden, "The Sense of Mastery in the Childbirth Experience," pp. 87–105 in Malkah T. Nortman and Carol C. Nadelson, eds., *The Woman Patient: Medical and Psychological Interfaces,* vol. 1, New York: Plenum, 1978, p. 92.

34. Doering and Entwisle, 1975, p. 835.

35. Bing, 1972, p. 72.

36. H. Lloyd Miller, Francis E. Flannery, and Dorothy Bell, "Education for Childbirth in Private Practice: 450 Consecutive Cases," *American Journal of Obstetrics and Gynecology* 63 (1952): 798.

37. Seiden, 1978, p. 87.

38. Ibid., p. 89.

39. Interprofessional Task Force on Health Care of Women and Children, *Joint Position Statement on the Development of Family-Centered Maternity/ Newborn Care in Hospitals,* Chicago: American College of Obstetricians and Gynecologists, June, 1978, p. 3.

40. Ibid., p. 4.

41. Committee on Perinatal Health, *Toward Improving the Outcome of Pregnancy: Recommendations for the Regional Development of Maternal and Perinatal Health Services,* White Plains, N.Y.: The National Foundation–March of Dimes, 1976; Committee on the Fetus and Newborn, *Standards and Recommendations for Hospital Care of Newborn Infants,* 6th ed., Evanston, Ill.: American Academy of Pediatrics, 1977.

42. Tupper, 1956, p. 737.

43. Herbert Thoms and Robert H. Wyatt, "One Thousand Consecutive Deliveries under a Training for Childbirth Program," *American Journal of Obstetrics and Gynecology* 61 (1951): 205.

44. Robert A. Bradley, *Husband-Coached Childbirth,* New York: Harper and Row, 1965.

45. Jeanette L. Samsor, "The Role of the Father in Labor and Delivery," pp. 277–80 in *Psychosomatic Medicine in Obstetrics and Gynaecology, Third International Congress, London, 1971,* Basel: Karger, 1972, pp. 277, 279.

46. Interprofessional Task Force, 1978, p. 4.

47. F. S. W. Brimblecombe, M. P. M. Richards, and N. R. C. Roberton, *Separation and Special-Care Baby Units,* London: Heinemann, 1978, p. 113.

48. George A. Little and L. Joseph Butterfield, "Regionalization of Perinatal Care," pp. 415–20 in Robert A. Hoekelman, Saul Blatman, Philip A. Brunell, Stanford B. Friedman, and Henry M. Seidel, *Principles of Pediatrics: Health Care of the Young,* New York: McGraw-Hill, 1978, p. 415. See also George A. Little, "Establishing and Maintaining Relationships with Community Hospitals and Health Professionals," pp. 16–26 in M. L.

Duxbury, S. N. Graven, R. E. Redmann, and J. G. Sommers, eds., *Proceedings of the Conference on Outreach Programs: Their Integral Parts and Processes*, White Plains, N. Y.: The National Foundation–March of Dimes, 1978.

49. John Van S. Maeck, "Obstetrician-Midwife Partnership in Obstetric Care," *Obstetrics and Gynecology* 37 (1971): 317, 319.

50. Ibid., p. 317.

51. C. Slome, H. Wetherbee, M. Daly, K. Christensen, M. Meglen, and H. Thiede, "Effectiveness of Certified Nurse-Midwives: A Prospective Evaluation," *American Journal of Obstetrics andGynecology* 124 (1976): 177–82.

52. T. Schley Gatewood and Richard B. Stewart, "Obstetricians and Nurse-Midwives: The Team Approach in Private Practice," *American Journal of Obstetrics and Gynecology* 123 (1975): 35–40.

53. Thomas F. Dillon, Barbara A. Brennan, John F. Dwyer, Abraham Risk, Alan Sear, Lynne Dawson, and Raymond Vande Wiele, "Midwifery, 1977," *American Journal of Obstetrics and Gynecology* 130 (1978): 918, 922.

54. I conducted a three-year evaluation of the Vermont/New Hampshire Regional Perinatal Program. The federal contract which sponsored the program restricted the medical center staff from extending its educational and staff development programs to all hospitals in the region but provided for the extension of all referral, consultation, and medical services to all community hospitals delivering babies in Vermont and New Hampshire. Hospitals in the "control" group (those that were part of the Program but that did not receive educational and developmental programs) and hospitals in the "intervention" group (those that received educational programs) were similar even though group assignment was not random. Low birth-weight (500–2499 grams) mortality declined over the course of the program in intervention hospitals while it remained stable or increased slightly in the control hospitals. Normal birth-weight mortality remained unaffected overall. These results confirmed the expectation that regionalization would reduce mortality but that most reductions would come in the low birth-weight category, the category most likely to be affected by the provision of sophisticated technological services over large geographical areas. See Jerold F. Lucey, George A. Little, Alistair G. S. Philip, and William Ray Arney, *Vermont/New Hampshire Regional Perinatal Program: Final Report*, contract NO1-HR-52961, to Division of Lung Diseases, National Heart, Lung, and Blood Institute, National Institutes of Health, Bethesda, Md., 1979.

55. Alice Allgaier, "Alternative Birth Centers Offer Family-Centered Care," *Hospitals, Journal of the American Hospital Association* 52 (1978): 106.

56. John S. Tomkin, "Discussion" of Dillon, Brennan, Dwyer, et al., 1978, p. 924.

57. Frederick P. Zuspan, "Discussion" of Dillon, Brennan, Dwyer, et al., 1978, pp. 924–25.

58. Interprofessional Task Force, 1978, p. 4.

59. William Young, "The Birth Process: The Setting," pp. 425–27 in Robert A. Hoekelman, Saul Blatman, Philip A. Brunell, Stanford B. Friedman, and Henry M. Seidel, *Principles of Pediatrics: Health Care of the Young,* New York: McGraw-Hill, 1978, pp. 425–26.

60. Vermont Educational Television, "Home Birth in Vermont: New Odds for an Old Gamble?" 1978. Quote is from Jerold F. Lucey.

61. Diana Scully, *Men Who Control Women's Health: The Education of Obstetricians and Gynecologists,* Boston: Houghton Mifflin, 1980.

62. Graham, 1977, p. 33.

63. Dick-Read, 1956, pp. 30, 32, ix.

64. Michel Foucault, *Discipline and Punish: Birth of the Prison,* London: Allen Lane, 1977, pp. 202–3; emphasis added. See also Michel Foucault, "The Eye of Power," pp. 146–65 in Colin Gordon, ed., *Power/Knowledge: Selected Interviews and Other Writings, 1972-1977,* New York: Pantheon, 1980.

65. Michel Foucault, *The History of Sexuality,* vol. 1: *An Introduction,* New York: Pantheon, 1978, pp. 21, 26.

66. Ibid., p. 24.

67. Thoms and Wyatt, 1951, p. 206.

68. Tupper, 1956, p. 739.

69. Thoms and Wyatt, 1951, p. 206.

70. Samsor, 1972, p. 279.

71. Nettelbladt, Fagerstrom, and Uddenberg, 1976, p. 220.

72. Tupper, 1956, p. 735.

73. Susan G. Doering, Doris R. Entwisle, and Daniel Quinlan, "Modeling the Quality of Women's Birth Experience," *Journal of Health and Social Behavior* 21 (1980): 13; emphasis added.

74. J.-P. Clerc, "Fifteen Years of Obstetrical Prophylaxis in Private Practice," pp. 74–77 in *Psychosomatic Medicine in Obstetrics and Gynaecology, Third International Congress, London, 1971,* Basel: Karger, 1972, p. 76.

75. Ibid.

76. See ibid., but also see H. A. Brant, "Preparation of Multigravid Patients," pp. 78–80 in *Psychosomatic Medicine in Obstetrics and Gynaecology, Third International Congress, London, 1971,* Basel: Karger, 1972.

77. Tupper, 1956, p. 739.

78. A. Blankfield, "Conflicts Created by Childbirth Methodologies," pp. 87–89 in *Psychosomatic Medicine in Obstetrics and Gynaecology, Third International Congress, London, 1971,* Basel: Karger, 1972, p. 89.

79. Tupper, 1956, p. 739.

80. Marion D. Laird and Margaret Hogan, "An Elective Program on Preparation for Childbirth at the Sloane Hospital for Women, May, 1951,

to June, 1953," *American Journal of Obstetrics and Gynecology* 72 (1956): 646.

81. Dick-Read, 1956, pp. 140ff.

82. Weiss and Meadow, 1979, p. 113, emphasis added.

83. Destounis, 1972, p. 69; emphasis added.

84. Allan G. Charles, Kathleen L. Norr, Carolyn R. Block, Suzanne Meyering, and Ellen Meyers, "Obstetric and Psychologic Effects of Psychoprophylactic Preparation for Childbirth," *American Journal of Obstetrics and Gynecology* 131 (1978): 44.

85. Melvin Zax, Arnold J. Sameroff, and Janet E. Farnum, "Childbirth Education, Maternal Attitudes, and Delivery," *American Journal of Obstetrics and Gynecology* 123 (1975): 190.

86. Niles Newton, "Interrelationships between Sexual Responsiveness, Birth and Breast Feeding," pp. 77–98 in Joseph Zubin and John Money, eds., *Contemporary Sexual Behavior: Critical Issues in the 1970s*, Baltimore: The Johns Hopkins University Press, 1973, p. 96.

87. Foucault, 1978, pp. 31–32. The title of the French version of *The History of Sexuality* translates as "The Will to Knowledge." My "rush to knowledge" borrows unashamedly from this title.

88. See, for example, Doering, Entwisle, and Quinlan, 1980, or Norr, Block, et al., 1977. These papers present path analytic models of the childbirth experience. Even though the models are constructed from cross-sectional data, they have a temporal, processual character to them. Some analysts, the authors of these two articles included, use path analytic models to develop dynamic explanations of behavior that can be used to design behavioral management and experience optimizing schemes.

89. Jere B. Faison, R. Gordon Douglas, Gene S. Cranch, and Ruth Watson Lubic, "The Childbearing Center: An Alternative Birth Setting," *Obstetrics and Gynecology* 54 (1979): 527, 528.

90. Ibid., p. 531.

91. Ina May Gaskin, *Spiritual Midwifery,* Summertown, Tenn.: The Book Publishing Company, 1978, p. 11.

92. Ina May Gaskin, "Spiritual Midwifery on the Farm in Summertown, Tennessee," *Birth and the Family Journal* 5 (1978): 102–4.

93. Ibid., p. 103.

94. See n. 22 above.

95. Sheila Kitzinger, "The Woman on the Delivery Table," pp. 91–111 in Margaret Irene Laing, ed., *Woman on Woman,* London: Sedgwick and Jackson, 1971, pp. 92, 93.

96. Ibid., p. 105; emphasis added.

97. Foucault says this of "humanism": "By humanism I mean the totality of discourse through which Western man is told: 'Even though you don't exercise power, you can still be a ruler. Better yet, the more you deny yourself the exercise of power, the more you submit to those in power, the

more this increases your sovereignty.' Humanism invented a whole series of subjected sovereignties: the soul (ruling the body, but subjected to God), consciousness (sovereign in a context of judgment, but subjected to the necessities of truth), the individual (a titular control of personal rights subjected to the laws of nature and society), basic freedom (sovereign within, but accepting the demands of an outside world and 'aligned with destiny'). In short, humanism is everything in Western Civilization that restricts the desire for power" (Michel Foucault, "Revolutionary Action: 'Until Now,' " pp. 218–33 in Donald F. Bouchard, ed., *Michel Foucault: Language, Counter-Memory, Practice: Selected Essays and Interviews,* Ithaca, N.Y.: Cornell University Press, 1977, p. 221).

98. Young, 1978, p. 425; emphasis added.

99. Foucault, "Revolutionary Action," 1977, pp. 230–31.

100. Woolf, 1927, p. 235.

Index

Abortion, 182–83
Acid-base balance, 104
Adoption studies, support for bonding in, 157–58
Alternatives, arising within flexible systems rule, 237–40
American Academy of Pediatrics, 201
American Board of Obstetrics and Gynecology, 59
American College of Nurse-Midwives, 221
American College of Obstetricians and Gynecologists, 101, 221
American Gynecological Society, 46
American Journal of Obstetrics and Gynecology, 54
American Journal of Obstetrics and the Diseases of Women and Children, 46
American Medical Association, 45–46; and ethical reform, 202; and specialists, 52

American Nurses' Association, 221
American Society for Psychoprophylaxis in Obstetrics, 215
American Society of Human Genetics, 187
Amniocentesis, 80, 181–83; and abortion, 267n; cost-benefit analyses, 184; impact of, 183–84; investigations of, 181–84
Amnioscope, 104
Analysis: and control, 130; sustaining, 132
Anspach, Brooke, 70
Antenatal literature, 212–13
Apgar scores, 112, 114, 117
Apothecaries, 34
Arluke, Arnold, 193
Armstrong, David, 87, 122
Atelectasis, 188
Attachment. *See* Maternal-infant bonding
Aveling, James Hobson, 36

Baggish, Michael S., 110–14
Baker, R. Alan, 120
Banta, H. David, 108, 120
Barber surgeons, 25; Barber Surgeons Company, 26; instruments and operations, 246n; relationship with midwives, 9–10, 23–24; technology used by, 23–24
Barnes, Barry, 11, 14
Barnes, Robert, 37
Baudelocque, 28, 44
Bell, W. Blair, 76–77
Bellevue Hospital, 46
Bias, 266n
Bing, Elisabeth, 215
Biofeedback, 216
Birth: as moral crisis, 23; normal/ abnormal conceptualization, 23–26, 60–61; rational-scientific approach to, 24–26; strategic importance of, 33. See also Home birth; Hospital birth; Normal birth
Birthing center, 226–27, 237–38
Birthing rooms, 167
Birthing stools, 250n
Birth position, 62–69; and asepsis as justification, 66; changes in, 66–67; and development of American obstetrics, 64–65; and instinct, 63; and natural childbirth, 69; and perineal tears, 70; and professional organization, 64–65
Bishop's score, 79
Body: as machine, 8; and scientific approach to birth, 26
Bonding. See Maternal-infant bonding
Bosk, Charles, 16, 193
Boundary, 21; defense, 21; destruction by monitoring, 153–54. See also Demarcation
Boundary strength: and diffusion of professional practices, 52, 62; and professional rhetoric, 51–52

Boveri, Theodor, 178
British Medical Association, 36–37
British Nurses' Association, 37–38
Butter, Alexander, 28

Caldeyro-Barcia, Roberto, 101, 215n
Callahan, Daniel, 197
Cambridge University, 22
Campbell, A. G. M., 202, 205
Carnegie Foundation, 47
Central Midwives' Board, 38, 97, 227
Cervical dilation, 144–45, 148
Cesarean section, 114–17; absolute and relative indications, 145; family-centered, 146–47, 195; in fetal monitor studies, 114–17
Chalmers, Iain, 82
Chamberlen, Dr. Peter, 30; family of, 26; Hugh, 25; Peter the Elder, 25, 30; Peter the Younger, 30; William, 26
Chapman, Edmund, 26–27; and ethics, 34
Chertok, Leon, 215
Child abuse, 165
Church, and ecclesiastical oversight of midwives, 22, 39
Cianfrani, Theodore, 2–4
Clarke-Stewart, Alison, 160
Clinical judgment, 95–96, 121–22, 143
Clinical science, 122
Clouser, K. Danner, 194, 197
Cohen, Mandel, 212, 217
Collaborative Perinatal Study, 73–74
Committee on Medical Education, 47
Community of consensus, 199
Confessional, as metaphor, 233–35
Confinement, 123, 127
Contingent sovereignty, 95–97
Control: of birth, 229–42; normative and analytical questions, 229; by

obstetricians, 229–30; by women, 217–20. *See also* Panopticon

Cord compression, 103

Cord prolapse, 106

Corometrics, 107

Cost containment, 107, 227

Cottle, Thomas, 12

Coventry, Charles B., 42

Cranbrook Report, 126–28

Criteria lists: critical reaction, 199–201; ethics' reaction, 200–201

Culpepper, Nicholas, 27; *Directory* of, 27, 247n

Daly, Mary, 5

Darling, Rosalyn, 200–201

Death, in childbirth, 33

Deceleration, of fetal heart, 102–4

Decision-making: parents and, 203–5; by physicians in ethically complex situations, 198–99

DeLee, Joseph B., 249n; on birth position, 64–66; on episiotomy, 71; and form of profession, 53; on home deliveries, 61; on induction, 77–78; pathological dignity of pregnancy, 47; and pathological potential, 54–59; on professional organization, 58–59; on professional practices, 58–59; prophylactic forceps, 47; on statistics, 72

Deleuze, Gilles, 13

Delivery, modern, 106

Demarcation, 51–53, 125

De Maupertuis, Pierre Louis Moreau, 177

Demonstrative midwifery, 42

Dewees, William Potts, 43–44, 64

Dick-Read, Grantly, 210–11, 214–15, 230, 234; on birth position, 69

Dichotomies: abolition of, 139–40; rule of, 7

Diseases of nonattachment, 165, 168–69

Distress. *See* Fetal distress

Doctor-patient relationship, 8–9; and demands of research, 196; and family, 204–7; as joint adventure, 199; and professional boundary, 207; reformulation of, 199–207; and role obligations, 203–4; women in, 218–19

Donegan, Jane, 25, 41

Donnison, Jean, 35

Donzelot, Jacques, 171

Down's syndrome, 180–81, 183

Duff, Raymond, 202, 205

Dystocia, 146

Eastman, Nicholson, 71, 79

Ecological approach to care, 88–98

Ecological metaphor, 8, 87

Ecological perspective, 195–96, 199; harmony in, 196–97

Ehrenreich, Barbara, 3

Elective induction. *See* Induction, elective

Electronic fetal monitor. *See* Fetal monitor

Endocrinology, 158

Englemann, George, 62

English, Deidre, 3

Enjoyment, of childbirth, 212

Epidemiology: in America, 132–33; in Britain, 130–32; map of birth, 130–33

Episiotomy, 69–75; and "average man" argument, 74; in Britain, 74–75; complications, 73; justification, 73–74; restrictive characterization, 74–75; scientific justification, 72–74; and sexual interests, 71–72; as sign of abnormality, 74

Ergot, 44; in second stage, 76; in third stage, 76

Ether, 44

Ethical discourse, 191–97

Ethical neutrality, 96–97
Ethical review, committees for, 206
Ethics: as early device for professional organization, 34; and ecological view, 193–94; and harmony, 196–97; as internal organizing device, 196–97; and technology, 176
Ethology, support for bonding, 156–58
Eugenics, 178
Euthanasia, 202; active and passive, 202
Experimental studies: of maternal-infant bonding, 157–60; of monitoring 110–13, 116–18

Family: as conservator of culture, 171–72; as patient concept, 204–7
Family commons, 205
Family-centered care, 221–23; as management scheme, 235–36
Farm, The, 237–39
Father absence, in maternal-infant bonding theory, 172
Fathers, and cesarean sections, 146
Fear, and pain, 211
Female Medical Society, 35
Feminism, radical, 5
Feminist scholarship, 3, 173
Fetal advocacy, 136–37
Fetal distress, 101–4, 123; and cesarean sections, 114–17; changing meaning of, 134–35, 139–41; disappearance of, 139–40
Fetal ecology, 99
Fetal heart-rate patterns, 102–5
Fetal heart sounds, detecting, 101
Fetal monitor, 101–23; and cord prolapse, 80; and cost containment, 101, 107; cost-benefit analyses, 107–8, 257n; as cause of increased cesarean sections, 262n; as focus of debate, 99; government regulation, 108–9; interventions averted with, 137; limiting women's freedom, 106; mandatory monitoring, 121; obstetricians' response to criticism of, 120–21; radiotelemetry of, 149–50; risks of, 114; studies, 257n
Fetal scalp-blood sampling, 104
Fetus: discovery of, 134–38; as focal point of obstetrical ecology, 94; as second patient, 134–35
Flexible systems rule, 220, 226–27, 237–40
Flexner Report, 41, 47
Forceps, 25–27; in America, 44
Foucault, Michel, 11–16, 87, 94, 130, 150–51, 196, 230–32, 236
Fraiberg, Selma, 92, 168
Freeman, John, 203
Freeman, Roger, 120–21
Friedman, Emanuel, 143–45
Friedman curve. See Partograph

General Medical Council, 36, 38; reorganization of 1858, 37
General practitioners, 37, 125
Genetic inheritance, 177–81
Genetic Research Group, 207
Genetic screening programs, 184–86; and normality and abnormality, 186
Gilman, Chandler, 42
Goodlin, Robert, 141
Gordon, Alexander, 44
Gordon, Charles, 58
Gordon, Myron, 73
Graham, Hilary, 212–13, 229
Greenhill, J. P., 65, 78

Habermas, Jürgen, 99
Haksteen, John, 42
Harvard Medical School, 41
Hauerwas, Stanley, 203–4

Haverkamp, Albert, 116–18, 150, 151
Health Systems Agency, 196
Heart rate, 101–4
History: obstetrics' own, 2–4; writing of, 1–2
Hobbins, John, 120–21
Hodge, Hugh, 43
Hoekelman, Robert A., 89–92
Hoerner, J. K., 78
Hofbauer, J., 78
Hollingsworth, Leta S., 170–71
Holmes, Oliver Wendell, 44
Holmes, Rudolph, 57
Home birth, 127–28, 213
Hon, Edward, 101, 107
Hooker, Worthington, 45
Hospital: as center of surveillance network, 125–26; as sponsor of program for midwives, 46; as strategic resource, 28–29
Hospital birth, 124–29, 228–29; alternatives to, 237–40
Hospital practices, changes in, 165–68
Hotel-Dieu, 24, 246n
Humane care, 89, 241, 278n
Humanism, 278n
Hunt, Harriot, 41
Hunter, William, 28, 29
Husband, as labor coach, 215–16, 223
Hyperalimentation, 189
Hypoxia, 103–4

Idealism, 11
Inborn error of metabolism, 178, 182–83, 189–90
Individual, importance of in ecological metaphor, 91–92
Individualization of birth, 123
Induction of labor, 75–85; in Britain, 81–85; change in rhetoric, 84; early

criticism of, 77; elective, 80–81; and normal/abnormal boundary, 77–78; old means for effecting, 76; prematurity and, 77; by prostaglandins, 84; public reaction to increase, 81–82
Informed consent, 206
Inglefinger, Franz J., 198–99
Innate behavior, 165
Integrated systems of control, 147–49
Integration, of obstetrical services, 126–27. See also Regionalization
Intellectual, role of, 13–14
Intensive care, 188–91; orientation of, 152
Interprofessional Task Force on Health Care of Women and Children, 221, 223, 228
IQ, 71, 159

Johns Hopkins case, 191–92
Johns Hopkins University, 41
Joint adventure, birth as, 97, 199, 220, 230

Karmel, Marjorie, 215
Kelso, Ian, 118
Kennell, John, 157–72
Kitzinger, Sheila, 216, 239
Klaus, Marshall, 157–72

Labor, monitoring: partographic control of, 145. See also Fetal monitor; Induction of labor
Lamaze, Fernand, 215
Lannec, R. T. H., 101
Lasch, Christopher, 172
Lateral delivery: in America, 65; in Britain, 68
Lee, Wing K., 110–14
Legal reform, 201–3
Legislative-ethical solution, 201–3
Leifer, A. D., 161–62

Levret, 24, 28
Liberation, by maternal-infant bonding theory, 171
Licensing, in America, 45
Licensure, of physicians, 22
Lithotomy position, 64–66; in Britain, 68–69
Litoff, Judy Barrett, 45, 47–48
Loomis, Horatio, 42
Lorber, John, criteria lists, 199–201
Lucey, Jerold, 228

Maeck, John Van S., 225–26
Male midwives, 7
Management schemes, 89, 232–33
Mapping birth, 129–34
Mariceau, 25
Masters, John C., 161
Materialism, 11
Maternal instinct, 171
Maternal-infant bonding, 155–74; classical study described, 159–60; defined, 156; dependent variables in, 159; effects of, 164–65; and fetal monitors, 150; methodological flaws in research on, 160–65. See also Diseases of nonattachment
Meaning of obstetrical work, 134–38, 208–9
Mechanical metaphor, 87
Meconium aspiration syndrome, 189
Medical education, 47
Medical ethics, 202–3
Medical genetics, 178–81; and control of health professionals, 186–87
Medicalization, 5, 99, 107, 123, 229
Medical Register, 35; and removal of midwives, 38
Medical schools: as confessional, 234–35; for women, 41
Medical societies, 45

Medicine: "regular," 41, 45; colonial, 39; and society, isolationist position, 198–99
Membranes, rupture of, 106
Mendel, Gregor, 177–78
Mental retardation, 108–9
Metaphor, and episiotomy, 70–71. See also Body, as machine; Mechanical metaphor
Middlesex Hospital, 29
Midwife, 3, 7, 20–50; in America, 40–41, 47–48; change in traditional role, 21–22; colonial, 40–41; confrontation with scientific obstetrics, 30–33; as monitor, 150; municipal and private, 131–32; organization of, 30; under regionalization in Britain, 127–29; registration of, 37; return of, 225–26; support of upper-class women in Britain for, 36–37; as team member, 227; and theoretical knowledge, 29; traditional training of, 22–23; ultimate decline of, 47–48. See also Male midwives; Midwives' Act of 1902; Royal College of Midwives; Demonstrative midwifery
Midwives' Act of 1902, 20, 38
Midwives' Institute, 36
Milunsky, Aubrey, 198
Modeling childbirth experiences, 278n
Modesty and decorum, 25
Mongolism, See Down's syndrome
Monitoring, 9, 89; effect on staff, 123; extension to minutiae of life, 133; as structure of control, 9, 100, 123. See also Fetal monitor; Surveillance
Monitoring concept, 90, 100, 122–23, 151–52, 209, 230, 255n
Monitrices, 215, 223

Monthly nurses, 29
Mortality: and fetal monitors, 108–9; in fetal monitor studies, 111–13; studies in eighteenth-century England, 32–33
Mother, as means of surveillance, 141
Multiple indicator criticism, 161

National Center for Health Care Technology, 101
National Health Service, 125
Natural childbirth, 122, 208–23; under ecological perspective, 138; and maternal infant bonding theory, 166; and meaning of obstetrical intervention, 135–37; and monitoring, 149–50; as means of controlling birth, 230–36; methodological critique of studies, 217; profession's response to, 216–18; studies of, 217–18; as threat to obstetricians' work, 219–20; values espoused by, 219–21
Negotiation, 91; of medicine and ethics, 197–207
Neural tube defects, 181, 190
Neutra, Raymond R., 119
Newborn intensive care. See Intensive care
Nightingale, Florence, 35
Nihell, Elizabeth, 30–31
Niswander, Kenneth, 73
Nonstress test, 141
Normal birth, 8; blurring boundary, 25–26; elimination of concept, 129; and female midwife, 25–26; re-emergence of concept, 137–38
Normality and abnormality, and genetic screening programs, 16
Normal maternal behavior, as comparison in bonding research, 162
Normalization, 9, 90–91, 138

Normalizing gaze, 88–89
Nugent, Fred, 72–73
Nurses. See British Nurses' Association; Monthly nurses
Nurses Association of the American College of Obstetricians and Gynecologists, 221
Nutrition, 189

Oakley, Ann, 5, 16
Obstetrical alternatives, 9
Obstetrical anatomy of communities, 131–33
Obstetrical Association of Midwives, 36
Obstetrical case, the: in America, 59–60; in Britain, 61; integration into system of care, 128
Obstetrical forceps. See Forceps
Obstetrical material: as social impediment to male practitioners, 28–29; women as, 59
Obstetrical Society, 34–36
Obstetrical space, 91, 234; as infected, 129; partitioning of, 124
Obstetrical training, segregated by sex, 28
Obstetrics, French, 24
Office of Technology Assessment, 108
Organization, 58–59, 125, 209; and birth position, 64–65; and rhetoric, in Britain, 57–58. See also Regionalization
Ould, Sir Fielding, 70
Ovariotomy, 45
Oxford, 22
Oxytocin challenge test, 141

Pain: and childbirth, 209–16; in ecological perspective, 211–12; and ecstasy, 218–19; treatment of, 211–12; two-dimensional, 209–18

Palfyn, Jean, 26
Pamphleteering, 30–31
Panoptic control, 230–31
Panopticon, 87, 94; and control of controllers, 150–51
Parenteral nutrition, 189
Parents, as decision-makers, 204–6
Parsons, Talcott, 268n
Partograph, and control of labor, 144–45
Pathological potential, 52–54
Pathology, pregnancy as: and American obstetrics, 42–44; in England, 33; and innovation, 44–45; and science, 42; strengthening image of, 37–38. See also DeLee, Joseph B.
Patient, changed concept of, 90
Paul, Richard, 107–8, 115
Pavlov, Ivan Petrovich, 215
Peel Report, 126, 128–29
Pelvimetry, 24
Perinatal concept, 152–53
Person-oriented philosophy of care, 205
Phenylketonuria (PKU), 184
Physician: as decision-maker, 198–99; "average," 58; as monitor, 90; new conceptualization of, 90
Pituitary extract, 76–77; artificial, 79; control through nasal administration, 78; infusion pump, 79; intravenous administration, 78
Platonov, K., 215
Pomeroy, Ralph, 70, 73
Population Investigation Committee, 130–31
Pregnancy, conceptual refinement of, 138–47. See also Pathology, pregnancy as
Prematurity: caused by induction, 77; tests for, 80

Professional boundary. See Boundary
Professional Service Review Organization (PSRO), 196
Pseudoscience, 169
Psychological aspects of birth, 209–13, 228–29
Psychoprophylaxis, 215–16
Psychosexual approach to birth, 216, 235, 239
Public opinion: and boundary strength, 82, 84; professional reaction to, 84
Puerperal fever, 44

Quasi-experimental studies: of maternal-infant bonding, 158–59; of monitoring, 110–16
Queenan, John, 120–21
Quilligan, Edward, 107–8, 115, 135, 138

Rachels, James, 203
Radical vision, and sociobiology, 92–93
Radiotelemetry, of fetal heart sounds, 102, 149–50
Ramsey, Paul, 199
Randall, Clyde, 217
Randomized controlled trials, 116–18
Record, obstetrical, 151
Record reviews, of monitoring, 110, 119
Reflexive control, 150–54, 230, 233–35
Reform, 165–69, 209–29, 237–40
Regionalization, 97; in America, 224–29; in Britain, 127; effectiveness, 224–27, 276n
Reid, Duncan, 212, 217
Renou, Peter, 118
Research, and doctor-patient relationship, 196

Residual knowledge, 67–68
Residual normalcy, 51
Respiration, 188–89
Respiratory distress syndrome, 188
Risk: as continuum, 143; disappearance of high-risk concept, 141–43; high-risk pregnancy, 140; individualizing, 133; at-risk populations, 132–33
Risk scoring, 142–43; and regionalization, 261n
Role obligations, 203–4
Romanticism, and natural childbirth, 212
Rosenthal, Miriam K., 161
Rossi, Alice, 92, 173
Roux, Jacques, 151
Royal College of Midwives, 20
Royal College of Obstetricians and Gynecologists, 126, 130
Royal College of Physicians, 26, 30
Royal Colleges, 34–35, 39
Rush, Benjamin, 43

Savage, woman as, 63
Schroeder, Karl, 70
Science: as force for professional expansion, 3–5; as ideology in midwife debate, 31; and midwifery, 25; and privileged knowledge, 173; and professional vulnerability, 95–96; and social organization of medicine, 42–43
Scientism, 96, 121, 155; and autonomy, 167
Screening legislation, 184
Scully, Diana, 16, 229
Seidel, Henry M., 89–92
Semmelweis, Ignaz P., 44
Sensitive period, 157–58, 160; and hospital practices, 166
Separation studies: of animals, 157; of humans, 158–60

Shaw, Anthony, 206
Shippen, William, 39–40
Sickle cell anemia, 185
Sickle cell screening, 268n
Sims, J. Marion, 45
Smellie, William, 27–28, 30, 242; on birth position, 69; and ethics, 34; and the forceps, 27; and the scientific approach to birth, 28; as teacher, 28
Social order, 91, 170–73
Social policy, 168–70
Social theory, 10–11; and social history, 14; and reform of institutions, 169–70. See also Theory
Sociobiology, 92–93, 165
Sociology of knowledge, 11
Spina bifida. See Neural tube defects
Stahl, F. A., 70
Stander, Henricus J., 79
Stewart, David, 167
Stinchcombe, Arthur L., 14
Stress test. See Oxytocin challenge test
Support, as mechanism of control, 232–33
Surgery, 190
Surgico-prophylaxis, 217–18
Surveillance, 8, 100, 123, 141; of medical practitioners, 152–53
Sutton, Walter S., 178
Systematic desensitization, 216

Task Force on Predictors of Fetal Distress, 108–9; recommendation on fetal monitoring, 121
Tay-Sachs disease, 184–85
Team approach to care, 8–9, 92, 129, 152–53, 227
Team, genetic counselor on, 186–87
Technical criteria fallacy, 201
Technology, 147–50; of control, 210; simplification of, 149–50

Telemetry. *See* Radiotelemetry
Tetanic contraction, control of, 78
Thacker, Stephen B., 108, 120
Theory: classical notions of, 92; as practice, 12
Therapeutic options, 195
Thickness, Philip, 29
Thoms, Herbert, 223, 232
Tomkinson, John, 97, 227
Trisomy syndromes, 180
Turnbull, A. C., 82, 182
Two-dimensional childbirth, 209–19

Univocal discourse, 208–42
Utero-placental insufficiency, 104

Value conflicts, 176
Value-neutral medicine, 198
Vaughan, Kathleen, 249n, 252n
Veatch, Robert, 201
Vellay, Pierre, 215
Velvovsky, I. Z., 215

Watson, B. P., 59
Wellman, Henry M., 161
Wertz, Richard W., and Dorothy C., 24, 124–25
White, Charles, 32
White, James P., 42
Williams, J. Whitridge: on birth position, 66; on cesarean sections, 145–46; and clinical judgment, 95; and form of profession, 53; on induction, 77–80; and pathological potential, 56; and state of the profession, 47
Wilson, E. O., 92, 157
Witches, 22
Women, as vehicles for conveying obstetrical material, 210
Woolf, Virginia, 218, 242

X-linked disorders, 178–79

Young, William, 241